The Infectious Disease Diagnosis

Michael David • Jean-Luc Benoit

Editors

The Infectious Disease Diagnosis

A Case Approach

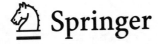 Springer

Editors
Michael David
Department of Medicine
University of Chicago
Chicago, IL
USA

Jean-Luc Benoit
Department of Medicine
University of Chicago
Chicago, IL
USA

The original version of the book was revised. The "Index" and "Appendix" were modified as requested by the editors of the book.

ISBN 978-3-319-87899-7   ISBN 978-3-319-64906-1   (eBook)
https://doi.org/10.1007/978-3-319-64906-1

Printed on acid-free paper

This Springer imprint is published by Springer Nature
The registered company is Springer International Publishing AG
The registered company address is: Gewerbestrasse 11, 6330 Cham, Switzerland

We would like to dedicate this book to Dr. David Pitrak—teacher, section chief, and friend

Introduction

This volume is intended to be a resource for all health-care providers interested in infectious diseases and also an educational reference for medical students, residents, fellows, nursing students, and students in training programs for physicians' assistants and other allied health professional fields. This is neither a textbook nor a manual for use in clinical practice. Instead, it is a review of common and uncommon infectious diseases that are often in the differential diagnosis for patients in any medical setting.

We intend for the cases in this book to enable us to share the excitement of infectious diseases practice and to inspire students and other trainees who are deciding upon a career path to choose infectious diseases. This field is fascinating and always presents new challenges in diagnosis, prognosis, and therapy. Humans are surrounded by potentially deadly pathogens, but they cause infections in only very specific circumstances. The diagnosis of an infection often requires knowledge of pathogens and host risk characteristics. Each human infection presents a detective story to the physician, and as clues are assembled in many cases, the most likely diagnosis becomes clear, sometimes quickly and sometimes gradually.

In order to diagnose and treat an infectious diseases patient, the clinician must consider many facets of the individual's life and behavior. The infectious diseases doctor has to determine what environmental, pathogen, and host factors may have aligned to create the "perfect storm" that changed an environmental or commensal microorganism into the cause of a clinically significant infection in a patient. In other cases, epidemic spread of a pathogen, such as influenza, may lead to an infection. The clinician must take account of changing pathogen epidemiology, shifting host immunologic status, and environmental change. Social and biological factors are constantly altering the balance between a commensal and a pathological interaction between people and the microorganisms in their environment. No other field of medicine requires as close an examination of environmental and behavioral factors in the determination of a diagnosis and in the choice of an empiric plan for therapy.

While we have many tools to diagnose and treat patients with viral, bacterial, fungal, and parasitic infections, we do not always succeed. While we have many excellent and effective vaccines and prophylactic strategies, some infections cannot yet be prevented. While we have many antimicrobial drugs, there are some infections we still cannot cure. Infectious diseases still kill many millions of people each year around the world, and thus there are exciting opportunities for new experts in clinical and basic research to pursue novel preventative measures, diagnostic modalities, and treatments for infectious diseases. In some of the cases presented in this book, the limits of our therapeutic armamentarium are discussed.

The goal of this book is to present a broad, although not comprehensive, range of cases in infectious diseases, with representation of tropical diseases, arthropod-borne diseases, human immunodeficiency virus (HIV)/acquired immune deficiency syndrome (AIDS) medicine, infections arising as a complication of medical care, and general infectious diseases. These types of cases are all frequently encountered at a typical tertiary medical center in the United States such as ours. Many of the disease processes described are common, "bread-and-butter" cases, but there are also more unusual cases in patients who have had rare exposures or specific vulnerabilities. We included cases of infection in children and adults, infections arising in the community, and others arising in the health-care setting.

In each chapter, the author or authors describe the case of different patients, most of whom were treated at our tertiary care medical center. These cases were nearly all presented by a clinical fellow at our weekly Thursday afternoon case conference in the Section of Infectious Diseases and Global Health of the Department of Medicine of the University of Chicago between 2004 and 2016. The cases thus have benefited from discussion by a group of experts with many decades of combined experience in the field. As it was in our conference, each case is presented here as an unknown, and the reader is invited to develop a differential diagnosis as he or she reads it. The history of the illness, relevant past medical history, family history, social history, exposures, travel, behaviors, medications, allergies, physical findings, laboratory test results, and findings on imaging studies are presented. One or more radiographic, clinical, gross pathological, histological, entomologic, or environmental image is shown in nearly every chapter to enhance the educational impact of the case.

We hope that the reader of our book will gain a greater understanding of the pathogenic microorganisms that infect humans; the social, biological, and behavioral factors associated with increased risk of infection or outcome of an infection; the interaction of infectious diseases with other comorbidities; the approaches to diagnosis of infectious diseases (including by means of the history, signs and symptoms, cultures, and serologic, radiographic, molecular, histological, and surgical data); the considerations in the selection of medical and surgical treatment modalities; the variety of clinical manifestations of human infections with the pathogens discussed; the pathogenesis of infectious diseases within specific organs and organ systems; the vectors associated with vector-borne diseases; the problems of antimicrobial resistance; and the geographic distribution of the described pathogens. However, while all of these fascinating aspects of infectious diseases are included in most of the cases, the primary focus of this book and at the center of each case is the differential diagnosis.

Often before the diagnosis is revealed in each case, the reader's attention is importantly directed to a table listing the relevant differential diagnosis. In most of the cases, the authors also provided in the text a discussion of the differential diagnosis as applied to the specific circumstances of the patient presented, examining the factors that make certain diagnoses more or less likely. This teaching exercise is meant to enhance the reader's skills of deductive reasoning in clinical medicine. This is the detective work of infectious diseases.

An index is provided in an appendix at the end of the book that includes each diagnosis listed in the tables of differential diagnosis from all chapters. This "differential diagnosis index" is a very unusual and important resource. For each pathogen, by consulting this index, it is possible to review all cases in the book for which that pathogen was a diagnostic consideration. Thus, from the cases in this book, the reader is able to review the potential presentations of many pathogens and to understand how to narrow the differential diagnosis rapidly and efficiently and how to distinguish that pathogen from others with a similar clinical presentation. This index expands the value of our book because it can be used to shape the clinician's approach to considering a specific diagnosis in a number of different clinical circumstances.

The editors have attempted to reproduce much of the teaching value of our case conference in this volume. The 47 cases presented have been drawn from more than 12 years of our weekly case discussions. During those 12 years in the first part of the twenty-first century, clinicians in our inpatient and outpatient services provided care for many thousands of patients. Among these, more than 450 patients were chosen by clinical fellows and faculty for case presentations at our weekly conferences. The editors chose approximately 10% of these presented cases to represent the breadth of the pathology as well as some of the most intriguing and confusing patients whom we have encountered at out medical center. Many "generations" of pediatric and adult clinical fellows have contributed to this effort, some overlapping in their time at our medical center and others not. Many of them have now practiced elsewhere and enhanced their knowledge of infectious disease in a variety of practices across the United States. These authors are responsible for the rigorous and stimulating content of this book.

It is our hope that once the reader has finished the cases presented here, the volume can later be consulted as an adjunct to preparation for clinical rotations in infectious diseases, board examinations, teaching in the clinical context, and a quick and fairly comprehensive reference to concise descriptions of the key elements related to a pathogen, a syndrome, or a differential diagnosis.

We hope that in the cases presented in this volume, we can transmit to you some of our great enthusiasm for the dynamic and exciting field of infectious diseases. If you are considering choosing infectious diseases as a specialty, we encourage you to do this! The field provides constant challenges and fascinating problems affecting all organ systems in the human body, a broad range of human behaviors, data derived from almost innumerable sources, a fascinating view of humanity's interaction with the microbial world surrounding us, a unique perspective on humanity's interaction with the environment, a succession of mysteries almost everyday to solve, and the great satisfaction of often providing a successful cure.

Michael Z. David
Jean-Luc Benoit

Contents

Contributors

M. Ellen Acree, M.D. Section of Infectious Diseases and Global Health, Department of Medicine, University of Chicago, Chicago, IL, USA

Muayad Alali, M.D. Section of Infectious Diseases, Department of Pediatrics, University of Chicago, Chicago, IL, USA

Sara Hurtado Bares, M.D. University of Nebraska Medical Center, Omaha, NE, USA

Jean-Luc Benoit, M.D. Section of Infectious Diseases and Global Health, Department of Medicine, University of Chicago, Chicago, IL, USA

Eric Bhaimia, D.O. Department of Medicine, NorthShore University HealthSystem, Evanston, IL, USA
University of Chicago Medicine, Chicago, IL, USA

Jennifer L. Burns, C.P.N.P. Section of Infectious Diseases, Department of Pediatrics, University of Chicago, Chicago, IL, USA

Fredy Chaparro-Rojas, M.D. Delaware Valley Infectious Diseases Associates, Wynnewood, PA, USA

Dima Dandachi, M.D. Baylor College of Medicine, Houston, TX, USA

Michael Z. David, M.D., Ph.D. Section of Infectious Diseases and Global Health, Department of Medicine, University of Chicago, Chicago, IL, USA

Vinny DiMaggio, M.D. Department of Medicine, University of Chicago, Chicago, IL, USA

Leona Ebara, M.D. Section of Infectious Diseases and Global Health, Department of Medicine, University of Chicago, Chicago, IL, USA

Daniel Glikman, M.D. Pediatric Infectious Diseases Unit, Galilee Medical Center, Nahariya, and The Faculty of Medicine in the Galilee, Bar-Ilan University, Safed, Israel

Kevin Gregg, M.D. University of Michigan Health System, Ann Arbor, MI, USA

Vagish Hemmige, M.D. Baylor College of Medicine, Houston, TX, USA

David Kopelman, M.D. Department of Medicine, University of Chicago, Chicago, IL, USA

Frances Lahrman, D.O. NorthShore University Health System, Evanston, IL, USA

Emily Landon, M.D. Department of Medicine, University of Chicago, Chicago, IL, USA

Kathleen Linder, M.D. University of Michigan Health System, Ann Arbor, MI, USA

Oana Denisa Majorant, M.D. University of Nebraska Medical Center, Omaha, NE, USA

Moira McNulty, M.D. Section of Infectious Diseases and Global Health, Department of Medicine, University of Chicago, Chicago, IL, USA

Kathleen Mullane, D.O. Section of Infectious Diseases and Global Health, Department of Medicine, University of Chicago, Chicago, IL, USA

Colleen B. Nash, M.D., M.P.H. Rush University Medical Center, Rush University Children's Hospital, Chicago, IL, USA

Margaret Newman, M.D. Section of Infectious Diseases and Global Health, Department of Medicine, University of Chicago Medicine, Chicago, IL, USA

Emily Obringer, M.D. Section of Infectious Diseases, Department of Pediatrics, University of Chicago, Chicago, IL, USA

Daniela Pellegrini, M.D. Section of Infectious Diseases and Global Health, Department of Medicine, University of Chicago, Chicago, IL, USA

Lindsay A. Petty, M.D. University of Michigan, Ann Arbor, MI, USA

Kenneth Pursell, M.D. Section of Infectious Diseases and Global Health, Department of Medicine, University of Chicago, Chicago, IL, USA

Amutha Rajagopal, M.D. Section of Infectious Diseases and Global Health, Department of Medicine, University of Chicago, Chicago, IL, USA

Matthew Richards, A.M., L.C.S.W., M.Div. Department of Pediatrics, University of Chicago, Chicago, IL, USA

Jessica Ridgway, M.D., M.S. Section of Infectious Diseases and Global Health, Department of Medicine, University of Chicago, Chicago, IL, USA

Stephen Schrantz, M.D. NorthShore University Health System, Evanston, IL, USA

Nirav Shah, M.D., M.P.H. Department of Medicine, NorthShore University HealthSystem, Evanston, IL, USA

University of Chicago Medicine, Chicago, IL, USA

Shirley Stephenson, R.N., F.N.P.-B.C. Department of Medicine, University of Chicago Medicine, Chicago, IL, USA

Ralph Villaran, M.D. Infectious Disease Specialists, Highland, IN, USA

Linda J. Walsh, N.P. Section of Infectious Diseases, Department of Pediatrics, University of Chicago Medicine, Chicago, IL, USA

Connor Williams, A.M., L.C.S.W. Department of Pediatrics, University of Chicago, Chicago, IL, USA

Karl O.A. Yu, M.D., Ph.D. Center for Infectious Diseases and Immunology, Rochester General Hospital Research Institute, Rochester General Hospital, Rochester, NY, USA

Traveler to Uganda

Nirav Shah and Eric Bhaimia

A 25-year-old, otherwise healthy female who traveled to Uganda 2 weeks prior to presentation complained of dyspnea on exertion and cough productive of clear sputum. Notably, she was concerned that several colleagues who traveled with her were displaying similar symptoms.

The patient was a graduate student who studied malaria in birds and mammals and had undertaken a research project in the rainforest of western Uganda near Fort Portal for the previous 2 months. The goal of the expedition was to collect and test the blood of various animals. She reported coming into contact with rats, mice, shrews, civets, bats, other small mammals, and various birds. She took part in capturing, drawing blood from, and skinning these animals. She did not use contact precautions consistently and did not use airborne precautions. Her team entered a large, hollow tree (Fig. 1.1) that housed insect-eating bats. In the cavity of the tree, she collected bats and bat droppings. Her team also placed traps for fruit-eating bats, and she drew their blood without the use of gloves. She did not skin any fruit-eating bats. Bat genera that she encountered on the trip included *Hipposideros*, *Epomops*, and *Epomophorus*.

N. Shah, M.D., M.P.H. (✉) • E. Bhaimia, D.O.
Department of Medicine, NorthShore University
HealthSystem, Evanston, IL, USA

University of Chicago Medicine, Chicago, IL, USA
e-mail: nshah2@northshore.org

There was a variety of monkeys inhabiting the area around the town where she lived, but she did not have direct contact with any of them.

The patient and her team swam in flowing streams but did not swim in ponds or other bodies of standing water. The patient reported that she took atovaquone/proguanil for malaria prophylaxis for only 6 weeks of the 8-week trip, and she recalled suffering from numerous mosquito bites. She consumed local dishes, which included meat from chickens and goats butchered by her research team. She also ate local fish dishes. All meat and fish she consumed were cooked. She denied any sexual activity during the trip. She was not aware of contact with anyone ill with tuberculosis.

Several weeks into the trip, the patient and the other members of her team developed high fevers, chills, malaise, and cough. The team was

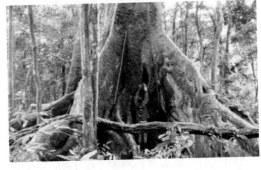

Fig. 1.1 Large, hollow tree filled with insect-eating bats

© Springer International Publishing AG 2018
M. David, J.-L. Benoit (eds.), *The Infectious Disease Diagnosis*,
https://doi.org/10.1007/978-3-319-64906-1_1

empirically treated for possible leptospirosis with a 12-day course of oral doxycycline. While on doxycycline, the patient discontinued taking the atovaquone/proguanil because she was concerned for toxicity and drug interactions. After starting doxycycline, she reported that the headaches, fevers, and chills resolved but the cough persisted. When she returned to Chicago from her trip, two of her colleagues fell ill. A Ugandan collaborator was diagnosed with pulmonary tuberculosis based on a chest x-ray (CXR) and was being empirically treated. A coworker from the United States developed shortness of breath and cough, and his physicians suspected that he had tuberculosis.

The patient had no significant past medical or surgical history. Her family history was not remarkable. She was a daily smoker and drank alcohol socially, but she did not use illicit drugs. Her only regular medication was oral contraceptive pills. She was up to date with her childhood vaccines, had a rabies vaccine 5 years prior to presentation, and had received the influenza vaccine within the year. She was allergic to penicillin, which caused anaphylaxis.

On physical examination, the temperature was 96.8 °F, heart rate was 75 beats per minute, blood pressure was 122/80 mmHg, respiratory rate was 16 breaths per minute, and oxygen saturation was 99% breathing room air. She was in no acute distress and breathing comfortably. She had no rash, no conjunctival pallor or injection, and no nasal discharge. Her oropharynx was without lesions or abnormality, and she had no lymphadenopathy. The heart demonstrated a regular rhythm with no murmur, and the lungs were clear to auscultation bilaterally. The abdomen was benign, and she had no edema in the lower extremities. The neurologic exam was nonfocal, and her thought process was clear.

The complete blood count and complete metabolic panel were normal. Her CXR (Fig. 1.2) revealed a diffuse miliary pattern throughout the lungs without pleural effusion or pneumothorax.

The differential diagnosis is presented in Tables 1.1 and 1.2. The differential diagnosis for a miliary pattern on CXR includes tuberculosis; endemic fungal pathogens; bacterial infections including psittacosis, tularemia, bartonellosis, and brucellosis; parasitic diseases including

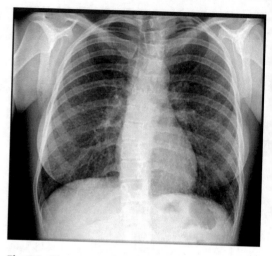

Fig. 1.2 Chest x-ray with bilateral miliary pattern

Table 1.1 Differential diagnosis for miliary infiltrates on chest x-ray

1. Micronodules can be seen in multiple infectious and noninfectious diseases

2. Miliary infiltrates refer to the presence of multiple pulmonary micronodules of millet-seed size (about 2 mm)

3. The distribution of micronodules can point to a range of diagnoses:

   (a) Random distribution (diffuse and uniform distribution) of micronodules is most often indicative of miliary tuberculosis, miliary fungal infection (histoplasmosis, coccidioidomycosis, blastomycosis, or cryptococcosis), hematogenous metastases, extensive sarcoidosis, or rarely Langerhans cell histiocytosis

   (b) Perilymphatic distribution (subpleural, septal, or peribronchovascular) of micronodules is most often indicative of sarcoidosis, silicosis, coal worker's pneumoconiosis, lymphangitic spread of carcinoma, or rarely lymphoid interstitial pneumonitis and amyloidosis

   (c) Centrilobular distribution (no pleural nodules) of micronodules is most often indicative of hypersensitivity pneumonitis, respiratory bronchiolitis, bronchoalveolar carcinoma, or infections with endobronchial spread (tuberculosis, nontuberculous mycobacterial infection, bacterial bronchopneumonia due to *Staphylococcus aureus*, beta-hemolytic streptococci, or *Mycoplasma pneumoniae*)

4. Also consider viral pneumonia (influenza, measles), psittacosis, Q fever (*Coxiella burnetii*), leptospirosis (*Leptospira* ssp.), bartonellosis (*Bartonella* spp.), brucellosis (*Brucella* spp.), strongyloidiasis (*Strongyloides stercoralis*), and toxoplasmosis (*Toxoplasma gondii*)

Table 1.2 Bat-associated infections

1.	Rabies: bite or direct contact of bat saliva with the mouth, eyes, nose, or fresh wound
2.	Histoplasmosis: grows in bat guano with pulmonary inhalation from aerosols generated when the soil and guano are disturbed
3.	Filovirus hemorrhagic fevers present in Africa:
	(a) Marburg hemorrhagic fever has a fruit bat reservoir (*Rousettus aegyptiacus*)
	(b) Ebola hemorrhagic fever may have a bat reservoir, likely fruit and insect-eating bats
4.	Henipavirus encephalitis
	(a) Nipah virus encephalitis associated with *Pteropus* fruit bats (flying foxes) in parts of Asia (documented human outbreaks in Malaysia, Singapore, India, and Bangladesh), with risk of person-to-person droplet transmission in the case of respiratory infections
	(b) Hendra virus encephalitis associated with fruit bats (flying foxes) in Australia; humans are infected only when exposed to Hendra virus-infected horses, without bat-to-human or human-to-human infection
5.	Some human coronavirus have originated from bats
	(a) The SARS (severe acute respiratory syndrome) coronavirus originated in Chinese horseshoe bats; person-to-person transmission is the major mode of infection
	(b) The MERS (Middle East respiratory syndrome) coronavirus may have originated from Saudi Arabian bats; however, human infections have been associated with direct exposure to camels

Table 1.3 Laboratory results in the present case

Test	Result
Interferon gamma release assay	Negative
AFB sputum culture × 2	Negative
Fungal sputum culture	Negative
Serum *Histoplasma* antibody	Negative initially, then positive
Serum *Blastomyces* antibody	Negative
Urine *Histoplasma* antigen	Positive

This patient had a large number of exposures during her travels, but initially the most worrying among them was the patient's dissection without wearing gloves of fruit-eating bats, specifically the genus *Epomops*. The *Epomops* fruit-eating bat has tested positive for Ebola virus IgG and is considered a potential reservoir of Ebola virus [2, 3]. Furthermore, Ebola outbreaks were previously reported in Uganda in 2000 and 2007 [4, 5]. Ebola was not a likely diagnosis, however, given that our patient and her fellow team members did not display any of the typical signs and symptoms of a hemorrhagic fever syndrome. Her case was part of a larger outbreak initially suspected to be tuberculosis because of dyspnea and a miliary pattern on CXR. However, arguing against this diagnosis was the lack of known specific exposures to tuberculosis.

Instead, with the common exposure of ill travelers within the bat-infested hollow tree, the outbreak was most consistent with histoplasmosis. This was particularly suggested by the typical pulmonary findings and the incubation period. The initial symptoms of headache, fever, chills, and malaise (initially empirically diagnosed as leptospirosis) most likely represented the initial symptoms of histoplasmosis after exposure inside the hollow tree. Our patient first developed symptoms 4 weeks prior to presentation, when the *Histoplasma* serology test was positive only at the lower limit of positivity, while subsequent serologic testing revealed high-level positivity, confirming the diagnosis. The patient's symptoms resolved completely with oral itraconazole therapy. This case demonstrates how an extensive history is vital in the returning traveler who has multiple high-risk exposures.

Interestingly, it appears that a similar histoplasmosis outbreak affecting 13 of 24 students on a biology field trip occurred when another group entered the hollow cavity of the very same tree

toxoplasmosis, strongyloidiasis, and schistosomiasis; and noninfectious etiologies including malignancy, sarcoidosis, hypersensitivity pneumonitis, and pneumoconiosis. On interviewing the patient, we provided her with a case series of biology students who entered into a bat-infested hollow tree in Uganda and who developed histoplasmosis [1]. The patient recognized the tree pictured in a figure in the manuscript and stated that it was the same tree that her team had entered. Further laboratory work-up included an interferon gamma release assay (IGRA), sputum culture for acid fast bacteria, fungal sputum culture, *Histoplasma* urine antigen, *Histoplasma* serum antibody, and *Blastomyces* serum antibody. Results from further work-up are shown in Table 1.3. The *Histoplasma* urine antigen was positive, confirming the diagnosis of histoplasmosis.

[1] visited by the patient in the present case. In that earlier outbreak, histoplasmosis was ultimately confirmed serologically but was also initially mistaken for tuberculosis.

1.1 Histoplasmosis

Histoplasma capsulatum var. *capsulatum* is a dimorphic fungus that displays characteristic narrow-based budding (Fig. 1.3). *Histoplasma* grows as a mold in the soil and proliferates best in soil contaminated with bird or bat droppings, which favors sporulation. Exposure occurs when soil or droppings with a high concentration of spores are disturbed as in a cave, in an attic or basement, or at a construction site [6].

Of note, there are two varieties of *Histoplasma capsulatum* pathogenic to humans, *Histoplasma capsulatum* var. *duboisii* (African histoplasmosis) and *Histoplasma capsulatum* var. *capsulatum* (classic histoplasmosis). African histoplasmosis is a rare, deep mycosis that usually occurs in the tropical belt of Africa and can involve the skin, subcutaneous tissues, lymph nodes, and bones [7]. It rarely affects the lungs and is rarely reported outside of Africa. Classic histoplasmosis is found worldwide, including Africa, and can cause pulmonary infection or disseminated infections.

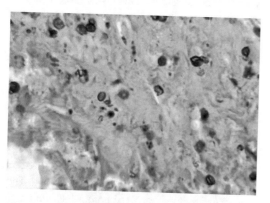

Fig. 1.3 Methenamine silver stain reveals *Histoplasma capsulatum* var. *capsulatum* fungi. Source: CDC. Available at https://phil.cdc.gov/phil/details.asp (Image ID#4220; Accessed on-line, June 21, 2017)

Pulmonary histoplasmosis has a broad spectrum of presentations, from asymptomatic infection to life-threatening pneumonia. Disseminated disease can involve many different organ systems including the skin, central nervous system, gastrointestinal tract, joints, and adrenal glands. It can also cause endocarditis, prostatitis, osteomyelitis, pancreatitis, cholecystitis, pericarditis, and chorioretinitis.

Acute pulmonary histoplasmosis typically occurs within 1–3 weeks of exposure and is usually self-limited. For patients with impaired cellular immunity, dissemination may occur and may be fatal. Diagnosis is made by *Histoplasma* polysaccharide antigen test in the urine or in the blood [8]. The antigen test peaks 4–6 weeks after infection but is usually negative in the first 4 weeks. For patients who are symptomatic, therapy is warranted as per Infectious Diseases Society of America guidelines [9]. Antifungal therapy with itraconazole is recommended in patients who have symptoms for longer than a month. Intravenous liposomal amphotericin B followed by oral itraconazole is recommended for patients with moderately severe to severe acute pulmonary histoplasmosis.

Key Points
- Histoplasmosis is an endemic dimorphic fungus with a worldwide distribution and is on the differential for a returning traveler with lower respiratory symptoms.
- Activities associated with histoplasmosis exposure include cleaning attics, barns and chicken coops, caving, construction, and demolition.
- An outbreak with the same exposure may point to the diagnosis.
- *Histoplasma* polysaccharide antigen testing may be negative within 4 weeks of onset of infection in acute pulmonary histoplasmosis, so a repeat test may be necessary to confirm the diagnosis.
- Symptomatic patients and patients with moderate to severe disease warrant antifungal therapy.

References

1. Cottle LE, Gkrania-Klotsas E, Williams HJ, Brindle HE, Carmichael AJ, Fry G, et al. A multinational outbreak of histoplasmosis following a biology field trip in the Ugandan rainforest. J Travel Med. 2013;20(2):83–7.

2. Gonzalez JP, Pourrut X, Leroy E. Ebolavirus and other filoviruses. Curr Top Microbiol Immunol. 2007;315:363–87.

3. Pourrut X, Délicat A, Rollin PE, Ksiazek TG, Gonzalez J-P, Leroy EM. Spatial and temporal patterns of Zaire ebolavirus antibody prevalence in the possible reservoir bat species. J Infect Dis. 2007;196(Suppl 2):S176–83.

4. Borchert M, Mutyaba I, Van Kerkhove MD, Lutwama J, Luwaga H, Bisoborwa G, et al. Ebola haemorrhagic fever outbreak in Masindi District, Uganda: outbreak description and lessons learned. BMC Infect Dis. 2011;11:357.

5. MacNeil A, Farnon EC, Wamala J, Okware S, Cannon DL, Reed Z, et al. Proportion of deaths and clinical features in Bundibugyo Ebola virus infection, Uganda. Emerg Infect Dis. 2010;16(12):1969–72.

6. Cano MV, Hajjeh RA. The epidemiology of histoplasmosis: a review. Semin Respir Infect. 2001;16(2):109–18.

7. Tsiodras S, Drogari-Apiranthitou M, Pilichos K, Leventakos K, Kelesidis T, Buitrago MJ, et al. An unusual cutaneous tumor: African histoplasmosis following mudbaths: case report and review. Am J Trop Med Hyg. 2012;86(2):261–3.

8. Wheat LJ, Kohler RB, Tewari RP. Diagnosis of disseminated histoplasmosis by detection of *Histoplasma capsulatum* antigen in serum and urine specimens. N Engl J Med. 1986;314(2):83–8.

9. Wheat LJ, Freifeld AG, Kleiman MB, Baddley JW, McKinsey DS, Loyd JE, et al. Clinical practice guidelines for the management of patients with histoplasmosis: 2007 update by the Infectious Diseases Society of America. Clin Infect Dis. 2007;45(7):807–25.

Visual Loss in a Hematopoietic Stem Cell Transplant Recipient

Kathleen Linder and Kevin Gregg

A 58-year-old man with a history of chronic lymphocytic leukemia (CLL) presented with vision loss in his left eye, decreased depth perception, and gait imbalance 7 weeks after undergoing an allogeneic hematopoietic stem cell transplant (HSCT). His pre-transplant course had been complicated by a mild loss of visual acuity. Immediately after transplant, his blurry vision persisted. He was seen by the ophthalmology consultation service and diagnosed with a refractive disorder with no other ocular pathology discovered. His visual symptoms persisted, however, and acutely worsened over the 2 weeks prior to presentation with emergence of gait imbalance. The patient denied any fevers, chills, rigors, neck pain or stiffness, spots or "floaters" in his vision, eye pain, syncope, or falls.

In addition to CLL, the patient's medical history was notable for hypertension, hyperlipidemia, oral herpes, and intermittent sinusitis. Pre-HSCT evaluation demonstrated that the patient was seronegative for cytomegalovirus (CMV) but seropositive for herpes simplex virus (HSV) and Epstein-Barr virus (EBV); the stem cell donor was seronegative for CMV and HSV but seropositive for EBV. The patient had no relevant surgical or family history. He was a non-

smoker and did not drink alcohol or use illicit drugs. He worked as a custodian. His only remarkable travel history was to Southeast Asia when he was in the military decades earlier; he had been exposed to the dioxin-containing herbicide and defoliant Agent Orange at that time. His medication regimen after HSCT included prophylactic valacyclovir, fluconazole, and trimethoprim/sulfamethoxazole (two double-strength tablets twice weekly). His immunosuppression regimen consisted of tacrolimus 1 g every 12 h.

On admission, the patient had a temperature of 36.9 °C, a heart rate of 79 beats per minute, and a blood pressure of 109/69 mmHg. He was alert and oriented to person, place, and time. Pertinent exam findings included pupils that were equal and reactive to light, unremarkable cardiopulmonary and abdominal exams and presence of a Hickman central venous catheter on his right upper chest without erythema or induration at the insertion site. The patient's neurologic examination was grossly abnormal. Cranial nerve exam revealed a left homonymous hemianopsia. Reflexes were symmetric and normal throughout. The patient had 5/5 strength in all extremities but had a left-sided pronator drift. Sensation to pain and light touch was diminished in the left lower extremity. The patient was noted to have left-sided hemi-neglect. His gait was narrow-based and unsteady. Coordination was impaired, and the patient was unable to complete finger-to-nose

K. Linder, M.D. • K. Gregg, M.D. (✉)
University of Michigan Health System,
Ann Arbor, MI, USA
e-mail: kvngregg@med.umich.edu

© Springer International Publishing AG 2018
M. David, J.-L. Benoit (eds.), *The Infectious Disease Diagnosis*,
https://doi.org/10.1007/978-3-319-64906-1_2

and heel-to-shin maneuvers with the left arm and leg, respectively.

Laboratory testing demonstrated a white blood cell count of 2300 cells/μL (normal range, 4500–11,000/μL) (61% neutrophils, 16% lymphocytes, 19% monocytes), hemoglobin of 9.1 g/dL (13.5–17.5 g/dL), and platelet count of 43,000/μL (150,000–450,000/μL). The patient's basic metabolic panel and hepatic function panel were normal. Serum tacrolimus level was 9.0 mg/dL, within the desired therapeutic range.

The differential diagnosis of acute neurologic symptoms in an HSCT recipient patient is broad and is shown in Table 2.1. Central nervous system infections, particularly opportunistic infections such as cerebral aspergillosis and reactivation of herpesvirus infections (CMV, HSV, varicella zoster virus [VZV], and human herpesvirus-6 [HHV-6]), need to be excluded promptly. These infections are of particular concern in the first 3 months after transplant, when there is absence or reduced function of the innate immune system (i.e., neutropenia), cell-mediated immunity, and humoral immunity. The likelihood of herpesvirus infections is affected by the pre-transplant serologies of the patient and donor. In this case, the patient and donor were seronegative for CMV, so this infection was of much lower likelihood as primary CMV infection would be unusual in this setting. Early consideration of neurologic side effects of medications is also important, as withdrawal of any offending agents is likely necessary to alleviate the symptoms.

To evaluate this patient's neurologic symptoms, a magnetic resonance imaging (MRI) study of the brain was performed that demonstrated focal areas of edema, most prominent in the right occipital lobe (Fig. 2.1). A lumbar puncture was completed for diagnostic purposes. Tube 4 demonstrated 452 red blood cells/μL and 2 white blood cells/μL. Glucose was 71 mg/dL (normal) and protein was 41 mg/dL (low). The cerebrospinal fluid (CSF) polymerase chain reaction (PCR) tests were negative for HSV, VZV, enterovirus, CMV, EBV, HHV-6,

Table 2.1 Differential diagnosis of acute neurologic symptoms in hematopoietic stem cell transplant recipients

Infectious etiologies
Encephalitis
• Cytomegalovirus (CMV)
• Epstein-Barr virus (EBV)
• Other human herpesviruses (e.g., HHV-6)
• Herpes simplex virus
• Varicella-zoster virus (VZV)
• JC virus (progressive multifocal leukoencephalopathy [PML])
• West Nile virus and other arthropod-borne encephalitides
• Toxoplasmosis (*Toxoplasma gondii*)
Invasive fungal infection
• Aspergillosis (*Aspergillus* spp.)
• Cryptococcosis (*Cryptococcus* spp.)
• Blastomycosis (*Blastomyces dermatitidis*)
• Coccidioidomycosis (*Coccidioides immitis*)
• Histoplasmosis (*Histoplasma capsulatum*)
Bacterial meningitis
Pyogenic brain abscess
Tuberculosis
Noninfectious etiologies
Posterior reversible leukoencephalopathy syndrome (PRES)
Cerebral hemorrhage (hemorrhagic stroke)
Cerebrovascular accident (CVA, ischemic stroke)
Chemotherapy-related neurotoxicity
Acute disseminated encephalomyelitis (ADEM)
Central nervous system lymphoma

and *Mycobacterium tuberculosis*. Oligoclonal bands were not present. Three days after lumbar puncture, JC virus (JCV) PCR returned positive in both the CSF (>25 million copies/mL) and serum (372,000 copies/mL), establishing a diagnosis of progressive multifocal leukoencephalopathy (PML).

Following the diagnosis of PML, immune suppression was decreased by discontinuing tacrolimus. Interferon-α was administered for 2 weeks without any clinical improvement. In fact, the patient's neurologic symptoms progressed to left hemi paresis and development of confusion during this time. Ultimately, the patient and his family elected to transition to home hospice, and he expired shortly thereafter.

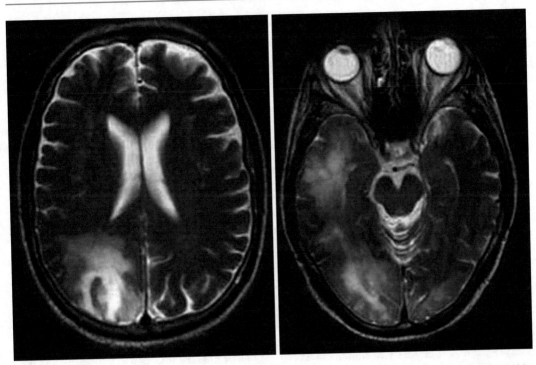

Fig. 2.1 T2-weighted MRI brain images obtained on presentation with unilateral vision loss depicting abnormal white matter enhancement of the right occipital and parietal lobes

2.1 Progressive Multifocal Leukoencephalopathy (PML)

PML is a rare acute-to-subacute demyelinating disorder of the central nervous system caused by reactivation of the JC polyomavirus. This disorder was first reported in 1958 in a cohort of patients with CLL and Hodgkin's disease [1]. Approximately 85% of cases occur in patients with human immunodeficiency virus (HIV) infection/AIDS, but it also occurs in patients after HSCT or solid organ transplant (SOT) and in other disorders causing lymphopenia [2]. The monoclonal antibody therapies rituximab and natalizumab have also been associated with an increased risk of PML [3, 4], and a similar association has been found with dimethyl fumarate and fingolimod, two drugs used in the management of multiple sclerosis.

JCV is a double-stranded DNA virus and is a member of the *Polyomaviridae* family. There is an estimated seroprevalence of anti-JCV antibodies of over 80% in the adult population [5]. Infection is

generally asymptomatic in immunocompetent hosts. Primary infection typically occurs in childhood, and the virus remains latent in the bone marrow and lymphoid tissues. In the setting of pronounced immunosuppression, the neurotropic virus reactivates and infects both astrocytes and oligodendrocytes. The latter are predominantly located in the white matter where they are involved in myelin synthesis. JCV causes astrocytes to enlarge, to develop multiple nuclei, and to take on a bizarre appearance but causes a lytic infection of oligodendrocytes, leading to widespread demyelination with concomitant development of neurologic deficits corresponding to the affected parts of the brain [6].

PML is uncommon in transplant recipients but carries a grave prognosis. In a review of 69 cases of PML after SOT and HSCT, the incidence after heart or lung transplant was estimated to be 1.24 cases per 1000 post-transplant person-years, a higher risk than seen in HIV patients on effective antiretroviral therapy, and mortality was 84% [2]. The most common symptoms of post-transplant

PML in this study were cognitive deficits (47%), weakness (42%), visual changes (24%), cerebellar symptoms (19%), and dysarthria (17%) [2].

The gold standard for diagnosis of PML is detection of viral DNA or proteins by in situ hybridization or immunohistochemistry on a brain biopsy specimen, as well as the presence of the typical histopathologic triad of demyelinization, bizarre astrocytes, and enlarged oligodendroglial nuclei [6, 7]. Given the potential risks of brain biopsy, a positive PCR assay for JCV in the cerebrospinal fluid in the setting of consistent clinical and radiographic findings has largely replaced brain biopsy to establish a diagnosis of PML [2, 7]. Sensitivity and specificity of JCV PCR for diagnosing PML are 74% and 95.8%, respectively [8]. A negative CSF PCR for JCV is not sufficient to rule out the diagnosis of PML, and brain biopsy should be pursued if suspicion is high despite a negative CSF PCR assay. Serum JCV antibody testing is not a reliable test for PML given the high prevalence of anti-JCV antibodies in the normal population resulting in a low positive predictive value of positive tests [5].

The mainstay of therapy for PML is improvement in host immune function. In HIV patients, this is accomplished with antiretroviral therapy. In HSCT recipients, however, reconstitution of the immune system is limited to withdrawal of any immune suppressing medications, which is often insufficient for resolution of infection. Multiple experimental therapies have been attempted, including cidofovir, cytarabine, and mefloquine, but none showed significant improvement in patient outcomes [9–11]. There are case reports suggesting a benefit with interferon-α or interleukin-2 therapy [12, 13], but there are no robust studies that show benefit of these medications.

PML is a grave diagnosis, with a 1-year mortality of >50% in all patient populations despite the beneficial effects of antiretroviral therapy for HIV patients and plasmapheresis for patients with natalizumab-associated PML [14, 15]. However, the prognosis for PML is even poorer after HSCT and SOT with an associated mortality of >80% [2].

Key Points/Pearls
- Progressive multifocal leukoencephalopathy (PML) is a demyelinating disease caused by reactivation of JCV in the setting of profound immunosuppression, with lytic infection of oligodendrocytes.
- Patients may present with diffuse neurologic findings, but the most common are cognitive deficits, weakness, and visual changes.
- Diagnosis is made by characteristic triad of demyelinization, bizarre astrocytes, and enlarged oligodendroglial nuclei on brain biopsy along with positive JCV PCR or by a positive JCV PCR on the CSF with an appropriate clinical syndrome.
- Treatment of transplant-associated PML requires reduction in immunosuppression, but prognosis is poor.
- JCV can cause various neurological syndromes: Classic PML is the most common and is associated with HIV infection in >80%. PML in non-HIV-infected patients has been associated with immunosuppression, stem cell and solid organ transplant, the monoclonal antibodies rituximab (used in non-Hodgkin lymphoma, CLL, and rheumatoid arthritis) and natalizumab (used in multiple sclerosis and Crohn's disease), and the agents dimethyl fumarate and fingolimod (both used in multiple sclerosis).
- On MRI, classic PML appears as T1 hypointense and T2 hyperintense lesions in the subcortical white matter without enhancement.
- When HIV-infected patients with PML are treated with antiretroviral therapy, immune-reconstitution inflammatory syndrome PML (IRIS-PML) may present with paradoxical worsening of symptoms and the presence on MRI of peripheral or rim enhancement with mass effect and vasogenic edema.
- JCV also can cause granular cell neuropathy (GCN) due to infection of the cerebellar granule cell neurons with cerebellar ataxia and dysarthria, aseptic meningitis, and encephalopathy when it infects extensively the pyramidal cell neurons with little infection of oligodendrocytes, leading to abnormalities of higher CNS functions without focal neurologic deficit.

References

1. Astrom KE, Mancall EL, Richardson EP Jr. Progressive multifocal leuko-encephalopathy; a hitherto unrecognized complication of chronic lymphatic leukaemia and Hodgkin's disease. Brain. 1958;81(1):93–111.

2. Mateen FJ, Muralidharan R, Carone M, et al. Progressive multifocal leukoencephalopathy in transplant recipients. Ann Neurol. 2011;70(2):305–22.

3. Kleinschmidt-DeMasters BK, Tyler KL. Progressive multifocal leukoencephalopathy complicating treatment with natalizumab and interferon beta 1-a for multiple sclerosis. N Engl J Med. 2005;353:369–74.

4. Carson KR, Evens AM, Richey EA, et al. Progressive multifocal leukoencephalopathy after rituximab therapy in HIV-negative patients: a report of 57 cases from the Research on Adverse Drug Events and Reports project. Blood. 2009;113:4834–40.

5. Weber T, Trebst C, Frye S, et al. Analysis of the systemic and intrathecal humoral immune response in progressive multifocal leukoencephalopathy. J Infect Dis. 1997;176(1):250–4.

6. Tan CS, Koralnik IJ. Progressive multifocal leukoencephalopathy and other disorders caused by JC virus: clinical features and pathogenesis. Lancet Neurol. 2010;9(4):425–37.

7. Berger JR, Aksamit AJ, Clifford DB, et al. PML diagnostic criteria: consensus statement from the AAN neuroinfectious disease section. Neurology. 2013;80(15):1430–8.

8. Fong IW, Britton CB, Luinstra KE, Toma E, Mahony JB. Diagnostic value of detecting JC virus DNA in cerebrospinal fluid of patients with progressive multifocal leukoencephalopathy. J Clin Microbiol. 1995;33(2):484–6.

9. Gasnault J, Kousignian P, Kahraman M, et al. Cidofovir in AIDS-associated progressive multifocal leukoencephalopathy: a monocenter observational study with clinical and JC virus load monitoring. J Neurovirol. 2001;7:375–81.

10. Hall CD, Dafni U, Simpson D, et al. Failure of cytarabine in progressive multifocal leukoencephalopathy associated with human immunodeficiency virus infection. N Engl J Med. 1998;338(19):1345–51.

11. Clifford DB, Nath A, Cinque P, et al. A study of mefloquine treatment for progressive multifocal leukoencephalopathy: results and exploration of predictors of PML outcomes. J Neurovirol. 2013;19:351–8.

12. Geschwind MD, Skolasky RI, Royal WS, McArthur JC. The relative contributions of HAART and α-IFN for therapy of PML in AIDS. J Neurovirol. 2001;7:353–7.

13. Przepiorka D, Jaeckle KA, Birdwell RR, et al. Successful treatment of PML with low-dose interleukin-2. Bone Marrow Transplant. 1997;20:983–7.

14. Marzocchetti A, Tompkins T, Clifford DB, et al. Determinants of survival in progressive multifocal leukoencephalopathy. Neurology. 2009;73:1551–8.

15. Clifford DB, DeLuca A, Simpson DM, et al. Natalizumab-associated progressive multifocal leukoencephalopathy in patients with multiple sclerosis: lessons from 28 cases. Lancet Neurol. 2010;9(4):438–46.

Like Mother, Like Daughter

Emily Obringer

A 32-year-old pregnant woman presented to an outside hospital at 25 weeks gestation with complaints of back pain, fever, and decreased fetal movement for one day. She had recently been diagnosed with gestational diabetes, which was being managed with dietary modification; otherwise, she had no medical problems. She denied any history of urinary tract, yeast, or sexually transmitted infections, including herpes simplex virus (HSV). There were no sick contacts or pets at home, and she denied any recent travel. Her review of systems was negative for rhinorrhea, nasal congestion, cough, loose stools, dysuria, or vaginal discharge. For the past several hours, she had had intermittent abdominal pains consistent with contractions.

Her initial vital signs were temperature 101.4 °F, pulse 104 beats per minute, respiratory rate 18 breaths per minute, and blood pressure 104/61 mmHg. She was in moderate distress related to contractions, and a closed, minimally effaced cervix was noted on pelvic examination. The fetal heart rate was 140 beats per minute with moderate variability and occasional variable decelerations. Table 3.1 shows initial maternal laboratory results. She was started on intravenous (IV) ceftriaxone for presumed pyelonephritis. Within hours, the contractions became more regular and frequent. Due to concerns for progression to active labor, she was given magnesium, betamethasone, penicillin, and indomethacin, and she was transferred to our tertiary care facility. Upon arrival she was fully dilated, and the baby was promptly delivered via Cesarean section due to breech presentation and premature labor.

The 25 2/7-week female was born pale and limp with Apgar scores of 1, 1, and 6 at 1 minute, 5 minutes, and 10 minutes, respectively. Resuscitation included chest compressions, intubation, and vasopressor support. Her initial examination was notable for a diffuse, faint, erythematous rash with papules and pustules most prominent across her upper torso. She was also found to have passed meconium in the delivery room. Other physical exam findings were consistent with gestational age. Her initial laboratory studies were significant for a white blood cell count of 6900/μL (normal range, 6500–30,600/μL) with 27% bands, platelet count of 89,000/μL (150,000–450,000/μL), and an arterial blood gas with pH <6.8. A complete metabolic panel showed an elevated aspartate aminotransferase of 101 U/L (normal range, 8–37 U/L) but was otherwise unremarkable for gestational age. A blood culture was collected and broad-spectrum antimicrobials were started.

E. Obringer, M.D.
Section of Infectious Diseases, Department of Pediatrics, University of Chicago,
Chicago, IL, USA
e-mail: emily.obringer@gmail.com

Table 3.1 Maternal laboratory results

Laboratory test (units)	Result	Reference range
Prenatal		
HIV antibody/antigen	Negative	Negative
Rubella IgG serology	Positive	Result suggests immunity
Hepatitis B surface antigen, blood	Negative	Negative
Rapid plasma reagin (RPR), blood	Nonreactive	Nonreactive
Chlamydia and gonorrhea DNA PCR, urine	Negative	Negative
Group B *Streptococcus* culture, vaginal	Unknown	Negative
At presentation		
Complete blood count		
WBC (per µL)	16,300	4100–11,300
Neutrophils (%)	83.7	41.9–75.7
Lymphocytes (%)	10.8	13.7–42.9
Monocytes (%)	5.2	3.7–11.3
Hemoglobin (g/dL)	11.0	11.6–14.4
Platelets (per µL)	257,000	145,000–368,000
Complete metabolic panel	Within normal limits	
Urinalysis		
Specific gravity	1.020	1.005–1.030
pH	6.0	5.0–9.0
Nitrites	Negative	Negative
Leukocyte esterase	Positive	Negative
Ketones	Positive	Negative
WBC (per hpf)	5	None seen
Red blood cells (per hpf)	0	None seen
Epithelial cells (per hpf)	2	None seen

DNA deoxyribonucleic acid, *HIV* human immunodeficiency virus, *hpf* high-power field, *PCR* polymerase chain reaction, *WBC* white blood cells

Additional maternal history was obtained after delivery. She had immigrated from Mexico several years prior and lived with her husband and 14-year-old daughter in Chicago. She denied eating any new or unusual foods, undercooked meats or shellfish. She did report consumption of soft cheeses, particularly "queso fresco," throughout the pregnancy. She was uncertain whether the cheese was pasteurized. She had never been screened for tuberculosis.

Early-onset sepsis due to intrauterine infection was suspected given the baby's presentation at delivery and the maternal history of fever. The differential diagnosis for such infection is broad and includes bacteria, viruses, and fungi (see Table 3.2). Organisms may cause ascending infection through the maternal genitourinary tract, particularly if rupture of membranes is pro-

longed or fetal monitoring devices are used. Alternatively, a systemic maternal infection may allow for certain pathogens to cross the placenta leading to intrauterine infection. Open communication between the obstetrician and pediatrician is essential to ensure that all confirmed or suspected maternal infections are considered in the evaluation and treatment of the infant.

As in this case, the maternal history and presenting signs in the neonate may provide clues to the clinician as to the etiology of neonatal sepsis. Group B *Streptococcus* and *Escherichia coli*, two of the most common pathogens that cause early-onset sepsis, may be suspected if the mother has a positive screening vaginal culture or a urinary tract infection, respectively. A history of HSV infection at any time prior to delivery, but

Table 3.2 Differential diagnosis of early-onset neonatal sepsis

Gram-positive bacteria
Group B *Streptococcus*
Viridans group streptococci
Staphylococcus aureus
Enterococcus spp.
Listeria monocytogenes
Other *Streptococcus* spp.
Gram-negative bacteria
Escherichia coli
Haemophilus influenzae
Enterobacter spp.
Citrobacter spp.
Klebsiella spp.
Viruses
Herpes simplex virus (HSV)
Enteroviruses
Coxsackieviruses
Echoviruses
Parechoviruses
Influenza
Parainfluenza
Varicella zoster virus (VZV)
Chikungunya virus
Dengue virus
Fungi
Candida spp.

particularly if the mother has active lesions, should warrant further investigation of the neonate. Other common viral infections, such as influenza, parainfluenza, and enterovirus, may be considered if the mother has upper respiratory, gastrointestinal, or influenza-like symptoms. If the mother has varicella or herpes zoster, congenital varicella should be in the differential diagnosis of the ill neonate. A recent travel history may increase the likelihood of chikungunya and dengue. *Candida* is the most common fungus that causes neonatal sepsis and may be considered if the mother has had vaginal candidiasis. Infectious etiologies for rash in the newborn may include HSV, enterovirus, and *Candida* infections, as well as chikungunya and dengue viruses. A negative maternal history or lack of a specific exam finding in the newborn does not rule out a particular pathogen.

Twenty-four hours after delivery, the baby's blood culture grew Gram-positive rods, which later speciated to *Listeria monocytogenes*. Additional blood cultures were negative; a lumbar puncture could not be performed. She was treated with IV ampicillin for 21 days. Gentamicin was initially included as part of synergistic therapy, but after the baby clinically stabilized it was discontinued due to concern for nephrotoxicity in the presence of unrelated renal anomalies.

The mother's urine culture showed no growth, and blood cultures had not been obtained. She defervesced promptly after delivery and antibiotics were not continued. Placental pathology was consistent with severe acute chorioamnionitis. Placental culture was not performed. The mother's acute febrile illness was likely caused by transient *Listeria* bacteremia, which was then transmitted through the infected placenta to her daughter, leading to preterm labor and neonatal sepsis. A possible source for this foodborne infection may have been contaminated soft cheese given the mother's dietary history.

3.1 Listeriosis

Listeria monocytogenes is a facultatively anaerobic Gram-positive rod that grows readily on blood agar (Fig. 3.1). Ideal incubation temperatures range from 30 to 37 °C; however, the organism is also known to grow better than other bacteria at refrigerator temperatures (4 to 10 °C) [1]. The organism may also have different morphology in clinical culture, including diphtheroid, coccoid, and diplococcoid appearance, which may contribute to initial laboratory misidentification [1]. Pulsed-field gel electrophoresis and whole genome sequencing are utilized to identify particular strains.

Listeria is widespread in the environment, and most clinical cases outside the neonatal period are due to ingestion of contaminated food. *Listeria* infection is nationally notifiable, and cases in the United States (USA) are tracked through the *Listeria* Initiative, a nationwide surveillance system directed by the US Centers for Disease Control and Prevention (CDC) [2].

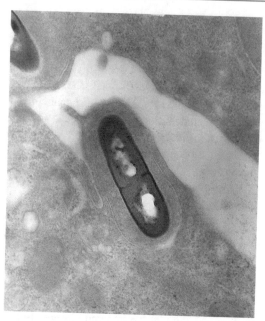

Fig. 3.1 Transmission electron microscope image of a *Listeria* bacterium in a tissue sample. Source: Public Health Image Library, CDC, https://phil.cdc.gov/phil/details_linked.asp?pid=10828 (Accessed June 21, 2017)

The incidence is low, with 0.29 cases of listeriosis per 100,000 individuals; however, the rate is higher in certain populations, including adults aged ≥65 years (1.3 per 100,000) and pregnant women (3.0 per 100,000) [3]. In particular, pregnant Hispanic women have a rate 24 times higher than the general population. Both sporadic cases and outbreaks occur and frequently involve unpasteurized soft cheese, raw produce, and processed meat, such as hot dogs and deli meat [3]. The largest known outbreak occurred in 2011, when 147 cases, 33 deaths, and 1 miscarriage were associated with consumption of contaminated cantaloupe [4].

Clinical presentation ranges from asymptomatic infection to bacteremia or meningitis, and in some cases infection can lead to death. Pregnant women, particularly those in the third trimester, may experience an acute febrile illness with diarrhea and influenza-like symptoms, such as myalgias, arthralgias, back pain, and headache. Bacteremia is the most common clinical presentation in this setting, unlike in other immunocompromised adults in whom meningitis predominates. Stillbirth and spontaneous abortion occur in approximately 22% of intrauterine infections, and neonatal listeriosis occurs in two thirds of surviving babies [1]. Preterm delivery is common, and amnionitis and brown staining of the amniotic fluid can occur [5]. Early-onset neonatal sepsis is usually due to in utero infection. However, those infants exposed (usually through maternal vaginal colonization) during the peripartum period may present up to 3 weeks of age.

Clinical presentation in the neonate is similar to other forms of bacterial sepsis, but purulent conjunctivitis and a disseminated papular rash may rarely be observed. The rash, more often seen in severe infection, is characterized histologically by granulomas and is also known as "granulomatosis infantisepticum" [5]. In older adults and in immunocompromised hosts, meningitis is the most common clinical presentation. *Listeria* has a predilection for the brain parenchyma, in addition to the meninges, and symptoms are often consistent with meningoencephalitis [1]. Other manifestations in immunocompromised hosts include endocarditis and rarely, localized infection. Noninvasive illness can occur in immunocompetent individuals, who usually present with febrile gastroenteritis.

Prompt diagnosis and treatment of listeriosis are essential as the mortality is approximately 20% overall and up to 36% for neonatal disease [1, 3, 6]. The diagnosis should be considered especially for those at highest risk including immunocompromised, elderly and pregnant patients. A thorough dietary history is recommended for all patients. Isolation of the organism from a sterile body fluid site, such as blood or cerebrospinal fluid, confirms the diagnosis. The treatment of choice is IV ampicillin. Combination therapy with an aminoglycoside, such as gentamicin, is generally recommended for severe cases such as meningitis and endocarditis although evidence supporting this practice is limited [7]. Trimethoprim-sulfamethoxazole could be considered as an alternative antibiotic in patients with penicillin allergy; however, some experts recommend desensitization to penicillin in these cases [7].

Listeriosis prevention methods include washing hands, knives, and cooking surfaces that have been exposed to uncooked, raw foods. In addition, raw foods derived from animal sources should be thoroughly cooked prior to consumption. Pregnant women and the immunocompromised should avoid certain foods, including soft cheeses, raw or unpasteurized milk, and deli meats. People at high risk should also thoroughly wash raw produce and cook hot dogs and other ready-to-eat foods until steaming before eating. The US Food and Drug Administration has established regulatory standards to reduce the risk of contamination of refrigerated and ready-to-eat foods with *Listeria monocytogenes*. Also, active surveillance has helped to limit the impact of outbreaks.

Key Points/Pearls

- *Listeria* can grow at standard refrigerator temperatures, contaminating ready-to-eat foods that are not cooked before eating, such as unpasteurized soft cheese, raw produce, hot dogs, and deli meat.
- Exposure to *Listeria* is common, but the risk of invasive listeriosis after exposure is very low.
- Listeriosis is a foodborne illness that may rarely cause serious morbidity and mortality, including meningoencephalitis and neonatal sepsis.
- Certain populations are at particular risk for invasive disease, including fetuses and neonates, pregnant women, immunocompromised patients, and older adults.
- Early-onset neonatal sepsis may be caused by a variety of pathogens; a thorough review of the maternal history may reveal clues as to possible exposures.
- Rash and meconium-stained amniotic fluid in a critically ill premature newborn may be signs of listeriosis.

- Pregnant women and immunocompromised hosts should avoid certain foods, such as soft cheeses, raw or unpasteurized milk, and deli meats.
- Ampicillin is the preferred therapy, with or without the addition of gentamicin.
- Trimethoprim-sulfamethoxazole is an alternative antibiotic in patients with penicillin allergy although some experts recommend desensitization to penicillin in these cases.

References

1. Lorber B. Listeria monocytogenes. In: Mandell GL, Bennett JE, Dolin R, editors. Mandell, Douglas, and Bennett's: principles and practice of infectious diseases, vol. 2. 7th ed. Philadelphia: Elsevier; 2010. p. 2707–14.
2. CDC. National enteric disease surveillance: the *Listeria* initiative. 2016. http://www.cdc.gov/listeria/pdf/listeriainitiativeoverview_508.pdf. Accessed 3 Feb 2017.
3. CDC. Vitals signs: *Listeria* illnesses, deaths, and outbreaks—United States, 2009-2011. MMWR Morb Mortal Wkly Rep. 2013;62(22):448–52.
4. CDC. Multistate outbreak of listeriosis associated with Jensen Farms cantaloupe—United States, August-September 2011. MMWR Morb Mortal Wkly Rep. 2011;60(39):1357–8.
5. American Academy of Pediatrics. *Listeria monocytogenes* infections. In: Kimberlin DW, Brady MT, Jackson MA, Long SS, editors. Red book: 2015 Report of the Committee on Infectious Diseases. 30th ed. Elk Grove Village: American Academy of Pediatrics; 2015. p. 513–6.
6. Farber JM, Peterkin PI. *Listeria monocytogenes*, a food-borne pathogen. Microbiol Rev. 1991;55(3):476–511.
7. Hof H, Nichterlein T, Kretschmar M. Management of listeriosis. Clin Microbiol Rev. 1997;10(2):345–57.

From the Lungs to the Brain: A Case of Pneumonia in an Immunocompromised Patient

4

Fredy Chaparro-Rojas

A 59-year-old Hispanic male from Mexico with a past medical history of type 2 diabetes mellitus, hypertension, and chronic renal disease who had undergone a kidney transplant 4 years prior to presentation was admitted to the hospital. He complained of a 1-and-a-half month history of progressive fatigue, diminished appetite, and weight loss of about 25 lb associated with diaphoresis and left pleuritic chest pain. His initial evaluation was negative for acute coronary syndrome or pulmonary embolism. A chest X-ray and computed tomography (CT) of the chest revealed a small left pleural effusion and left lower lobe atelectasis. No additional testing was performed, and he was discharged home on analgesics.

A week later, he returned, reporting persistence of symptoms, including pain and subjective fevers associated with continued weight loss and new onset of a dry cough. He denied any sick exposures or recent travel. He also denied prior exposure or treatment for tuberculosis. The patient was receiving immunosuppressive therapy with tacrolimus, prednisone, and mycophenolate mofetil, as well as prophylaxis with trimethoprim-sulfamethoxazole (TMP-SMX) before his symptoms started.

On physical examination, the patient was afebrile, but rales and diminished breath sounds in the lower left lung field were noted on auscultation. No skin lesions were seen. His initial laboratory tests showed a normal white blood cell (WBC) count but with a left shift (WBC 6300/µL, with differential showing neutrophils 55%, bands 21%, lymphocytes 7%, and monocytes 15%). A chest X-ray showed a left basilar consolidation and associated pleural effusion (Fig. 4.1a), and a CT of the chest revealed a large area of consolidation in the left lung, in the region of his reported thoracic pain (Fig. 4.1b). A CT-guided biopsy of the lesion was obtained. The material was sent for bacterial, mycobacterial, and fungal stains and cultures (Fig. 4.2). The results were positive for modified acid-fast variable, branching filamentous bacteria, consistent with *Nocardia* species.

The patient received treatment with high-dose TMP-SMX and imipenem for *Nocardia asteroides* complex. After an induction phase, he was continued on therapy with high-dose TMP-SMX only, with improvement of his symptoms and resolution of his chest CT findings.

The patient returned 3 months after starting therapy complaining of headaches, lethargy, falls (especially when climbing in or out of his truck), and forgetfulness (he sometimes forgot to take his medications). On physical examination, he was found to have a wide-based gait, foot slapping, and a right temporal visual field defect.

F. Chaparro-Rojas, M.D.
Delaware Valley Infectious Diseases Associates,
Wynnewood, PA, USA
e-mail: freddych6@yahoo.com

© Springer International Publishing AG 2018
M. David, J.-L. Benoit (eds.), *The Infectious Disease Diagnosis*,
https://doi.org/10.1007/978-3-319-64906-1_4

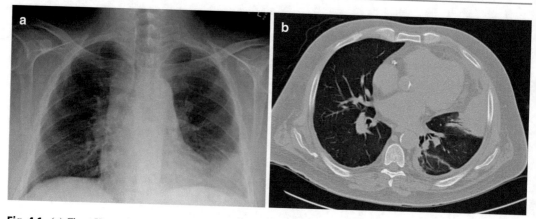

Fig. 4.1 (**a**) Chest X-ray showing left basilar infiltrate and blunting of the costophrenic angle, suggestive of pleural effusion. (**b**) CT of the chest revealing pulmonary consolidation and a small pleural effusion

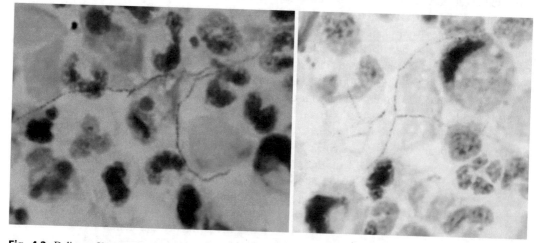

Fig. 4.2 Delicate filamentous Gram-positive branching rods, acid-fast stain positive, consistent with *Nocardia* species

A CT scan of the head followed by a magnetic resonance imaging (MRI) of the brain showed a large (3.4 × 3.4 cm), cystic mass in the left temporoparietal region. A brain biopsy was performed by the neurosurgical service, and a brain tissue specimen grew *Nocardia transvalensis/wallacei*, consistent with central nervous system (CNS) nocardiosis. The cultured isolate remained susceptible to TMP-SMX and ceftriaxone but had intermediate susceptibility to minocycline (minimum inhibitory concentration [MIC] 2 μg/mL) and resistant to imipenem (MIC 16 μg/mL).

The patient was initially treated with intravenous (IV) ceftriaxone and oral minocycline, but this was changed to IV ceftriaxone and oral TMP-SMX when the susceptibilities were reported. After 18 months of therapy, he was transitioned to suppressive oral TMP-SMX therapy alone. He had serial head CT scans, and 28 months after his presentation with neurological symptoms, the CT scan showed a stable lesion <1 cm in each dimension. At his 30-month follow-up visit to the infectious diseases clinic, he had no residual neurologic deficits.

4.1 Pulmonary Infections in the Solid Organ Transplant Patient

Pulmonary infections in transplant recipients are diverse, and rapid and aggressive evaluation and treatment are recommended to improve clinical outcomes. Community-acquired bacterial and viral infections, as well as opportunistic infections of relevance only in immunocompromised hosts need to be considered. The clinical presentation and classic manifestations of medical conditions are usually atypical in immunocompromised patients due to an impaired inflammatory response. The lungs are one of the most common sites of infection in transplant recipients more than 6 months after transplantation. These infections can progress rapidly and may constitute medical emergencies. Common causes of respiratory infections in immunocompromised patients include *Pneumocystis jirovecii*, *Nocardia asteroides*, *Aspergillus* spp., *Cryptococcus neoformans*, cytomegalovirus (CMV), varicella-zoster virus (VZV), influenza, respiratory syncytial virus (RSV), *Rhodococcus equi*, and *Legionella* spp., as shown in Table 4.1 [1].

4.2 *Nocardia* spp.

Nocardia spp. are ubiquitous microorganisms that can be found in soil, decomposing vegetation, and other organic matter, as well as in fresh and salt water, with more than 50 different species isolated to date. They tend to infect mainly immunocompromised patients; less than a third of infections have been reported in immunocompetent individuals. Nocardiosis occurs in patients with different types of cell-mediated immunodeficiencies including those with human immunodeficiency virus (HIV) infection, with lymphoma, or with long-term treatment with steroids, other immunomodulators, or immunosuppressive therapy for solid organ or hematopoietic stem cell transplantation. The incidence of nocardiosis in such patients has been estimated to be 140–340-fold higher than in the general population. Early recognition and therapy are imperative for successful outcomes [2].

Nocardia is a Gram-positive bacterial genus that grows aerobically and appears as a filamentous organism with branching on direct microscopy. It may express varying degrees of acid-fastness, depending on the mycolic acid composition of the cell wall and type of stain used. The modified Kinyoun acid-fast stain uses 1% sulfuric acid as a decolorizer instead of the more potent hydrochloric acid used in the decoloration step in the Ziehl-Neelsen staining procedure that enhances the ability of *Nocardia* to retain the colored fuchsin [3]. *Nocardia* has a "beaded" acid-fast appearance on microscopy, unlike *Mycobacteria*. It may resemble *Actinomyces* species on Gram stain. However, *Nocardia* can be distinguished because *Actinomyces* species are not acid-fast and only grow under anaerobic conditions.

Table 4.1 Differential diagnosis in an immunocompromised patient after solid organ transplantation with a pulmonary consolidation

Community-acquired pneumonia
Mycobacterium tuberculosis
Nontuberculous *Mycobacterium* spp.
Fungal pneumonia • Aspergillosis (*Aspergillus* spp.) • Mucormycosis • Histoplasmosis (*Histoplasma capsulatum*) • Blastomycosis (*Blastomyces dermatitidis*) • Cryptococcosis (*Cryptococcus* spp.)
Nocardiosis (*Nocardia* spp.)
Actinomycosis
Pneumocystis jirovecii pneumonia
Rhodococcus equi
Legionella spp.
Mycoplasma pneumoniae
Chlamydia
Viral pneumonia • Influenza • Cytomegalovirus (CMV) • Varicella zoster virus (VZV) • Respiratory syncytial virus (RSV)
Lung malignancy

Nocardia is not part of the normal human flora, and thus any isolate from a clinical culture must be carefully evaluated. However, patients with structural lung disease, such as bronchiectasis and cystic fibrosis, may develop colonization of the airways by these microorganisms [4]. Alveolar proteinosis is uniquely associated with pulmonary nocardiosis. Although there is no internationally accepted disease classification scheme for nocardiosis, commonly accepted clinical categories include pulmonary, disseminated, and primary cutaneous nocardiosis. Cutaneous nocardiosis is caused mostly by inoculation by *N. brasiliensis*. Immunocompetent patients with traumatic inoculation may develop superficial cutaneous disease or primary cutaneous nocardiosis, which can progress to lymphocutaneous disease or actinomycetomas. Primary infection of the skin or subcutaneous tissues often presents as a localized, nodular process but may progress to a more severe condition involving joints and bones [5].

The respiratory tract is the most common system involved. Respiratory *Nocardia* infection is usually acquired via aerosolization of the microorganism and secondary invasion of the respiratory tract. The clinical presentation of pulmonary nocardiosis is typically indolent, with symptoms often present for a period of weeks. Pulmonary nocardiosis induces a variety of inflammatory responses ranging from granulomatous to purulent reactions. Radiological evaluation can demonstrate abnormalities ranging from irregular nodular lesions, which may progress to cavitation, to diffuse pneumonic infiltrates or consolidative lesions with pleural effusions. Both local and hematogenous spreads of *Nocardia* infections are common with extrapulmonary disseminated disease complicating up to 40–50% of cases [6]. The diagnosis of pulmonary *Nocardia* infection should prompt a search for disseminated disease, including MRI of the brain to exclude cerebral abscess.

Ocular, endovascular, renal, osteoarticular, and other localized diseases have been described in rare cases in immunosuppressed patients and less frequently in the immunocompetent.

Among patients with a history of solid organ transplantation (SOT), *Nocardia* infection has a frequency of 0.6–3% and has been described in kidney, heart, liver and lung recipients. Lung transplant recipients have the highest incidence of *Nocardia* infection, followed by recipients of heart, small bowel, kidney, and liver transplants. A global decrease in the incidence of nocardiosis among transplant patients has been observed in recent years. This trend may be in part due to the introduction of TMP-SMX prophylaxis, although there are no data demonstrating the efficacy of this antibiotic for prevention of *Nocardia* infections. Based on the largest series of nocardiosis cases in SOT, 63% of patients were diagnosed within the first year following transplantation, and 14% had this diagnosis >5 years after SOT [7].

4.3 Treatment of Nocardiosis

The treatment of nocardial infections needs to be individualized. Optimal antimicrobial treatment regimens have not been established in part because *Nocardia* displays variable in vitro antimicrobial susceptibility, but empiric therapy should not be delayed. *Nocardia* isolated from clinically significant infections should undergo antimicrobial susceptibility testing. Common drug susceptibility patterns for major *Nocardia* species are listed in Table 4.2. Among the *Nocardia* species, *N. farcinica*, *N. brasiliensis*, and *N. otitidiscaviarum* tend to have a higher degree of multidrug resistance.

Sulfonamides are the drugs of choice to treat nocardiosis; TMP-SMX is the most commonly used sulfonamide in the USA. Alternative agents include amikacin, imipenem, meropenem, ceftriaxone, cefotaxime, minocycline, moxifloxacin, levofloxacin, linezolid, tigecycline, and amoxicillin/clavulanic acid. Imipenem is more active than other carbapenems against most *Nocardia* species. Ertapenem should not be used [9]. Of the tetracyclines, minocycline has the best activity against *Nocardia* and is an alternative agent in patients allergic to sulfonamides. Linezolid is active against virtually all known pathogenic *Nocardia* species and has successfully been used in patients with disseminated and CNS nocardiosis, however, its high cost and concern for toxicities have limited its use [10].

Table 4.2 Antimicrobial susceptibility of selected *Nocardia* species

Antimicrobial	N. cyriacigeorgica	N. farnica	N. nova complex	N. brasiliensis	N. transvalensis
Trimethoprim-sulfamethoxazole	S	R	S	S	S
Amoxicillin-clavulanate	R	V	R	V	S
Ceftriaxone	S	R	S	S	R
Imipenem	S	S	S	S	R
Amikacin	S	S	S	R	S
Minocycline	V	R	V	R	R
Moxifloxacin	V	S	R	ND	R
Clarithromycin	R	R	R	S	R
Linezolid	S	S	S	S	S

Adapted from [8]
ND no data, *R* generally inactive, *S* generally active (some isolates may be resistant), *V* may be active but resistance common

Combination therapy is usually recommended. Combinations of imipenem and cefotaxime, amikacin and TMP-SMX, imipenem and TMP-SMX, amikacin and cefotaxime, or amikacin and imipenem may provide enhanced activity [11]. In CNS disease, therapy should include drugs with favorable CNS penetration including TMP/SMX (e.g., TMP-SMX and ceftriaxone) [12]. Combination therapy should continue at least until clinical improvement occurs, and *Nocardia* species identification and antimicrobial susceptibility information are available. Immunocompetent patients with pulmonary or multifocal (non-CNS) nocardiosis may be successfully treated with 6–12 months of therapy. Immunosuppressed patients and those with CNS disease should receive at least 12 months of therapy.

Key Points/Pearls
- Nocardiosis can cause localized or disseminated disease in at risk patients, including those with advanced HIV infection, alveolar proteinosis, chronic granulomatous disease, and other immunodeficiencies including solid organ transplant recipients.
- Microscopically, *Nocardia* appear as Gram-positive, beaded, weakly acid-fast, branching rods.
- Cerebral imaging, preferably magnetic resonance imaging, should be performed in all cases of pulmonary and disseminated nocardiosis to rule out subclinical CNS disease.
- The microbiology laboratory should be informed about the suspicion of nocardiosis at the time a culture specimen is submitted.
- Species identification is necessary to determine the appropriate treatment, and susceptibilities should be performed; however, this should not delay empiric therapy.
- Branching Gram-positive rods include the anaerobe *Actinomyces* (actinomycosis) and aerobic actinomycetes including *Nocardia*, *Rhodococcus equi*, *Gordonia*, *Tsukamurella*, and *Streptomyces*.
- Lung-brain syndromes include nocardiosis, tuberculosis, nontuberculous mycobacterial infections, and fungal infections (cryptococcosis, histoplasmosis, coccidioidomycosis, mucormycosis, aspergillosis, and infection with *Scedosporium apiospermum*)

References

1. Fishman JA. Infections in solid organ transplant recipients. N Engl J Med. 2007;357(25):2601–14.
2. Wilson JW. Nocardiosis: updates and clinical overview. Mayo Clin Proc. 2012;87(4):403–7.
3. McNeil MM, Brown JM. The medically important aerobic actinomycetes: epidemiology and microbiology. Clin Microbiol Rev. 1994;7(3):357–417.
4. Ferrer A, Llorenç V, Codina G, de Gracia-Roldán J. Nocardiosis and bronchiectasis. An uncommon

association? Enferm Infecc Microbiol Clin. 2005; 23(2):62–6.

5. Lebeaux D, Morelon E, Suarez F, et al. Nocardiosis in transplant recipients. Eur J Clin Microbiol Infect Dis. 2014;33:689–702.

6. Minero MV, Marín M, Cercenado E, Rabadán PM, Bouza E, Muñoz P. Nocardiosis at the turn of the century. Medicine (Baltimore). 2009;88(4):250–61.

7. Peleg AY, Husain S, Qureshi ZA, et al. Risk factors, clinical characteristics, and outcome of *Nocardia* infection in organ transplant recipients: a matched case–control study. Clin Infect Dis. 2007;44(10):1307–14.

8. Sorrell TC, Mitchell DH, Iredell JR, Chen SC. *Nocardia* species. In: Bennett JE, Dolin R, Blaser MJ, editors. Mandell, Douglas, and Bennett's principles and practice of infectious diseases. 8th ed. Philadelphia: Churchill Livingstone/Elsevier; 2015. p. 2853–63. Table 255–3.

9. Cercenado E, Marin M, Sanchez-Martinez M, Cuevas O, Martinez-Alarcon J, Bouza E. In vitro activities of tigecycline and eight other antimicrobials against different *Nocardia* species identified by molecular methods. Antimicrob Agents Chemother. 2007;51(3):1102–4.

10. Moylett EH, Pacheco SE, Brown-Elliott BA, et al. Clinical experience with linezolid for the treatment of *Nocardia* infection. Clin Infect Dis. 2003;36(3): 313–8.

11. Gombert ME, Aulicino TM. Synergism of imipenem and amikacin in combination with other antibiotics against *Nocardia asteroides*. Antimicrob Agents Chemother. 1983;24(5):810–1.

12. Anagnostou T, Arvanitis M, Kourkoumpetis T, et al. Nocardiosis of the central nervous system. Medicine. 2014;93(1):19–27.

Student with Fever and Rash

5

Moira McNulty

A previously healthy 23-year-old male presented with 3 days of fever, chills, headache, and 1 day of rash. He was studying in the Midwestern United States (USA) but recently traveled home to the Southern United States for the winter holiday, returning 1 week prior to presentation. He noted a lack of appetite and was very fatigued, sleeping most of the afternoons and evening. He was taking acetaminophen and ibuprofen with temporary relief in his symptoms. He noticed an erythematous rash on his trunk and face 1 day prior to presentation. It was not pruritic or painful. He was unsure where the rash started on his body. He did not report conjunctivitis, rhinorrhea, cough, diarrhea, nausea, vomiting, muscle pain, or joint pain. He was not sexually active and had no known sick contacts. He spent time outdoors while home but did not recall any tick or insect bites. He did not use tobacco, alcohol, or illicit drugs. He was not on any medications and had no drug allergies. Of note, he had received the first in the series of measles, mumps, and rubella (MMR) vaccine 3 weeks prior because he did not remember having received the vaccination as a child, and it was a requirement to study at his school.

M. McNulty, M.D.
Section of Infectious Diseases and Global Health, Department of Medicine, University of Chicago, Chicago, IL, USA
e-mail: moira.mcnulty@uchospitals.edu

On physical examination, he had a temperature of 38 °C. His heart rate was 121 beats per minute and blood pressure 138/85 mmHg. He was in no distress but appeared fatigued with a flushed face. His oropharynx was mildly erythematous without exudate. He had normal conjunctiva and no cervical adenopathy. He was tachycardic with regular rhythm and no murmurs. His breath sounds were normal. His abdomen was soft and non-tender, without hepatosplenomegaly. His skin was warm, and he had a diffuse maculopapular, blanching rash covering his trunk, extremities, and neck, including the palms of his hands. He had no petechiae or vesicles and no mucosal involvement. His joints were normal without pain or swelling.

His symptoms of maculopapular rash, fever, and fatigue were concerning for a viral exanthem, possibly from enterovirus or infectious mononucleosis caused by either Epstein-Barr virus (EBV) or cytomegalovirus (CMV). A monospot test was performed for heterophile antibodies, which was negative. Another cause of viral exanthem that could have been causing his symptoms included measles, and though he did not have cough, coryza, conjunctivitis, or Koplik's spots, he did not remember being vaccinated as a child and had recent travel on an airplane where he could have been unknowingly exposed to an ill person. He was asked to call his parents to determine his vaccination history, and his mother reported that he had received all recommended childhood immunizations, including MMR. This

© Springer International Publishing AG 2018
M. David, J.-L. Benoit (eds.), *The Infectious Disease Diagnosis*,
https://doi.org/10.1007/978-3-319-64906-1_5

made a diagnosis of measles much less likely, but since he had received the MMR vaccine 2 weeks prior, he could have been affected by a vaccine-associated reaction.

Also on the differential diagnosis were bacterial illnesses including scarlet fever caused by streptococcal pharyngitis, which was considered because of his erythematous posterior oropharynx although he did not describe a sore throat. A rapid streptococcal test was performed to detect the presence of group A streptococcal antigen and was faintly positive. A throat culture was performed. Additional causes of fever and maculopapular rash are listed in Table 5.1. Several of these diagnoses were considered less likely given the patient's age.

The patient was started on cephalexin for a 10-day course to treat streptococcal pharyngitis with associated scarlet fever. The day after starting cephalexin, his fatigue improved, and his face was no longer flushed. His throat culture was negative for group A β-hemolytic streptococci. He was seen in clinic again 3 days later, and his fever and rash had resolved. He completed the course of cephalexin with resolution of his symptoms.

5.1 Scarlet Fever

Scarlet fever is a diffuse erythematous rash caused by erythrogenic exotoxins produced by group A β-hemolytic streptococcal strains (*Streptococcus pyogenes*) [1]. It most frequently occurs following pharyngeal infection with group A *Streptococcus* but can also occur after streptococcal skin and wound infections as well as postpartum infections [1, 5]. Scarlet fever is seen most often in children 5–15 years of age but can occur in anyone [5].

The rash of scarlet fever usually appears on the second day of illness and is first noted on the upper chest, spreading to the trunk, neck, and extremities (Fig. 5.1). The palms and soles are often spared [1]. It begins as small red blotches that gradually develop into the texture of sandpaper due to occlusion of sweat glands [1, 5]. The face appears flushed with circumoral clearing. Areas of skin folds may appear deeper red, which are called Pastia's lines. The tongue may be swollen red (strawberry tongue), and small hemorrhagic spots may be presented on the hard and soft palates [1, 5]. The skin rash

Table 5.1 Differential diagnosis of maculopapular rash and fever [1–4]

| *Noninfectious* |
| Drug eruption |
| Kawasaki's disease, of unknown etiology |
| Vaccine-associated reaction |
| *Infectious* |
| Enteroviruses including Coxsackie virus may cause a variety of rashes; hand, foot, and mouth disease is seen with enteroviruses, especially with Coxsackie 16 in the United States and notably with enterovirus 71, which may also cause severe brainstem encephalitis |
| Adenovirus |
| Epstein-Barr virus (EBV) |
| Cytomegalovirus (CMV) |
| Erythema infectiosum (Parvovirus B19) |
| Roseola infantum (Human herpesvirus-6 [HHV-6]) |
| Measles |
| Rubella |
| Scarlet fever due to group A *Streptococcus*, streptococcal toxic shock syndrome |
| Staphylococcal toxic shock syndrome (sunburn rash) |
| Staphylococcal scalded skin syndrome (fluid-filled bullae) |
| *Haemophilus influenzae* (cellulitis in the setting of bacteremia) |
| *Arcanobacterium haemolyticum* (a cause of pharyngitis with rash) |
| Yersiniosis (*Yersinia enterocolitica*) |
| Acute human immunodeficiency virus (HIV) infection, often with oral erosions, lymphadenopathy, and fever |
| Secondary syphilis (*Treponema pallidum*) |
| Lyme disease (*Borrelia burgdorferi*) (erythema migrans and secondary erythema migrans) |
| Disseminated gonococcal infection (up to 20 hemorrhagic pustules along with tenosynovitis and arthritis) |
| Rocky Mountain spotted fever (*Rickettsia rickettsii*) and other rickettsioses |
| Southern tick-associated rash illness (STARI) (erythema migrans in areas of the United States without Lyme disease) |
| Anaplasmosis (*Anaplasma phagocytophilum*) and ehrlichiosis (*Ehrlichia chaffeensis* or *E. ewingii*) (may cause a rash) |
| Dengue fever (rash is usually delayed for a few days after onset of fever) |
| Zika virus (rash associated with conjunctivitis) |
| Typhoid fever (*Salmonella typhi*) (rose spots are sometimes seen) |
| Chikungunya virus (rash associated with prominent arthralgia) |

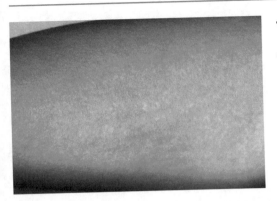

Fig. 5.1 Forearm demonstrating the rash of scarlet fever due to group A *Streptococcus*; the rash appears as tiny red bumps resembling sunburn with the texture of sandpaper. (Source: https://phil.cdc.gov/phil/details.asp (ID#5163, Accessed June 21, 2017))

resolves in about 1 week. Skin desquamation follows the rash and may last for several weeks [1, 5]. The early stages of the rash are often indistinguishable from other causes of exanthem.

Severe cases of scarlet fever may be complicated by sepsis and arthritis. Other noninfectious complications of streptococcal infections include acute rheumatic fever and post-streptococcal glomerulonephritis [1]. Treatment with antibiotics targeted at group A *Streptococcus* reduces duration of symptoms, infectivity, and risk of acute rheumatic fever but does not prevent the development of post-streptococcal glomerulonephritis [2, 5, 6].

Key Points/Pearls

- The rash of scarlet fever is caused by exotoxin-producing group A streptococcal species (*Streptococcus pyogenes*).
- Scarlet fever most often occurs in children ages 5–15 years of age but less frequently can occur in other age groups.

- Group A streptococcal pharyngitis most frequently precedes symptoms of scarlet fever.
- In the older literature, a syndrome of "malignant scarlet fever" now is referred to as streptococcal toxic shock syndrome, often due to a soft tissue infection followed by bacteremia and sepsis with a prominent exotoxin-mediated rash.
- Acute rheumatic fever is a dreaded complication of group A *Streptococcus* pharyngitis, especially when antibiotic treatment is delayed or not provided.
- Antibiotic treatment can prevent the development of acute rheumatic fever but does not prevent post-streptococcal glomerulonephritis.

References

1. Bisno AL, Stevens DL. *Streptococcus* pyogenes. In: Mandell GL, Dolin R, Bennett JE, editors. Mandell, Douglas, and Bennett's principles and practice of infectious diseases. Philadelphia: Churchill Livingstone; 2010. p. 2593–610.
2. Bisno AL, Gerber MA, Gwaltney JM, Kaplan EL, Schwartz RH. Practice guidelines for the diagnosis and management of group A streptococcal pharyngitis. Clin Infect Dis. 2002;35(2):113–25.
3. Garcia JJG. Differential diagnosis of viral exanthemas. Open Vaccine J. 2010;3:65–8.
4. Drago F, Paolino S, Rebora A, Broccolo F, Cardo P, Parodi A. The challenge of diagnosing atypical exanthems: a clinic-laboratory study. J Am Acad Dermatol. 2012;67(6):1282–8.
5. U.S. Centers for Disease Control and Prevention. Scarlet fever: group A streptococcal infection. Page last updated January 19, 2016. https://www.cdc.gov/features/scarletfever/. Accessed 21 June 2017.
6. Bisno AL. Nonsuppurative poststreptococcal sequelae: rheumatic fever and glomerulonephritis. In: Mandell GL, Dolin R, Bennett JE, editors. Mandell, Douglas, and Bennett's principles and practice of infectious diseases. Philadelphia: Churchill Livingstone; 2010. p. 2611–22.

Fever, a Rash, and a … "Bug Bite"?

6

Karl O.A. Yu and Jennifer L. Burns

A 3-year-old girl with no past medical history presented to the emergency department with fever, fatigue, rash, and eye redness. The patient's parents noted that, beginning 1–2 days prior to presentation, the child grew tired and had a tactile fever. Over the course of a day, she developed a whole body rash that involved her palms, generalized fatigue, cough, post-tussive vomiting, watery non-bloody diarrhea, and anorexia. There was also a large painful swelling over the child's right shin that developed over a few days and looked like a "bug bite" (Fig. 6.1).

The child's past medical and family history were noncontributory. Her immunizations were up-to-date. While the child and her family lived in a suburban area, there was recent and recurrent travel to a tick-endemic area in the midwestern United States and history of "backyard camping" by the child's older siblings. There was no specific report of a tick or other arthropod identified on the patient. She visited the southwestern United States 1 month prior to admission, where she had exposure to horses. She also had a pet guinea pig.

K.O.A. Yu, M.D., Ph.D. (✉)
Center for Infectious Diseases and Immunology,
Rochester General Hospital Research Institute,
Rochester General Hospital, Rochester, NY, USA
e-mail: KarlOliver.Yu@rochesterregional.org

J.L. Burns, C.P.N.P.
Section of Infectious Diseases, Department of Pediatrics, Comer Children's Hospital, University of Chicago Medicine, Chicago, IL, USA

On physical examination, the child's height and weight were normal for her age. Her temperature was 37.5 °C, with a daily maximum of 39.1 °C. The heart rate was 155 beats per minute, blood pressure 86/49 mmHg (5th percentile of systolic pressure for age, 76 mmHg), and respiratory rate 38 breaths per minute. She was briefly hypoxic (spO$_2$ 88%), requiring supplemental oxygen by nasal cannula, but was returned to room air quickly (spO$_2$ 97%). She was tired-appearing and interacted minimally with the examiner. Her sclerae and conjunctivae were injected with yellow exudate. Her eyelids appeared puffy. The tympanic membranes were normal. There was no pharyngeal erythema, but there appeared to be a "strawberry tongue." Kernig and Brudzinski signs were negative. Diffuse rales were intermittently heard on exam. There was tachycardia with regular rhythm but no murmur. Her abdomen was soft, nontender, and without organomegaly. There was subcentimeter nontender lymphadenopathy on the left anterior neck and right inguinal region and an erythematous generalized blanching maculopapular rash over the child's chest, back, face, abdomen, and extremities including the palms. There were no neurologic deficits. Capillary refill was delayed at 3 s. There was a 2-cm area of apparently painful induration over the child's right shin, with overlying erythema, and apparent scratches over both ankles. The child's parents later recalled a history of minor trauma about

© Springer International Publishing AG 2018
M. David, J.-L. Benoit (eds.), *The Infectious Disease Diagnosis*,
https://doi.org/10.1007/978-3-319-64906-1_6

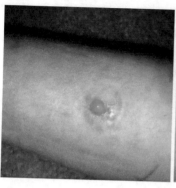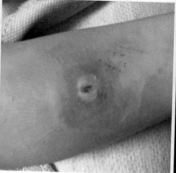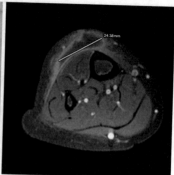

Fig. 6.1 *Left and center*, the patient's leg wound, shortly before and 4 days after incision and drainage. *Right*, T1-weighted magnetic resonance imaging scan axial image of the leg showing residual abscess 5 days after her initial incision and drainage. Line, 24 mm

1 week before presentation, when the patient hit her leg against a wooden chair's leg.

Laboratory studies were significant for leukocytosis at 18,300/mm³ (normal range, 3500–11,000/mm³) with a "left shift" differential count, with 50% segmented neutrophils, 43% band forms, 1% lymphocytes, and 4% monocytes. Platelets were low at 149,000/mm³ (150,000–450,000/mm³). Döhle bodies and large platelets were present on examination of a blood smear. Serum sodium was low at 129 mmol/L (134–149 mmol/L), albumin was low at 2.9 g/dL (3.5–5.0 g/dL), and alanine aminotransferase was elevated at 152 U/L (8–35 U/L). Blood urea nitrogen and creatinine were normal. Coagulation studies were prolonged, with prothrombin time 18 s, international normalized ratio 1.47, and activated partial prothrombin time 40.6 s (normal ranges, 9.4–12.5 s, 0.9–1.1 ratio, and 25–37 s, respectively). The erythrocyte sedimentation rate was 20 mm/h, and C-reactive protein and procalcitonin levels were elevated at 170 mg/L and 98.5 ng/mL, respectively (normal ranges, < 20 mm/h, < 8 mg/L and < 0.15 ng/mL). A chest X-ray showed interstitial and alveolar opacities, concerning for congestion or edema overlying an infectious process, such as pneumonia.

With tachycardia and delayed capillary refill, a systemic inflammatory response was suspected. This informed the differential diagnosis for mucocutaneous involvement in a sepsis-like picture (Table 6.1). Given the child's history of travel to a tick-borne disease-endemic area and exposure to animals, she was initially placed on a broad-spectrum empiric antibiotic regimen that included

Table 6.1 Differential diagnosis for pediatric mucocutaneous symptom complexes

"Conventional" bacterial infections
Streptococcal toxic shock due to *Streptococcus pyogenes* (group A Streptococcus)
Staphylococcal toxic shock due to methicillin-susceptible or -resistant *Staphylococcus aureus*
Staphylococcal scalded skin syndrome
Toxic shock-like disease due to *Streptococcus agalactiae* (group B Streptococcus) or *S. pneumoniae*
Other infections
Rocky Mountain spotted fever (*Rickettsia rickettsii*)
Ehrlichiosis (*Ehrlichia chaffeensis* or *E. ewingii*)
Anaplasmosis (*Anaplasma phagocytophilum*)
Leptospirosis (*Leptospira* spp.)
Epstein-Barr virus (EBV) mononucleosis
Common viral infections (e.g., adenovirus, enteroviruses)
Non-infectious disease
Kawasaki disease and the so-called Kawasaki shock syndrome
Stevens-Johnson syndrome (idiopathic, drug induced, or due to infections such as *Mycoplasma pneumoniae*)
Toxic epidermal necrolysis
Juvenile idiopathic arthritis
Behçet disease

doxycycline, a drug that would treat Rocky Mountain spotted fever (RMSF), ehrlichiosis, anaplasmosis, and Q fever. A number of laboratory tests were requested (Table 6.2). Despite antibiotics, the child became hypotensive, with her blood pressure declining to 64/35 mmHg, and her heart rate increased to 170 beats per minute. Neither responded to intravenous fluid boluses. The patient was therefore transferred to the intensive care unit

Table 6.2 Laboratory and other results for the present case

Initial testing	
Arterial blood gas	pH 7.32 (low), pCO$_2$ 23 mmHg (low), pO$_2$ 98 mmHg, [HCO$_3^-$] 11.6 mmol/L (low), base excess −12.7 mmol/L (excess negative)
C-reactive protein, plasma	170 mg/L (normal < 8 mg/L)
Uric acid, ferritin, and lactate dehydrogenase levels	Normal
Blood culture	Negative × 2
Urinalysis	Trace ketones, negative nitrites, small leukocyte esterase; white blood cells 11–20/high power field, red blood cells 0–5/high power field
Urine culture	> 100,000 CFU/mL *E. coli* and 50,000 CFU/mL Gram-positive cocci (likely contaminated with loose stool)
Urine culture (repeat)	Negative
Respiratory viral/bacterial multiplex polymerase chain reaction (PCR) panel	Negative
Stool culture	No *Salmonella, Shigella, Yersinia, Aeromonas,* or *Plesiomonas*; Shiga toxin test negative
Leg lesion aspirate	
Gram stain	Occasional Gram-positive cocci, no neutrophils
Aerobic culture	Moderate methicillin-susceptible *Staphylococcus aureus*
Anaerobic culture	Negative
Acid-fast bacilli stain and culture	Negative
Fungal stain and culture	Negative
Human immunodeficiency virus (HIV) antigen/antibody combination test, blood	Negative
Rapid plasma reagin	Negative
Cytomegalovirus IgM and IgG, blood	Negative
IgM and IgG to Epstein-Barr virus (EBV) capsid antigen and antibody to nuclear antigen, blood	Negative
Rocky Mountain spotted fever (RMSF) IgM and IgG, blood	IgM < 1:64 (negative)
	IgG 1:128 (low positive)
Borrelia burgdorferi IgM and IgG, blood	Screen borderline positive
	IgM and IgG Western blots negative
Coxiella burnetii IgM and IgG panel, blood	IgM phase I, IgM phase II, IgG phase II all negative
	IgG phase I positive
Brucella antibody, blood	Negative
Babesia, Ehrlichia, Anaplasma, and West Nile virus blood PCR	Negative
Tick-borne encephalitides and West Nile virus IgM and IgG, blood	Negative
Histoplasma, S. pneumoniae, and *Legionella pneumophila* urine antigens	Negative
Transthoracic echocardiogram	Limited study; left ventricular ejection fraction > 65%; pericardial fluid at the upper limits of normal; no apparent coronary artery dilation
Later in the hospital admission (hospital day 4 through discharge)	
C-reactive protein, plasma (trend)	Hospital day 4: 80 mg/L
	Hospital day 8: 15 mg/L
	Hospital day 11: 6 mg/L

(continued)

Table 6.2 (continued)

Lupus anticoagulant	Positive
Antiphospholipid antibodies	IgM positive, IgG negative
Factor V Leiden R506Q mutation	Negative
Prothrombin G21210A mutation	Negative
RMSF IgM and IgG, blood (repeat)	IgM < 1:64 (negative) IgG 1:128 (low positive)
Leg lesion aspirate (repeat)	
Gram stain	Occasional Gram-positive cocci, moderate neutrophils
Culture	Few methicillin-susceptible *Staphylococcus aureus*
Leg lesion aspirate (19 days post-presentation)	
Gram stain	No organisms, no neutrophils
Culture	Few Gram-positive rods/cocci. No *S. aureus*, *β*-hemolytic streptococci, or *Pseudomonas* isolated

(ICU) and started on a dopamine infusion and supplementary oxygen. An arterial blood gas suggested metabolic acidosis with respiratory compensation.

The lesion on the child's right leg was incised and drained. Gram stain of the recovered fluid showed no neutrophils, but there were Gram-positive cocci. Culture showed methicillin-susceptible *Staphylococcus aureus* (MSSA). Antibiotic therapy was narrowed accordingly, with the doxycycline stopped. As the most likely explanation for the child's presentation was staphylococcal toxic shock, the patient was given intravenous immune globulin at 500 mg/kg/day for 5 days. Repeat imaging (Fig. 6.1) showed residual abscess, which required repeated drainage. That culture again grew MSSA with identical antibiotic sensitivities.

On hospital day 4, the child's left arm showed mottling. Her arterial line was removed after Doppler ultrasound showed a partially obstructive acute thrombus in the radial artery, temporally associated with the platelet count dropping to a nadir of 43,000/mm³. At this time, the patient's serologic testing returned with a low positive for IgG against RMSF. Follow-up studies (Table 6.2) failed to substantiate a clear case for infection with this pathogen—but suggested the presence of a cross-reactive lupus anticoagulant or antiphospholipid antibody.

Given the difficulty of ruling out a rickettsial infection, and the child's tenuous state, doxycycline was restarted. Anti-staphylococcal therapy was narrowed to cefazolin. She contin-

ued to improve, and her leukocytosis and thrombocytopenia resolved. She was discharged on hospital day 8, on anticoagulation with enoxaparin and with plans to complete a course of oral cephalexin and doxycycline. She later required incision and drainage to fully evacuate a residual hematoma in her abscess site 19 days after her first presentation. Cultures this time were negative for *S. aureus*. On later follow-up, she was completely well.

6.1 A Mucocutaneous Disease Presentation

This patient's initial presentation included fever, fatigue, and findings on skin and at two mucus membranes—her mouth and her eyes. The differential diagnosis for this presentation is broad (Table 6.1) and includes both infectious and inflammatory diseases [1]. However, one may rank the differential diagnosis based on what other "clues" existed in the patient's history and physical examination.

An otherwise hemodynamically stable but irritable child, with prominent lymphadenopathy, a "strawberry tongue," lip cracking, and bilateral non-exudative conjunctivitis with peri-limbic sparing, may have Kawasaki disease. This is an inflammatory disease seen in young children that presents as a vasculitis with potential cardiac involvement. Laboratory findings in Kawasaki disease include elevated inflammatory markers, leukocytosis, hypoalbuminemia, transaminase elevation, and sterile pyuria—most of which the patient also had.

Alternatively, involvement of oral, ocular, and genital membranes in the setting of recent medication use (classically sulfa drugs), viral or *Mycoplasma* infection, or malignancy should raise suspicion for Stevens-Johnson syndrome and toxic epidermal necrolysis. These are severe, life-threatening dermatologic reactions that typically require management in a burn unit or ICU.

Hypotension, in the setting of fever and mucocutaneous findings, raises concern for staphylococcal and streptococcal toxic shock syndrome. A similar picture in a patient who has been in a tick-endemic region should lead one to presume infection with one of the severe tick-borne infections, in particular RMSF, until proven otherwise.

6.2 Staphylococcal Toxic Shock Syndrome

With hemodynamic shock as the prominent problem, and the isolation of MSSA from the child's leg abscess, the most likely diagnosis in this case is staphylococcal toxic shock syndrome—a rare, potentially lethal, bacterial toxin-mediated disease [1, 2]. While described as early as the 1920s, broad public awareness for staphylococcal toxic shock emerged in the late 1970s and early 1980s after a series of cases associated with use of certain brands of high-absorbency tampons during menstruation—though this only accounts for about half of cases of toxic shock [3]. The diagnostic criteria have been defined and revised by the US Centers for Disease Control and Prevention (CDC) (Table 6.3). This disease is classically caused by *S. aureus* strains that express either enterotoxin type B or toxic shock syndrome toxin-1 (genes *seb* and *tst1*, respectively) [4]. The latter is an exotoxin and superantigen that causes nonspecific T-cell hyperactivation and a systemic "cytokine storm," particularly in hosts lacking neutralizing antibodies against this toxin. Systemic signs occur even as the bacterial infection remains confined to a local space. Blood cultures are usually negative. Hypotension and

Table 6.3 2011 clinical case definition for non-streptococcal toxic shock syndrome

Clinical findings
Fever: temperature ≥ 38.9 °C
Rash: diffuse macular erythroderma
Desquamation: 1–2 weeks after onset
Hypotension: systolic blood pressure ≤ 90 mmHg for adults, < 5th percentile by age for children < 16 years old
Multisystem organ involvement: ≥ 3 of the following:
1. Gastrointestinal: vomiting or diarrhea at onset of illness
2. Muscular: severe myalgia or creatinine phosphokinase ≥ 2× upper limit of normal
3. Mucous membrane: vaginal, oropharyngeal, or conjunctival hyperemia
4. Renal: blood urea nitrogen or creatinine ≥ 2× upper limit of normal, or urine sediment white blood cells ≥ 5 per high-power field without infection
5. Hepatic: total bilirubin, aspartate aminotransferase, or alanine aminotransferase ≥ 2× upper limit of normal
6. Hematologic: platelets < 100,000/mm³
7. Central nervous system: disorientation or altered consciousness without focal neurologic signs when fever or hypotension is absent
Laboratory criteria
Negative results (if obtained):
1. Blood or cerebrospinal fluid cultures; blood culture may be positive for *S. aureus*
2. Serologic tests for Rocky Mountain spotted fever, leptospirosis, or measles
Case classifications
Probable: a case that meets laboratory criteria and in which four of five clinical findings are present
Confirmed: a case that meets laboratory criteria and all five of the clinical findings, including desquamation, unless the patient dies before desquamation occurs

Source: Adapted from https://wwwn.cdc.gov/nndss/conditions/toxic-shock-syndrome-other-than-streptococcal/case-definition/2011/ (Accessed on September 4, 2017)

involvement of skin (a diffuse, maculopapular "sunburn-like" erythroderma, with eventual desquamation), mucous membranes (vaginal, oropharyngeal, or conjunctival hyperemia), and the gastrointestinal tract (vomiting, diarrhea) are seen. Renal, hepatic, bone marrow, and central nervous system involvement may occur as well.

Interestingly, the current North American epidemic of community-associated methicillin-resistant *S. aureus* (MRSA), predominately driven by strains of the USA300 pulsotype, is not associated with toxic shock syndrome [2]. In the United States, the CDC receives 59–99 reports of staphylococcal toxic shock syndrome per year [5]. Projecting from local data in the Minneapolis/St. Paul area, DeVries *et al.* [6] estimated a stable incidence in 2000–2006 for staphylococcal toxic shock syndrome of 0.52 cases per 100,000 persons per year, the majority of which were caused by MSSA strains. Both statistics are a fall from a high of 13.7 per 100,000 women aged 15–24 during the peak of the tampon-associated epidemic in 1980–1981.

ICU management of toxic shock syndrome includes aggressive fluid repletion and anticipation of multisystem organ failure. Corticosteroids are not indicated. Aggressive care in burn units is needed for patients with > 10% skin loss. Bactericidal anti-staphylococcal antibiotics—such as an MSSA-active β-lactam (e.g., cefazolin, oxacillin, nafcillin, or piperacillin/tazobactam) and/or vancomycin (to cover MRSA)—are the mainstay of therapy. Certain bacteriostatic antibiotics, such as clindamycin, are also used to inhibit bacterial protein synthesis and decrease toxin production. Some experts suggest using intravenous immune globulin for its ability to neutralize toxin; its use has minimal support in the literature [1, 2]. Importantly, receipt of immune globulin at high doses warrants delaying the administration of live vaccines, such as the measles/mumps/rubella and varicella zoster virus vaccines, for 11 months [7].

6.3   A "Red Herring"

The diagnosis in the present case was muddled by a prominent distraction. The patient's pressor requirements increased, and her platelet count fell, once doxycycline was discontinued when a presumptive diagnosis of MSSA toxic shock syndrome was made. That the patient's serologies came back as a low positive for RMSF-specific IgG complicated matters as well, because positive serologies for RMSF are *pro forma* exclusionary criteria for toxic shock syndrome (Table 6.3). This is because of the similar

presentations of staphylococcal septicemia and RMSF [8]. However, coinfection of RMSF and "conventional" bacteria has been reported in the literature [9]—so the diagnosis of one should not necessarily rule out the possibility of the other.

As the consequences of not treating RMSF infection are dire, the decision was made to complete a course of treatment for RMSF with doxycycline, despite a few reasons why this diagnosis is likely incorrect. First, the test for RMSF-specific IgM was negative, and there was no increase of RMSF IgG in a follow-up blood sample. Second, the transient clinical regression when doxycycline was discontinued may have been due to resurgence of staphylococcal toxin production *in vivo*. Doxycycline, as a tetracycline analogue, blocks aminoacyl-tRNA/mRNA-ribosome interactions—hence, inhibiting bacterial protein synthesis. This is a mechanism of action similar to that of clindamycin—an antibiotic long known to be of utility in toxic shock. *In vitro* studies also suggest that doxycycline inhibits the inflammatory response of human blood mononuclear cells to the staphylococcal toxins [10]. These reasons may explain why discontinuation of this drug may have led to a transient relapse in symptomatology.

In hindsight, the child's positive or borderline positive serologies to RMSF, *Coxiella burnetii* (Q fever), and *Borrelia burgdorferi* (Lyme disease) may all have been due to cross-reacting autoantibodies. This phenomenon has been reported for both treponemal and rickettsial infection [11, 12, 13]. There are also reports of *S. aureus* infection being associated with a hypercoagulable state and antiphospholipid antibodies. One potential mechanism for this is a staphylococcal virulence factor, the second immunoglobulin-binding protein, Sbi [14]. That the child developed a bloodstream catheter-associated thrombus supports this possibility.

Key Points/Pearls

- Mucocutaneous presentation of disease in children has a broad infectious and noninfectious differential diagnosis.
- Staphylococcal and streptococcal toxic shock syndromes are managed with antibiotics and

supportive care, often requiring ICU admission; there is some evidence for the utility of therapy with intravenous immune globulin.

- Adding an antibiotic that inhibits protein synthesis, such as clindamycin or doxycycline, may decrease toxin production and improve outcomes.
- False-positive results may be seen with serologic testing.
- Thrombosis and antiphospholipid antibodies may be observed in the setting of severe infection.
- Staphylococcal toxic shock syndrome was associated with the use of highly absorbent tampons due to colonization with toxin-producing *Staphylococcus aureus*.
- Recurrences of menstrual toxic shock syndrome may occur in women with low titers of toxin-specific antibody.
- Staphylococcal toxic shock syndrome may also be associated with infection of the skin and soft tissues and with colonization or infection of surgical wounds; obvious signs of infection may not be present.
- A sunburn rash is typical of staphylococcal toxic shock.
- Bacteremia is uncommon in staphylococcal toxic shock syndrome; mortality is low with anti-staphylococcal antibiotics and supportive care in the ICU.

References

1. Long SS. Mucocutaneous symptom complexes. In: Long SS, Pickering LK, Prober CG, editors. Principles and practice of pediatric infectious diseases. 4th ed. New York: Elsevier; 2012. p. 109–13.
2. American Academy of Pediatrics. Staphylococcal infections. In: Kimberlin DW, Brady MT, Jackson MA, Long SS, editors. Red book: 2015 Report of the Committee on Infectious Diseases. 30th ed. Elk Grove Village: American Academy of Pediatrics; 2015. p. 715–32.
3. Centers for Disease Control. Follow-up on toxic shock syndrome. MMWR Morb Mortal Wkly Rep. 1980;29(37):441–5.
4. Spaulding AR, Salgado-Pabóna W, Kohler PL, Horswill AR, Leung DYM, Schlievert PM. Staphylococcal and streptococcal superantigen exotoxins. Clin Micro Rev. 2013;26(3):422–47.
5. Centers for Disease Control and Prevention. Notifiable diseases and mortality tables. MMWR Morb Mortal Wkly Rep. 2016;64(52):ND923–40.
6. DeVries AS, Lesher L, Schlievert PM, Rogers T, Villaume LG, Danila R, et al. Staphylococcal toxic shock syndrome 2000-2006: epidemiology, clinical features, and molecular characteristics. PLoS One. 2011;6(8):e22997.
7. Kroger AT, Sumaya CV, Pickering LK, Atkinson WL. General recommendations on immunization: recommendations of the Advisory Committee on Immunization Practices (ACIP). MMWR Morb Mortal Wkly Rep. 2011;60(2):1–60.
8. Milunski MR, Gallis HA, Fulkerson WJ. *Staphylococcus aureus* septicemia mimicking fulminant Rocky Mountain spotted fever. Am J Med. 1987;83(4):801–3.
9. Raczniak GA, Kato C, Chung IH, Austin A, McQuiston JH, Weis E, et al. Case report: co-infection of *Rickettsia rickettsii* and *Streptococcus pyogenes*: is fatal Rocky Mountain spotted fever underdiagnosed? Am J Trop Med Hyg. 2014;91(6):1154–5.
10. Krakauer T, Buckley M. Doxycycline is anti-inflammatory and inhibits staphylococcal exotoxin-induced cytokines and chemokines. Antimicrob Agents Chemother. 2003;47(11):3630–3.
11. Asherson RA, Cervera R. Antiphospholipid antibodies and infections. Ann Rheum Dis. 2003;62(5):388–93.
12. Helbert M, Bodger S, Cavenagh J, D'Cruz D, Thomas JM, MacCallum P. Optimizing testing for phospholipid antibodies. J Clin Pathol. 2001;54(9):693–8.
13. Koike T, Sueishi M, Funaki H, Tomioka H, Yoshida S. Anti-phospholipid antibodies and biological false positive serological test for syphilis in patients with systemic lupus erythematosus. Clin Exp Immunol. 1984;56(1):193–9.
14. Cervera R, Asherson RA, Acevedo ML, Gómez-Puerta JA, Espinosa G, De La Red G, et al. Antiphospholipid syndrome associated with infections: clinical and microbiological characteristics of 100 patients. Ann Rheum Dis. 2004;63(10):1312–7.

Primed for Pathogens

Shirley Stephenson

A 50-year-old female presented to the emergency department (ED) for right lower extremity pain, redness, and swelling. Her past medical history included congestive heart failure (CHF), atrial fibrillation, obstructive sleep apnea, morbid obesity, chronic lymphedema with ulceration, and multiple polymicrobial lower extremity soft tissue infections. She had been followed in the outpatient Infectious Diseases Clinic for several years and had been treated with lengthy courses of antimicrobials for *Actinomyces*, methicillin-susceptible *Staphylococcus aureus* (MSSA), *Pseudomonas aeruginosa*, and *Enterococcus avium* soft tissue infections of both lower extremities. Four months prior to this admission, all antibiotics were stopped with clinical resolution of the cellulitis. However, 1 month later she returned to clinic complaining of resumed warmth and tenderness in the right lower extremity. At that time, the patient was treated empirically with clindamycin and amoxicillin-clavulanate, which resulted in minimal improvement. Fluconazole was added to cover a possible fungal infection, but in the following days, her pain worsened, she experienced chills and subjective fevers, and she found it increasingly difficult to perform her activities of daily living. The limited mobility worsened her edema, which in turn contributed to increasingly tender and friable skin. Despite having had many past bouts of cellulitis, she stated that she did not recall ever feeling quite this ill.

The patient reported excellent adherence to all of her prescribed medications, including a diuretic and an anticoagulant prescribed because of atrial fibrillation. She had no known drug allergies and had not consumed alcohol for more than 20 years. She was not a smoker and denied recreational drug use. She was unemployed and lived in an urban setting with her husband, two children, and a cat that frequently slept on her lap and rubbed against her legs. She had suffered no animal or rodent bites. Her family history was notable for her deceased mother, who also had lymphedema; her father, who died of an unspecified cancer; and a brother, who had colon cancer. She had not taken any recent trips or been immobile for prolonged periods of time. She denied any traumatic injury or laceration of her legs. She had not visited any rural or forested areas, and she denied recent swimming. She had undergone no past surgical procedures on her legs.

In the ED, her temperature was 97.9 °F, blood pressure 141/69 mmHg, and heart rate 103 beats per minute. On physical examination, she was in no acute distress. Her respirations were unlabored, and her lungs were clear to auscultation. Her cardiac rhythm was regular, and no murmur was appreciated. She had massive bilateral lower

S. Stephenson, R.N., F.N.P.-B.C.
Department of Medicine, University of Chicago Medicine, Chicago, IL, USA
e-mail: sstephenson@medicine.bsd.uchicago.edu

extremity edema. A pretibial region of erythematous, fluctuant tissue on her right leg was without drainage but exquisitely tender to palpation. The intertriginous skin of her lower extremities was inflamed and cracked. Her lower extremities were warm, sensation was intact, and she had palpable pedal pulses. The remainder of her exam was normal.

The differential diagnosis for pain, swelling, and erythema in a lower extremity is listed in Table 7.1. The patient's history of lymphedema, cellulitis, and compromised skin integrity increased the likelihood of recurrent soft tissue infection, while her anticoagulated status made a blood clot less likely, as did the intact pedal pulses and the absence of numb or cold lower extremities. CHF may have contributed to her edema, but her cardiopulmonary examination did not indicate a CHF exacerbation. The pain and edema were distal to her knee with no evidence of arthritis or arthralgia, so rheumatoid arthritis, which affects the joints, was unlikely. The patient

lived in an urban area and had not spent a lot of time outdoors, reducing the likelihood of an arthropod-borne infection. Necrotizing fasciitis is a rapidly progressing, potentially fatal soft tissue infection. The pace of her symptom onset made necrotizing fasciitis unlikely. Close contact with a cat, particularly in the setting of compromised skin, suggested inoculation by pathogens of the normal flora of cats (*Pasteurella multocida* and *Bartonella henselae*).

A computerized tomography (CT) scan with contrast of the right leg showed a 7 × 3-cm fluid collection within the subcutaneous fat of the distal anterolateral leg, 8 cm below her knee. Inflammatory changes extended to the anterior tibial tuberosity. No osteomyelitis or deeper fluid collections were evident (Fig. 7.1). Before the start of intravenous (IV) vancomycin, cefepime, and metronidazole, the Interventional Radiology Service placed a drain into the fluid collection, and specimens from the suspected abscess were sent for bacterial and fungal cultures, which grew two strains of *Pasteurella multocida*, susceptible to both ceftriaxone and penicillin.

The patient's white blood cell count was within normal limits, and other laboratory test results, including the complete metabolic panel, were consistent with the patient's baseline. One of two blood cultures grew two strains of coagulase-negative *Staphylococcus*, which were likely contaminants. The presence of abscess,

Table 7.1 Differential diagnosis for pain, edema, and erythema in a lower extremity

Infections
Bacterial cellulitis, abscess, or other soft tissue infection
Pyomyositis
Necrotizing fasciitis
Atypical infection due to fungi (blastomycosis, cryptococcosis, and molds), nontuberculous mycobacteria (rapid growers, e.g., *M. marinum*), and higher bacteria (e.g., *Nocardia brasiliensis*)
Noninfectious etiologies
Arterial embolism
Deep venous thrombosis
Malignancy
Rheumatoid arthritis
Trauma
Arthropod bite
Venous insufficiency
Ruptured Baker's cyst
Ruptured medial head of the gastrocnemius
Lymphedema (many etiologies)
Pelvic tumor
Compartment syndrome
Reflex sympathetic dystrophy

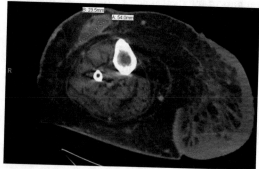

Fig. 7.1 Computerized tomography scan with contrast of the right leg showing a 7 × 3-cm fluid collection within the subcutaneous fat of the distal anterolateral leg, 8 cm below the knee; inflammatory changes extended to the anterior tibial tuberosity; no osteomyelitis or deeper fluid collections were observed

bacteremia, and past polymicrobial leg infections merited broad empiric IV antimicrobial coverage. A peripherally inserted central catheter was placed in her upper extremity, and she was treated with IV vancomycin and piperacillin-tazobactam for 6 weeks. This prolonged course was necessary because she had a persistent cellulitis. Had imaging indicated possible tumor, aspiration or biopsy with pathological examination would also have been indicated.

7.1 Pasteurella multocida

Pasteurella multocida is an aerobic or facultatively anaerobic pleomorphic Gram-negative, nonspore-forming coccobacillus that is part of the oral flora of cats and dogs. It is one of the most common commensal bacteria in domestic and wild animals around the world and the pathogen most frequently cultured from infected cat and dog bites [1]. It grows readily on blood and chocolate agar bacterial cultures. *Pasteurella* can cause cellulitis or an abscess at the site of a bite within hours of inoculation. Although a cat bite is a particularly efficient mode of transmission, *Pasteurella* can also be transmitted through nonbite contact [1]. In fact, in a study that compared patients with *Pasteurella multocida* infection either with or without a history of a bite, patients without a bite had higher rates of bacteremia and hospitalization [2]. Thus soliciting an accurate social history that includes questions not only about bites or scratches but also close contact with pets is of great utility.

Cellulitis may occur when a pathogen enters soft tissue through a break in the skin. Obesity, immunosuppression, a previous surgery or open wound, and lymphedema are risk factors for cellulitis and for polymicrobial infections [3–5]. The protein-rich tissue fluid associated with chronic lymphedema provides a favorable milieu for bacterial growth [6–8]. Once present, pathogens can chronically colonize the skin and soft tissues and be difficult to eliminate, perpetuating a cycle of cellulitis and increasingly impaired drainage. Each subsequent episode of cellulitis

further damages the lymphatic system [7], resulting in localized tissue compartments that are effectively immunocompromised [4]. Physical activity promotes drainage, yet as this patient's case illustrates, the discomfort and swelling of edema result in decreased mobility, exacerbating the edema and increasing a patient's vulnerability to infections.

Prophylactic antimicrobial treatment that covers aerobic and anaerobic bacteria, such as amoxicillin-clavulanate, is indicated after dog and cat bites for patients who have edema at the site of the bite [9]. Agents that do not offer coverage for *Pasteurella multocida* should not be used in cases of animal bites, scratches, or contact with broken skin. Because *Pasteurella* can result in deeper infections, it is important to rule out abscess and osteomyelitis. Tetanus toxoid should be given to anyone with an open wound after an animal bite, and other than those on the face, wounds from these bites should not be closed [9]. Broad antimicrobial coverage should be considered in patients with a history of multiple polymicrobial infections and risk factors for cellulitis. Management of recurrent cellulitis includes treating conditions that increase susceptibility to infection, such as obesity and lymphedema. Prophylactic antibiotics should be considered for patients with three or more episodes of cellulitis per year [9]. Management of lymphedema includes compression, treatment of compromised skin, and aggressive control of underlying conditions [8, 9].

Key Points/Pearls

- *Pasteurella multocida*, a common commensal bacterial species in the oral cavity of both cats and dogs, may be transmitted through a bite or other contact, resulting in potentially severe infections with a short incubation period.
- Obesity and lymphedema are risk factors for recurrent cellulitis, and each episode of cellulitis may further impair lymphatic drainage.
- Prevention of recurrent cellulitis may include prophylaxis with narrow-spectrum β-lactam antibiotics and should always address

underlying conditions that increase susceptibility to infection.

- Infections resulting from mammalian animal bites, or the combination of compromised skin and close contact with an animal, are an indication for antimicrobials that target *Pasteurella multocida*.

References

1. Lloret A, Egberink H, Addie D, Belak S, Boucraut-Baralon C, Frymus T, et al. *Pasteurella multocida* infection in cats: ABCD guidelines on prevention and management. J Feline Med Surg. 2013;15:570–2.
2. Giordano A, Dincman T, Clyburn BE, Steed LL, Rockey DC. Clinical features and outcomes of *Pasteurella multocida* infection. Medicine. 2015;94(36):1–7.
3. Dupuy A, Benchikhi H, Roujeau J-C, Bernard P, Vailllant L, Chosidow O, et al. Risk factors for erysipelas of the leg (cellulitis): case control study. BMJ. 1999;318:1591–4.
4. Soo JK, Bicanic TA, Heenan S, Mortimer PS. Lymphatic abnormalities demonstrated by lymphoscintigraphy after lower limb cellulitis. Br J Dermatol. 2008;158:1350–3.
5. Serdar ZA, Akcay SS, Inan A, Dagli O. Evaluation of microbiological spectrum and risk factors of cellulitis in hospitalized patients. Cutan Ocul Toxicol. 2011;30:221–4.
6. Baddour LM, Bisno AL. Non-group A beta-hemolytic streptococcal cellulitis. Association with venous and lymphatic compromise. Am J Med. 1985;79:155–9.
7. Collins PS, Villavicencio JL, Abreu SH, Gomez ER, Coffey JA, Connaway C, et al. Abnormalities of lymphatic drainage in lower extremities: a lymphoscintigraphic study. J Vasc Surg. 1989;9:145–52.
8. Mortimer PS, Levick JR. Chronic peripheral oedema: the critical role of the lymphatic system. Clin Med (Lond). 2004;4:448–53.
9. Stevens DL, Bisno AL, Chambers HF, Dellinger EP, Goldstein EJ, Gorbach SL, et al. Practice guidelines for the diagnosis and management of skin and soft tissue infections: 2014 update by the Infectious Diseases Society of America. Clin Infect Dis. 2014;59:e10–52.

The Gift That Keeps on Giving

8

Frances Lahrman and Stephen Schrantz

A 61-year-old female with a past medical history of genital herpes simplex virus type 2 (HSV-2) infection; idiopathic tenosynovitis treated with colchicine and hydroxychloroquine; myasthenia gravis (MG) treated with mycophenolate, prednisone, and pyridostigmine; and hypogammaglobulinemia receiving supplemental immune globulin every 6 weeks presented complaining of back pain. The patient reported that she had been unable to get out of bed due to pain and that any time she tried to walk she had a burning, tingling pain in her feet. Additionally, she reported difficulty urinating. She previously took valacyclovir for genital herpes but stopped 1 year prior to presentation because she had not had an outbreak for over a year, and her immunosuppressive therapy had been stopped for a short period. Prednisone was later restarted, but the valacyclovir was not restarted.

On presentation, her blood pressure was 148/86 mmHg, pulse 80 beats per minute, temperature 97.6 °F, respiratory rate 18 breaths per minute, and oxygen saturation 98% on room air. On physical examination, she demonstrated functional weakness and poor effort. Laboratory tests showed normal complete blood count, liver function tests, C-reactive protein, and erythrocyte sedimentation rate. On the night of admission, the patient noted blisters on her right leg, groin, and buttock (Fig. 8.1). A magnetic resonance imaging (MRI) scan of the thoracic and lumbar

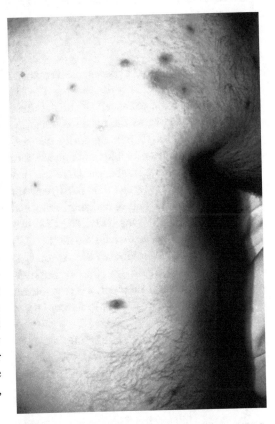

Fig. 8.1 Herpes simplex virus skin lesions. Source: CDC. (1963). *Herpes Simplex* [digital image]. Retrieved from http://phil.cdc.gov/phil/details.asp (ID#15563, Accessed on June 21, 2017)

F. Lahrman, D.O. • S. Schrantz, M.D. (✉)
NorthShore University Health System,
Evanston, IL, USA
e-mail: sjschrantz@gmail.com

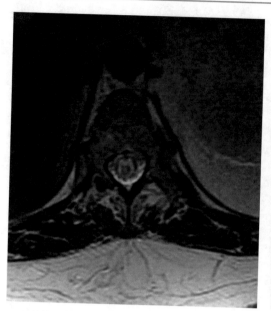

Fig. 8.2 Diffuse T2 hyperintense signal and expansion of the thoracic spinal cord

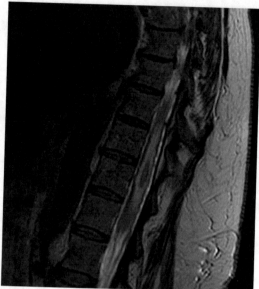

Fig. 8.3 Small focus of hyperintensity representing fluid collection or hemorrhagic component at the level of the T10–T11 disc space

spine showed diffuse T2 hyperintense signal and expansion of the thoracic cord spanning T3–T12 (Fig. 8.2) with focal enhancement of the distal spinal cord extending to the cauda equina. She also had a focus of T2 hyperintensity that was thought to represent a possible fluid collection or hemorrhage (Fig. 8.3). Lumbar puncture was performed and the cerebrospinal fluid (CSF) sent for Gram stain, bacterial culture and sensitivity, and West Nile virus (WNV) antibody. The CSF was also tested by polymerase chain reaction (PCR) for HSV, varicella zoster virus (VZV), cytomegalovirus (CMV), and enterovirus. Serological studies were performed for infection with the human immunodeficiency virus (HIV), *Mycoplasma*, and syphilis (IgG).

Later in the hospitalization, the patient's neurologic motor exam began to show weakness (2/5) of bilateral hip flexion, knee flexion, and knee extension with normal to decreased tone. Sensation was also decreased to light touch on the thighs bilaterally. The patient's urinary retention continued to progress requiring Foley catheter placement on the second day of admission. On the fourth day of admission, tests from the CSF and a skin lesion were positive

for HSV-2 by PCR. CSF showed high protein (272 mg/dL) and a lymphocyte-predominant pleocytosis. Given these findings, HSV-2 was thought to be the likely cause of the patient's myelitis.

Intravenous (IV) acyclovir was administered. Throughout the hospital admission, her lower extremity weakness showed daily improvement, but the pain persisted. At this point in the admission, the plan was to continue the patient on acyclovir for 3 weeks followed by lifelong suppressive valacyclovir. The patient was subsequently admitted to an inpatient rehabilitation facility on day 20 and then discharged to home on day 41 with a cane and a rolling walker. Unfortunately, her pain persisted after discharge.

8.1 Transverse Myelitis (TM)

Transverse myelitis (TM) is characterized by spinal cord dysfunction resulting in paresis, sensory abnormality, and autonomic impairment below the level of the lesion. TM can present as many different syndromes. Acute complete TM presents with paresis/plegia, sensory disturbance, and autonomic dysfunction below the level of the lesion. Acute partial TM presents with asymmetric manifestations. Longitudinally extensive TM extends over three or more vertebral segments. Secondary TM is related to a systemic inflammatory autoimmune disorder, and idiopathic TM does not have any identified etiology. Almost all TM patients experience some degree of bladder dysfunction that manifests as urinary retention and requires catheterization. Pain persists in many patients [1, 2].

The differential diagnosis of TM is long and requires a detailed history and physical examination (Table 8.1). The list includes idiopathic (compressive or noninflammatory), infectious, neoplastic, toxin-induced, autoimmune, and demyelinating diseases. MRI of the spinal cord is often the first step to exclude structural lesions. The next step is a lumbar puncture. If the CSF is noninflammatory, then vascular, toxic, metabolic, neoplastic, or neurodegenerative etiologies are more likely. If the CSF shows signs of inflammation, then the workup should be focused on infectious, demyelinating, or other inflammatory causes. If there are signs or symptoms of preceding infection, then the workup should include serology for various viruses (e.g., HSV, VZV, human T-cell lymphotropic virus-1 [HTLV-1], hepatitis A, B, or C virus, or HIV), bacterial pathogens (e.g., syphilis, *Borrelia burgdorferi*, or *Mycoplasma pneumoniae*), and rarely parasites (e.g., schistosomiasis or trypanosomiasis). CSF protein, glucose, and cell count should be analyzed for evidence of infection. Other systemic signs and symptoms include fever, adenopathy, meningismus, and rash (herpes zoster, enterovirus). Risk factors may include an immunocompromised state (herpes zoster, CMV). Recent travel (tuberculosis, parasitic infections), or genital infections (HSV) [4]. Hepatitis viruses cause TM via immune-mediated inflammatory mechanisms, and hepatitis C virus has been reported as the most common. Neurologic manifestations, such as TM, are the most common extrapulmonary complication of *Mycoplasma pneumoniae* infections [1, 2].

8.2   Herpes Simplex Virus (HSV)

HSV is a double-stranded DNA virus that is neurotropic, allowing for latency to develop. It is very common, with seroprevalence of HSV-2 estimated in the National Health and Nutrition Examination Survey (NHANES) at 15.7% and HSV-1 at 53.9% [5]. The incidence of HSV-1 is 63.6% for ages 40–49. The seroprevalence of HSV-2 is 1.2% at age 14–19, 9.9% at age 20–29, and 25.6% at age 40–49 [5]. This means that patients with primary HSV-2 infection often do have prior antibody to HSV-1, which offers some protection against severe symptoms of HSV-2 infection. As in our patient, most cases of HSV myelitis are due to HSV-2, whereas HSV-1, when it causes CNS infection, is mainly associated with encephalitis [6]. Klastersky et al. first described HSV myelitis in 1972 in a 45-year-old woman presenting with severe back pain. Throughout her hospital admission, the back pain persisted, and she developed weakness of the right psoas, gastrocnemius, and soleus muscles. Lumbar puncture demonstrated lymphocytic pleocytosis, and viral culture identified HSV-1. The patient developed facial paresis with impaired consciousness and subsequently died [7].

HSV-2 typically causes tender vesicles, pustules, and ulcers in genital areas of adults. Neurologic complications have been reported to be rare in immunocompetent individuals. However, Gobbi et al. described a case of a 70-year-old, otherwise healthy woman with three episodes of recurrent HSV-2 myelitis. The patient had a history of recurrent anogenital and gluteal herpetic skin lesions since youth. She presented with ascending numbness and progressive weakness of the right limb. MRI showed hyperintensity of T11–L1, and acyclovir and methylprednisolone therapy was started. Two weeks after discharge, she was readmitted with a gait disturbance and treated with the same two agents. One week later she was admitted for a third time, with diffuse numbness and weakness of the left lower extremity and skin lesions on the gluteal region. This time, she was treated with

Table 8.1 Differential diagnosis for transverse myelitis (TM) [2, 3]

Etiology	Key features
1. Demyelinating	
Multiple sclerosis	Most commonly presents with sensory disturbance
	Asymmetric lesions on MRI of spine
	Predilection for cervicothoracic cord
Neuromyelitis optica spectrum (NMO) (Devic's syndrome)	Optic neuritis and TM with MRI consistent with demyelinating lesions
Acute disseminated encephalomyelitis (ADEM)	Monophasic
	Associated with demyelinating peripheral neuropathy
	Multiple symmetric supratentorial and infratentorial lesions
	Post infectious or post immunization
	CSF pleocytosis
2. Systemic inflammatory	
Systemic lupus erythematosus	Only occurs in 1–2% of patients but has a poor prognosis
	Longitudinally extensive T2 hyperintense lesion
	Can present as gray (lower motor neuron) or white (upper motor neuron) matter myelitis
Sjögren's syndrome	Cervical cord affected and may be longitudinally extensive
	Only 20% of patients demonstrate seropositivity of SS-A or SS-B
	Cord involvement refractory to steroids
Behçet disease	Prevalence 2.5–30% of TM, with predilection for cervical or thoracic cord
	Longitudinally extensive and involves noncontiguous segments
Antiphospholipid syndrome (APL)	Prevalence less than 1% of TM
	Involves thoracic cord with sphincter involvement
	MRI may be normal in 40% of patients
Neurosarcoidosis	Predilection for cervical and thoracic cord and associated with back pain and radicular symptoms
	Half of patients have intracranial lesions
	CSF angiotensin-converting enzyme (ACE) levels are normal in more than half of patients
3. Paraneoplastic	
	CRMP-5-IgG antibody associated with small-cell lung cancer
	Subacute progressive motor myelopathy
4. Atopic	
	Majority occur in Japanese patients
	Predominantly sensory symptoms
	Rare motor or bladder involvement
	Posterior columns of cervical cord involved
5. Drugs and toxins	
	TNF-α inhibitors, sulfasalazine, chemotherapeutic agents, heroin, and general and epidural anesthesia

Table 8.1   (continued)

Etiology	Key features
6. *Idiopathic*	
	Centromedullary lesion
	Monophasic
	Criteria from the Transverse Myelitis Consortium Working Group:
	• Clinical evidence of bilateral sensory, motor, or autonomic dysfunction referable to the spinal cord
	• Neuroimaging that eliminates structural etiologies
	• Evidence supporting an inflammatory etiology by gadolinium enhancement within the cord or by CSF findings of pleocytosis or elevation of the immunoglobulin G (IgG) index
	• There must be no history of radiation near the spine for 10 years
	• No serologic evidence of connective tissue disease or infection
	• No brain MRI abnormalities
	• No clinical evidence of an anterior spinal artery infarction
7. *Parainfectious*	
West Nile virus (WNV)	Asymmetric flaccid weakness
	CSF shows pleocytosis with elevated protein and normal glucose
	MRI shows hyperintensity in anterior horn
Herpes simplex virus (HSV)	HSV-2 causes ascending myelitis
	Treat with acyclovir
Cytomegalovirus (CMV)	Usually causes myelitis in the immunocompromised
	Treat with ganciclovir or foscarnet
Epstein-Barr virus (EBV)	TM at the time of infection in immunosuppressed
Varicella zoster virus (VZV)	Necrotizing myelitis in immunosuppressed
Syphilis (*Treponema pallidum*)	Latency usually 6 years from infection to symptoms
	Inflammation involving the cervical cord
Human immunodeficiency virus (HIV)	HIV vacuolar myelopathy
	Posterior and lateral columns
Human T-cell lymphotropic virus type 1 (HTLV-1)	HTLV-1-associated myelopathy (HAM) also called tropical spastic paraparesis (TSP)
	Slowly progressive and spastic
	MRI usually shows atrophy and hyperintensity of the lateral cord (white and gray matter), but some patients have exacerbations with high T2 signal and swelling of the cord
	There are geographic areas of high endemicity (Japan, the Caribbeans, and Melanesia)
Poliomyelitis	Infects anterior horns with asymmetric flaccid weakness
Spinal schistosomiasis	*Schistosoma mansoni* and sometimes *S. japonicum* may cause transverse myelitis in travelers exposed to snail-infested freshwater when eggs released intravascularly are embolized into the cord
	MRI shows T2 hyperintensity and expansion of the distal cord and conus medullaris
Gnathostomiasis	Larvae of *Gnathostoma* spp. can enter the spine causing cord edema with high-signal intensity and later brain involvement with severe neurologic complications due to larvae migration
	Preceded by subcutaneous migratory swelling and associated with eosinophilia
	Most common in Southeast Asia
	May occur with ingestion of raw fish, eels, frogs, birds, or reptiles

(continued)

Table 8.1 (continued)

Etiology	Key features
Other bacterial, mycobacterial, and fungal infections	Spinal osteomyelitis and epidural abscess due to:
	• Pyogenic bacteria (especially *Staphylococcus aureus*)
	• Tuberculosis (*Mycobacterium tuberculosis*; Pott's disease)
	• Brucellosis (*Brucella* spp.)
	• *Aspergillus* spp.
	• *Candida* spp.
	• Histoplasmosis (*Histoplasma capsulatum*)
	• Blastomycosis (*Blastomyces dermatitidis*)
	• Cryptococcosis (*Cryptococcus* spp.)

CSF cerebrospinal fluid, *MRI* magnetic resonance imaging

long-term suppressive therapy with valacyclovir [8]. Symptoms of HSV-2 myelitis, as noted above, include pain, paresis, sphincter disturbances, and sensory loss [9]. Clinical manifestations of HSV myelitis can vary from mild cases with total recovery after several weeks to acute lethal ascending necrotizing myelitis [8].

In the past, diagnosis of HSV transverse myelitis was difficult because the virus was often not detected in CSF, but since the introduction of CSF HSV PCR, detection is more likely [10]. Patients also may or may not present with genital or other skin lesions at the time of neurological symptoms.

The pathogenesis of HSV myelitis begins with latent infection of the dorsal root ganglion at the lumbosacral spinal cord, which reactivates. Invasion of the spinal cord then occurs, causing necrotizing lesions. The length of spinal cord lesions varies, with diffuse enhancement and enlargement of the cord [4, 11]. HSV-1 more commonly causes myelitis involving the cervical and upper thoracic cord, while HSV-2 involves the entire spinal cord or the lumbosacral segment [12]. Nakajima reported nine cases of HSV myelitis, illustrating differences in clinical presentations between HSV-1 and HSV-2. MRI showed high signal on T2-weighted images with an ascending pattern in six cases with HSV-2. In the cases with an ascending pattern, lesions were continuous from the cervicothoracic spinal cord to the lumbosacral spinal cord, while cases without ascending patterns showed localization in the cervical or thoracic spinal cord. In the three cases that had a non-ascending pattern, HSV-1 was found via PCR.

Early treatment with acyclovir and possibly steroids to decrease ascending myelitis are essential to improve prognosis. Prolonged valacyclovir has also been recommended to prevent recurrence. Typically, IV acyclovir is continued until the CSF no longer contains HSV DNA [11]. However, Ganzenmueller et al. reported a case of prolonged detection of HSV-2 DNA in a patient who was highly immunocompromised, with HSV DNA in the CSF for 8 weeks. The patient's clinical symptoms resolved after 3 weeks of antiviral therapy. The authors speculated that the prolonged detectability might not indicate ongoing viral replication but rather neutralized virus [9].

Acyclovir-resistant HSV strains have also been isolated, usually in immunocompromised patients. Successful treatment with valacyclovir, foscarnet, and cidofovir has been reported with acyclovir resistance [11]. Prolonged detection of virus has been reported as a marker for poor outcome of HSV encephalitis, but its clinical significance in HSV-2 radiculomyelitis is not known. The risk factors associated with an unfavorable outcome of TM include rapidity of weakness onset, fever, a greater extent of MRI signal, and corticosteroid use [13]. The impact on treatment and outcome of the kinetics of HSV DNA levels in the CSF requires further investigation [9].

Key Points/Pearls
- HSV-2 is a neurotropic virus with latency.
- HSV-2 may cause severe neonatal encephalitis when vertically transmitted to the baby during delivery.
- HSV-2 may cause neurological syndromes in adults: acute aseptic meningitis, recurrent

aseptic meningitis (Mollaret's meningitis), transverse myelitis, and rarely encephalitis.

- HSV-2 is a known cause of transverse myelitis and often causes thoracic or lumbosacral ascending myelitis.
- Immunosuppressed individuals are more susceptible to HSV-associated transverse myelitis.
- Transverse myelitis has a broad differential including infectious, autoimmune, neoplastic, demyelinating, toxin-induced, and idiopathic etiologies.
- Diagnosis of the etiology of transverse myelitis is based on clinical findings, MRI, and CSF PCR.
- Treatment of HSV transverse myelitis is with acyclovir and is moderately successful in improving symptoms.

References

1. Borchers AT, Gershwin ME. Transverse myelitis. Autoimmun Rev. 2012;11(3):231–48.
2. Beh SC, Greenberg BM, Frohman T, Frohman EM. Transverse myelitis. Neurol Clin. 2013;31(1):79–138.
3. Ho E. Infectious etiologies of myelopathy. Semin Neurol. 2012;32(2):154–60.
4. West T. Transverse myelitis—a review of the presentation, diagnosis, and initial management. Discov Med. 2013;16(88):167–77.
5. Bradley H, Markowitz L, Gibson T, McQuillan G. Seroprevalence of Herpes simplex virus types 1 and 2—United States, 1999–2010. J Infect Dis. 2014;209(3):325–33.
6. Nakajima H, Furutama D, Shoji H, et al. Herpes simplex virus myelitis: clinical manifestations and diagnosis by the polymerase chain reaction method. Eur Neurol. 1998;39(3):163–7.
7. Klastersky J, Cappel R, Snoeck J, Flament J, Thiry L. Ascending myelitis in association with herpes-simplex virus. N Engl J Med. 1972;287(4):182–4.
8. Gobbi C, Tosi C, Städler C, Merenda C, Bernasconi E. Recurrent myelitis associated with herpes simplex virus type 2. Eur Neurol. 2001;46(4):215–8.
9. Ganzenmueller T, Karaguelle D, Heim A, et al. Prolonged detection of herpes simplex virus type 2 (HSV-2) DNA in cerebrospinal fluid despite antiviral therapy in a patient with HSV-2-associated radiculitis. Antivir Ther. 2012;17(1):125–8.
10. Petereit H, Bamborschke S, Lanfermann H. Acute transverse myelitis caused by herpes simplex virus. Eur Neurol. 1996;36(1):52–3.
11. Berger J, Houff S. Neurological complications of herpes simplex virus type 2 infection. Arch Neurol. 2008;65(5):596–600.
12. Figueroa D, Isache C, Sands M, Guzman N. An unusual case of acute transverse myelitis caused by HSV-1 infection. IDCases. 2016;5:29–31.
13. Kalita J, Misra U, Mandal S. Prognostic predictors of acute transverse myelitis. Acta Neurol Scand. 1998;98(1):60–3.

A Man with Heart Failure and Night Sweats

Amutha Rajagopal

A 72-year-old Caucasian man was admitted to the cardiology service for elective mechanical aortic valve revision for symptomatic, severe aortic regurgitation. On the day of admission, he described having drenching night sweats during the previous 2 weeks. He had experienced several months of gradually progressive palpitations, lightheadedness, orthopnea, dyspnea on exertion, and nonproductive cough. He reported an unintentional weight loss of 22 lb over 8 months. One month before hospitalization, an outpatient transesophageal echocardiogram (TEE) revealed severe aortic regurgitation with a paravalvular leak.

His past medical history was notable for St. Jude's mechanical aortic valve replacement 10 years before, coronary artery disease, ascending aortic aneurysm, transient ischemic attack, paroxysmal atrial fibrillation, gastrointestinal bleeding on anticoagulant therapy, asthma, anxiety, and obstructive sleep apnea. Due to a traumatic injury from a motor vehicle accident, he underwent splenectomy in childhood and received the appropriate immunizations.

A. Rajagopal, M.D.
Section of Infectious Diseases and Global Health, Department of Medicine, University of Chicago, Chicago, IL, USA
e-mail: Amutha.Rajagopal@uchospitals.edu

He lived in Chicago with his wife and three grandchildren. He was a retired power plant worker. He denied recent travel or sick contacts. He denied recreational drug or tobacco use. He took atorvastatin for hypercholesterolemia, warfarin for his heart conditions, clonazepam and bupropion for anxiety, and albuterol for asthma. His family history was notable for Parkinson's disease and coronary artery disease in first-degree relatives.

At presentation, the patient's vital signs were notable for blood pressure of 98/41 mmHg, lower than his chronic baseline (120–130s/50s). His physical examination was notable for a grade 3/6 diastolic murmur at the left upper sternal border and trace bilateral lower extremity edema. Laboratory results included a white blood cell count of 11,900/μL (normal range, 3500–11,000/μL), with 87% neutrophils, a normal comprehensive metabolic panel, and a normal urinalysis. A computed tomography (CT) scan of the chest without contrast revealed mild cardiomegaly, a small pericardial effusion, small bilateral pleural effusions, and a 4.7-cm ascending aortic aneurysm. A transthoracic echocardiogram showed a bi-leaflet mechanical prosthesis in the aortic position with severe paravalvular leak, malcoaptation of the mitral valve leaflets, and moderate mitral regurgitation. Microcavitations were noted in the left ventricle. No mass or thrombus was identified. The left ventricular ejection fraction was 50% with slightly reduced systolic function compared with his TEE 1 month prior.

While the patient remained afebrile and hemo-dynamically stable from the date of admission, he continued to report subjective fevers and chills and had a persistent, mild leukocytosis. On hospital day 3, 2 days prior to the planned surgical aortic valve replacement, the aerobic blood cultures from admission were positive for Gram-negative bacilli. The cardiac surgery was postponed, and intravenous (IV) piperacillin-tazobactam 4.5 g every 6 h was initiated on hospital day 3. A TEE was performed, but it did not show any valvular vegetation or abscess. An abdominal ultrasound was unremarkable. Daily blood cultures continued turning positive for Gram-negative bacilli until hospital day 5. Using matrix-assisted laser desorption/ionization time-of-flight mass spectrometry (MALDI-TOF MS), the Gram-negative bacilli were identified as *Bordetella trematum* on hospital day 6.

9.1   MALDI-TOF MS

In contrast to conventional speciation methods, which rely on biochemical tests and lengthy incubation procedures, MALDI-TOF MS identifies the species of bacteria or yeast within minutes directly from isolated colonies grown on culture plates.

In MALDI-TOF MS, first a single colony of bacteria or fungus is placed on a special metal plate (sample probe), and a photo-absorbing matrix solution (made of α-cyano-4-hydroxycinnamic acid dissolved in acetonitrile and trifluoroacetic acid) is added. The matrix solution is allowed to dry which leads to co-crystallization of the matrix and the biological sample. Second, the plate carrying the sample-matrix mixture is placed into the mass spectrophotometer, and an electromagnetic field is generated. The plate is charged positively compared to the detector. Third, laser-generated ultraviolet light pulses are beamed on the matrix-sample crystal, resulting in ionization of the photo-absorbing matrix molecules and transfer of protons to proteins from the pathogen

surface. This "soft ionization technique" ionizes the proteins without damaging them significantly (matrix-assisted laser ionization).

The positively charged proteins then are released from the surface of the crystal (desorption) and "fly" from the sample probe to the negatively charged detector, reaching it after a time of flight (TOF) that depends on the protein mass. Based on the degree of particle ionization and mass, ionized polypeptides have unique drift paths and times of flight in an electromagnetic field. Mass spectrophotometry identifies the time of flight of proteins, generating a mass spectrum that serves as species-specific fingerprints. Computer software automatically compares the results of the mass spectrum with a reference databank of medically relevant species to identify the pathogen with great accuracy, often to the species level [1].

9.2   Therapeutic Approach

After identification of *Bordetella trematum* from blood cultures on hospital day 7, IV azithromycin 500 mg every 24 h was added to piperacillin-tazobactam. Unfortunately, susceptibility testing, requested from an outside reference laboratory, could not be performed because the organisms did not grow. Serial blood cultures after hospital day 6 were negative, and the patient's symptoms and leukocytosis resolved. Piperacillin-tazobactam and azithromycin were recommended for a 2-week course prior to valve surgery. On the day of his surgery, a full repeat median sternotomy was performed. The surgeons identified a dehisced aortic valve and a 50% dehisced annulus, with an abscess in the annulus that measured about 10 mm in diameter (Fig. 9.1). There were no signs of active infection, but there was evidence of resolving endocarditis complicated by an aortic root abscess. A secundum atrial septal defect was also found, with a left-to-right cardiac shunt. The aortic valve was replaced with a bioprosthetic valve, and the surgeons performed a left ventricular outflow tract reconstruction and closure of a patent foramen ovale.

The abscess culture showed no organisms on Gram stain and had no growth. The patient was

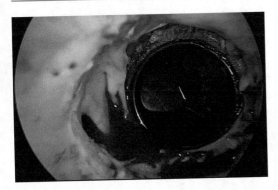

Fig. 9.1 Intraoperative photograph demonstrating dehiscence of St. Jude's mechanical aortic valve from infective endocarditis

discharged with a 6-week course of IV piperacillin-tazobactam and oral doxycycline 100 mg twice per day. This regimen was chosen instead of azithromycin due to prolongation of the QTc on the patient's electrocardiogram and concern for further prolongation.

9.3   *Bordetella* Species

Bordetella spp. are Gram-negative, encapsulated, nonsporulating coccoid bacilli. The genus *Bordetella* consists of nine species: *B. bronchiseptica, B. holmesii, B. avium, B. hinzii, B. pertussis, B. parapertussis, B. petrii, B. ansorpii,* and *B. trematum*. Most diagnosed infections caused by this genus are from *B. pertussis*, the etiological agent of whooping cough. *B. trematum* was initially described in 1996 in ten cases of wound and ear infections [2]. The root *trema* comes from the Greek, meaning *hole* or *perforation*, because the bacterium was initially isolated from skin wounds [2].

Since its description, few cases of human *B. trematum* infections have been published in the literature, with only three patients who have been diagnosed with bacteremia. The patients with *B. trematum* bacteremia included a Moroccan patient with severe burns [3], a 61-year-old male with septic shock from a soft tissue infection of the leg [4], and a 7-month-old infant in India with fever, vomiting, and abnormal hand movements [5]. To our knowledge, the present case is the first

report of infective endocarditis associated with *B. trematum* bacteremia. Details of our patient's infection and the three other reported cases of bacteremia caused by this species are shown in Table 8.1.

The reservoir and risk factors for infection with *B. trematum* are unknown. Comorbidities reported in published cases included diabetes mellitus, vascular disease, and impaired renal function. With respect to diagnosis, MALDI-TOF MS has been a rapid and reliable method for the identification of *B. trematum*, while 16S rRNA sequencing is the reference standard in many laboratories for final confirmation.

In most published cases, *B. trematum* was covered neither in the empiric nor in the initial directed antibiotic regimen [6]. Isolates of *B. trematum* have shown variable resistance patterns to commonly used antibiotics for skin and soft tissue infections, including amoxicillin-clavulanate, third-generation cephalosporins, fluoroquinolones, and aminoglycosides. Based on the few available case reports, imipenem, cefepime, and piperacillin-tazobactam may represent effective options for treatment. Further investigation is needed to guide empiric antibiotic therapy. If *B. trematum* is isolated, antimicrobial testing should be performed to guide treatment.

9.4   MALDI-TOF MS Identification of Unfamiliar Pathogens in Clinical Practice

With the availability of MALDI-TOF MS, it is increasingly common that unfamiliar species of bacteria are identified and speciated from clinical cultures. This creates an interesting challenge for infectious disease consultants who need to review the sometimes scant literature to determine optimal therapy. Our case is an example of the benefits and challenges of MALDI-TOF MS. The technique was instrumental in rapidly and accurately identifying the species of an unusual pathogen, preventing delays or mistakes in identification and also preventing the selection of an ineffective initial therapy. In our case, it was just as important that the infectious disease consul-

Table 8.1 Summary of reported cases of *Bordetella trematum* bacteremia

Ref.	Clinical data	Clinical diagnosis	Antimicrobial treatment prior to isolation	Infection isolates	Targeted treatments	Clinical outcome
[3]	60-year-old male with severe thoracic burn injuries	Sepsis and burn wound infection	Imipenem, netilmicin plus colistin	*B. trematum* and *Enterobacter cloacae* in blood cultures	None (patient expired)	Patient expired
[4]	61-year-old transgender male with mechanical fall and left leg wound	Sepsis and necrotizing fasciitis of left leg	Piperacillin/tazobactam plus vancomycin	*B. trematum* in blood cultures	Piperacillin/tazobactam, vancomycin, clindamycin, ciprofloxacin, and tobramycin	Patient expired
[5]	7-month-old female with fever, vomiting, and hand tremors	Sepsis, with unclear source of bacteremia	Ceftriaxone	*B. trematum* in blood cultures	Piperacillin/tazobactam plus amikacin, followed by ciprofloxacin plus azithromycin	Improved
Current case	72-year-old male with night sweats and heart failure	Prosthetic valve infective endocarditis	Piperacillin/tazobactam	*B. trematum* in blood cultures	Piperacillin/tazobactam and azithromycin	Improved

Ref. Reference

tant conducted a thorough review of the literature to select the best antibiotic treatment regimen. Rare species identified by MALDI-TOF often have no published guidelines for susceptibility testing. This means that examination of previous literature on the specific bacterial species identified in such cases is very important.

The increasingly common use of MALDI-TOF MS in hospital clinical microbiology laboratories is beneficial to the efficiency of patient care. It might decrease the duration of hospitalization because it speeds the identification of bacterial species in clinical samples [1, 7].

Key Points/Pearls

- *Bordetella trematum* is increasingly being recognized as an etiology of bacteremia and may cause infective endocarditis.
- 16S rRNA sequencing is the reference standard method for identification of *B. trematum*.
- Further study and susceptibility testing are needed to guide antimicrobial therapy.
- Matrix-assisted laser desorption/ionization time-of-flight mass spectrometry (MALDI-TOF MS) commonly identifies pathogens from clinical cultures that were previously rarely identified by traditional laboratory techniques; this approach often requires a review of the literature to determine the best antimicrobial therapy.
- MALDI-TOF MS is an extraordinary small-scale technique that allows the rapid, accurate, and cost-effective mass spectrum analysis of the proteins of a single bacterial or fungal colony to identify the pathogen to the species level.
- Early detection of an infecting species is important because patients can be treated appropriately earlier, improving survival and morbidity; accurate detection of uncommon pathogens by MALDI-TOF MS allows research and discovery to enhance our knowledge of infectious agents and the search for better therapies.

- Infectious diseases is an unusual field because novel pathogens continuously emerge.
- In many cases, emerging pathogens are a part of our environmental or commensal flora but are newly recognized because of improved detection methods, while in other cases a pathogen was already known to exist, but its pathogenicity was only recently recognized.

References

1. Wieser A, Schneider L, Jung J, et al. MALDI-TOF MS in microbiological diagnostics—identification of microorganisms and beyond (mini review). Appl Microbiol Biotechnol. 2012;93:965–74.
2. Vandamme P, Heyndrickx M, Vancanneyt M, et al. *Bordetella trematum sp. nov.*, isolated from wounds and ear infections in humans, and reassessment of *Alcaligenes denitrificans* Rüger and Tan 1983. Int J Syst Bacteriol. 1996;46(4):849–58.
3. Halim I, Ihbibane F, Belabbes H, Zerouali K, El Mdaghri N. Isolation of *Bordetella trematum* from bacteremia. Ann Biol Clin (Paris). 2014;72:612–4.
4. Majewski L, Nogi M, Bankowski M, Chung H. *Bordetella trematum* sepsis with shock in a diabetic patient with rapidly developing soft tissue infection. Diagn Microbiol Infect Dis. 2016;86:112–4.
5. Saksena R, Manchanda V, Mittal M. *Bordetella trematum* bacteremia in an infant: a cause to look for. Indian J Med Microbiol. 2015;33:305–7.
6. Almagro-Molto M, Eder W, Schubert S. *Bordetella trematum* in chronic ulcers: report on two cases and review of the literature. Infection. 2015;43:489–94.
7. Angeletti S. Matrix assisted laser desorption time of flight mass spectrometry (MALDI-TOF MS) in clinical microbiology. J Microbiol Methods. 2016. pii: S0167-7012(16)30253-6.

Seizure and Confusion in an Elderly Woman with Bacteremia

10

Leona Ebara

An 89-year-old female with a past medical history significant for chronic obstructive pulmonary disease (COPD), sick sinus syndrome requiring placement of a pacemaker, atrial fibrillation, hypertension, a cerebrovascular accident (CVA) approximately 5 months prior, ischemic colitis requiring colectomy, and Parkinson's disease that was well controlled on carbidopa-levodopa presented after seizure-like activity. She had been in her usual state of health until the day of admission when she developed sudden-onset whole-body shaking, foaming at the mouth, eye rolling, tachycardia, blurry vision, headache, and flushing for 1 min. She had a recent admission to an outside hospital where she initially was treated with intravenous (IV) cefepime and vancomycin for suspected hospital-acquired pneumonia. Both intravenous antibiotics were discontinued after a few days of treatment. Vancomycin-resistant *Enterococcus* (VRE) bacteremia was diagnosed, and her antibiotic therapy was then changed to oral linezolid. She was discharged to home from the outside hospital. On admission to our tertiary care medical center, she had been taking linezolid for 8 days for bacteremia. Her medications are listed in Table 10.1.

According to her housekeeper, following the seizure activity, she exhibited confusion for 2–3 min and was more lethargic than usual.

Vital signs on admission were temperature 37.3 °C, blood pressure 112/55 mmHg, heart rate 117 beats per minute, and oxygen saturation 100%. Laboratory tests showed white blood cell count 11,300/μL (normal range, 3500–11,000/μL), platelet count 423,000/μL (150,000–450,000/μL), hemoglobin 9.7 g/dL (11.5–15.5 g/dL), hematocrit 29.9% (36–47%), creatinine 1.8 mg/dL (0.5–1.4 mg/dL) (elevated from her baseline of 0.9), blood urea nitrogen 53 mg/dL (7–20 mg/dL), creatine kinase 70 U/L (9–185 U/L), and lactic acid 1.7 mmol/L (0.7–2.1 mmol/L).

The diagnostic evaluation for her condition was extensive. The Neurology Service was consulted to assess if her symptoms were consistent with a CVA; however this was determined to be unlikely. Two days following her seizure, the patient exhibited clonus on physical examination. A computed tomography (CT) scan of the head showed no intracranial hemorrhage or acute abnormalities, and magnetic resonance imaging (MRI) scan of the brain could not be performed due to her pacemaker. An electroencephalogram (EEG) performed 1 day after admission revealed no seizure activity. A workup for other potential causes of seizure, including metabolic abnormalities and psychiatric disease, was also unrevealing. The nursing staff initially reported that the patient had mild

L. Ebara, M.D.
Section of Infectious Diseases and Global Health, Department of Medicine, University of Chicago, Chicago, IL, USA
e-mail: Leona.Ebara@uchospitals.edu

© Springer International Publishing AG 2018
M. David, J.-L. Benoit (eds.), *The Infectious Disease Diagnosis*,
https://doi.org/10.1007/978-3-319-64906-1_10

Table 10.1 Medications of the patient prior to admission

Acetaminophen (PO 650 mg every 4 h as needed)
Aspirin (81 mg daily orally [PO])
Atorvastatin (PO 40 mg every evening)
Budesonide-formoterol (2 inhalations every 12 h)
Carbidopa-levodopa (PO 25–100 mg every 8 h)
Cefepime (IV 1 g every 12 h)
Furosemide (IV 20 mg every 12 h)
Heparin (subcutaneous 5000 units every 8 h)
Ipratropium-albuterol (1 inhalation every 4 h as needed)
Lidocaine patch (daily)
Metoprolol tartrate (PO 50 mg every 12 h)
Ondansetron (PO 2 mg every 8 h as needed)
Pantoprazole (PO 40 mg daily)
Sevelamer (PO 400 mg three times daily with meals)
Tiotropium (1 inhalation daily)
Tramadol (PO 50 mg every 12 h as needed)

confusion and agitation following admission, which improved throughout her hospital stay. She recovered to her baseline mental status on the third hospital day.

Upon admission to our hospital, linezolid therapy was stopped given suspicion for an adverse effect of this recently initiated drug. The patient, however, was continued on her home regimen of carbidopa-levodopa. She had been receiving carbidopa-levodopa for the previous 6 years, and according to her family, her symptoms were very well controlled. During the admission, she was transitioned to IV daptomycin to treat the previously diagnosed VRE bacteremia. An infectious diseases consultation was obtained. After review of the culture results from the outside hospital, it was noted that only one of two blood cultures there had been positive with VRE. Furthermore, VRE had grown only after 5 days of incubation, and all subsequent blood cultures were negative. Given the lack of a likely source and the scant evidence for a true bacteremia, the Infectious Diseases Service recommended that all antibiotic therapy be discontinued. She had no additional seizures during the admission, and she was discharged to home after 3 days with no more symptoms of infection.

10.1 Linezolid

Linezolid is a member of the oxazolidinone group of antibiotics that also includes tedizolid. Linezolid is a protein synthesis inhibitor that was first discovered in the 1990s and approved by the United States (US) Food and Drug Administration (FDA) for use in 2000. It is used to treat a variety of Gram-positive infections, including VRE. Linezolid is administered orally or IV in a dose of 600 mg every 12 h, and there is no dose adjustment necessary for renal or hepatic dysfunction.

Linezolid acts by inhibition of the first step of protein synthesis, thereby stopping the growth and reproduction of bacteria by disrupting translation by the ribosome of messenger RNA (mRNA) into proteins. In addition, it exhibits weak nonselective monoamine oxidase inhibition (MAOI). Suppression of the bone marrow, and most commonly thrombocytopenia, is a well-known side effect occurring with long-term use, but it is uncommon in patients who receive the drug for ≤14 days. Thrombocytopenia occurs much more frequently in patients who receive longer courses or who have renal failure. There are case reports of seizures resulting from linezolid use, but this is not common.

Linezolid also has a number of important drug-drug interactions that put patients at risk for serotonin syndrome (described below). This syndrome may occur when linezolid is combined with other pharmacologic agents having any of the following characteristics: (1) MAOI activity; (2) serotonergic effects, especially selective serotonin reuptake inhibitors (SSRIs); (3) adrenergic effects; or (4) dopaminergic effects. Linezolid also should not be used concomitantly if patients consume large amounts of tyramine-rich foods (e.g., pork, aged cheeses, alcohol, or smoked and pickled foods) because of the risk of serotonin syndrome. In 2011, the US FDA released a warning concerning the risk of serotonin syndrome when linezolid is combined with the antidepressant drug classes serotonin and norepinephrine reuptake inhibitors (SNRIs) or SSRIs, recommending that when possible these combinations should be avoided. Linezolid may also enhance the blood pressure-increasing effects of sympathomimetic drugs such as pseudoephedrine.

Tedizolid, a newer oxazolidinone antibiotic approved by the US FDA in 2014, in its registration trials had fewer drug-drug interactions than linezolid, was administered once per day, and was less likely to cause myelosuppression than linezolid. However, the much greater cost and lack of experience with tedizolid are the major downsides of this new drug.

10.2   Serotonin Syndrome

Serotonin syndrome is a potentially severe adverse effect that may occur when linezolid is combined with agents with the characteristics noted above. Clinical manifestations of serotonin syndrome include the following: (1) neurobehavioral symptoms (e.g., confusion, agitation, coma, or seizures); (2) autonomic abnormalities (e.g., hyperthermia, diaphoresis, tachycardia, or hyper- or hypotension); and (3) neuromuscular signs and symptoms (e.g., myoclonus, rigidity, tremor, ataxia, shivering, or nystagmus). There are two often-cited sets of criteria used to diagnose serotonin syndrome, the Hunter Criteria and Sternbach's Criteria (Table 10.2). Serotonin syndrome can develop 1–20 days following co-administration of linezolid with interacting agents. Signs and symptoms can last 1–5 days following discontinuation of the offending agents. To our knowledge, there are no previously published reports of serotonin syndrome resulting from the combination of linezolid and carbidopa-levodopa, but we concluded that this was the most likely drug interaction in our patient. There are no specific recommendations to avoid the combination of linezolid and carbidopa-levodopa. However, caution is advised, given the theoretical risk of combining a dopamine agonist (levodopa) which can increase serotonergic activity in the central nervous system with linezolid. There are reported cases of levodopa causing serotonin syndrome when combined with serotonergic agents.

In the case described here, our patient developed signs and symptoms consistent with the

Table 10.2   Criteria for diagnosing serotonin syndrome

Hunter Serotonin Toxicity Criteria
Patient must be receiving a serotonergic agent and meet one of the five following criteria:
1.   Spontaneous clonus
2.   Inducible clonus plus agitation or diaphoresis
3.   Ocular clonus plus agitation or diaphoresis
4.   Tremor plus hyperreflexia
5.   Hypertonia plus temperature >38 °C plus ocular clonus or inducible clonus
Sternbach's Criteria
Addition of or increase in a dose of a serotonergic agent and at least three of the following criteria:
1.   Mental status changes
2.   Agitation
3.   Myoclonus
4.   Hyperreflexia
5.   Shivering
6.   Tremor
7.   Diarrhea
8.   Incoordination
9.   Fever
10.   Other etiologies have been ruled out
11.   Neuroleptic agent has not been recently added or increased prior to symptom onset

Hunter Criteria for serotonin syndrome, with inducible clonus and agitation. She also met several of Sternbach's Criteria, with altered mental status, agitation, and myoclonus. The onset of the reaction 8 days after starting linezolid is also consistent with reports of serotonin syndrome in the literature. Our patient's symptoms resolved quickly. No further symptoms were observed after day 3 following discontinuation of linezolid. This fell within the expected range of 1–5 days for the resolution of serotonin syndrome following cessation of an offending agent.

Clinically, there may be situations in which the benefit of linezolid therapy may supersede the potential risk of serotonin syndrome in the setting of the use of an interacting medication. Discontinuation of the interacting medication is recommended. However, alternatives to linezolid should be considered in cases when stopping the other, potentially interacting, agent is not clinically appropriate, as in our patient who had Parkinson's disease well controlled on carbidopa-levodopa.

Key Points/Pearls

- Clinicians should be aware of the risk of serotonin syndrome and what signs and symptoms to monitor.
- Clinical manifestations of serotonin syndrome include neurobehavioral symptoms, autonomic abnormalities, and neuromuscular signs and symptoms.
- Linezolid use in combination with drugs that have MAOI, serotonergic, dopaminergic, and/or adrenergic activity should generally be avoided given the risk of serotonin syndrome.
- If the combination cannot be avoided, discontinuation of potentially interacting agents is recommended.
- Unusual symptoms occurring soon after initiation of a new drug should always prompt a review of possible drug-drug interactions and adverse reactions.
- Linezolid covers almost all Gram-positive bacteria, including *Nocardia*, *M. tuberculosis* and other mycobacteria, and especially important antibiotic-resistant pathogens, such as methicillin-resistant *Staphylococcus aureus* (MRSA), penicillin-resistant *Streptococcus pneumoniae* (PRSP), and vancomycin-resistant enterococci (VRE).

- Unfortunately, increasing resistance to linezolid is seen with VRE and also occurs in still rare cases of MRSA.
- Linezolid inhibits the synthesis of proteins and is bacteriostatic; it is a good antibiotic for pneumonia and osteomyelitis, but it is not recommended as sole therapy for bacteremia and endocarditis.
- Serious adverse effects of linezolid include the serotonin syndrome, severe thrombocytopenia (onset after at least 2 weeks), lactic acidosis, interstitial nephritis, and, with long-term use only, both peripheral neuropathy and sight-threatening optic neuritis.

Bibliography

1. Ramsey TD, Lau TT, Ensom MH. Serotonergic and adrenergic drug interactions associated with linezolid: a critical review and practical management. Ann Pharmacother. 2013;47:543–60.
2. Frank C. Recognition and treatment of serotonin syndrome. Can Fam Physician. 2008;54:988–92.
3. Sternbach H. The serotonin syndrome. Am J Psychiatry. 1991;148:705–13.
4. Dunkley EC, Isbister GK, Sibbrit D, Dawson AH, Whyte IM. The Hunter Serotonin Toxicity Criteria: simple and accurate diagnostic decision rules for serotonin toxicity. Q J Med. 2003;96:635–42.

Don't Toss Your Turtle! Seizures and Fever in an Infant

Muayad Alali

A previously healthy, 10-month-old male presented with new-onset seizure activity and fever of unknown origin (FUO) for 6 weeks. The child's mother reported tonic-clonic movements that lasted for about 15 min. The seizure-like activity resolved with one dose of lorazepam given at the emergency department of an outside hospital. At the well-child clinic visit at 9 months of age, his primary physician noticed an increase in the patient's head circumference above the 97th percentile. The child was referred for magnetic resonance imaging (MRI) of the brain, which showed a left-sided frontoparietal subdural fluid collection, approximately 12 mm in size, consistent with a subdural hematoma. Because the patient was asymptomatic without any neurologic deficit, there was no intervention. Three weeks later, a repeat MRI of the brain showed a stable appearance of the collection.

The patient's mother stated that her son had recurrent fevers that started a few days after his 9-month well-child visit. The fever was initially low grade, at 100–101 °F for the first 2 weeks, then had increased to 103–104 °F during the previous 3 weeks, with minimal response to acetaminophen and ibuprofen. The mother also recalled that the infant had a small-to-moderate amount of intermittent, watery, and non-bloody diarrhea during the previous 3 weeks. This had been attributed to an antibiotic-related diarrhea associated with empiric treatment with amoxicillin. The patient was evaluated by many physicians, including in three emergency departments, and on multiple occasions for his prolonged fever. A diagnosis of viral upper respiratory infection was made twice and managed by acetaminophen. Acute otitis media was diagnosed on another occasion and managed by a course of amoxicillin. Physicians who treated the child did not feel that he required hospital admission during the 6-week illness prior to his presentation to our center.

The history was complicated because it was suspected that the subdural hematoma was a result of non-accidental trauma. His mother had reported that he fell off his bed and hit his head a few months before and that she was unaware of any additional head trauma. The Department of Children and Family Services was involved in the case. A skeletal survey and ophthalmology examination at the time of the initial trauma were normal.

On arrival to an outside hospital prior to transfer to our center, the mother denied any history of sick contacts or exposures to tuberculosis, pets, or other animals. However, additional history taken 2 days after admission revealed that the child had direct contact with his maternal grandmother's two small turtles. Furthermore,

M. Alali, M.D.
Section of Infectious Diseases, Department of Pediatrics, University of Chicago, Chicago, IL, USA
e-mail: Muayad.Alali@uchospitals.edu

there was suspected exposure to chicken bones at a recent family barbecue. The patient's mother worked as a food handler in a restaurant.

The patient was transferred to our tertiary care medical center's pediatric emergency department. His initial vital signs were temperature 103 °F, pulse 174 beats per minute (normal range for age, 80–140), respiratory rate 35 breaths per minute (normal range for age, 20–30), and blood pressure 88/46 mmHg (normal range for age, 75–100/50–70). Once the seizure activity was aborted, no subsequent episodes were reported. The physical examination demonstrated fever, irritability, congestion, rhinorrhea, and macrocephaly. The anterior fontanelle was bulging but not tense. The patient was alert and had normal strength, and the rest of the physical examination was normal.

Computed tomography (CT) of the brain revealed a subacute cerebral convexity abnormality consistent with a subdural hematoma in the left frontoparietal region, as well as some acute hemorrhage with midline shift and mild subfalcine herniation. The previously identified subdural fluid collection had grown in size. The thickness of the collection had increased to approximately 30 mm compared with 14 mm 2 weeks before, and there was mass effect (Fig. 11.1). Initial laboratory studies were significant for leukocytosis with bandemia and an elevated C-reactive protein (Table 11.1). Further work-up in the setting of FUO including virologic studies was normal. A lumbar puncture could not be performed given the findings on the CT of the brain.

The differential diagnosis for the patient's prolonged febrile illness was broad. Given fever for 6 weeks in the setting of a chronic subdural hematoma complicated by new-onset seizures, subdural empyema was considered likely. Other possible diagnoses are listed in Table 11.2.

The patient received parental antibiotics, including ceftriaxone and vancomycin, as empiric, broad spectrum coverage for meningitis. He was then transferred to the pediatric intensive care unit and underwent an emergent neurosurgical procedure to drain the fluid collection, which was described as a mixture of

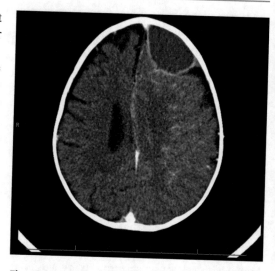

Fig. 11.1 CT of the brain with contrast at the time of presentation showing a large left convexity abnormality consistent with a subacute subdural hematoma measuring 30 mm in greatest thickness and causing localized mass effect and minimal midline shift

Table 11.1 Laboratory results from admission

Laboratory study	Result
Complete blood count	
WBC (per μL) (ref. 6000–17,300/μL)	18,000
Neutrophils (%)	60%
Lymphocytes (%)	30%
Monocytes (%)	7%
Hemoglobin (g/dL) (ref. 10.3–13.2 g/dL)	7.7
Platelets (per μL) (ref. 150,000–450,000/μL)	570,000
C-reactive protein (mg/L) (ref. <3 mg/L)	224
Complete metabolic panel[a]	Within normal limits
Blood culture	Negative
Urinalysis	Normal
Urine culture	Negative
Respiratory viral panel (by polymerase chain reaction)[b]	Rhinovirus/enterovirus positive

[a]Complete metabolic panel includes glucose, calcium, albumin, total protein, electrolytes, blood urea nitrogen, creatinine, alkaline phosphatase, alanine aminotransferase, aspartate aminotransferase, and bilirubin
[b]Pathogens in the respiratory viral panel: adenovirus, coronavirus (229E, HKU, NL63, and OC43 subtypes), human metapneumovirus, rhinovirus/enterovirus, influenza A (H1 2009, H1, and H3 subtypes), influenza B, parainfluenza 1, respiratory syncytial virus, *Bordetella pertussis*, *Chlamydophila pneumoniae*, and *Mycoplasma pneumoniae*

11 Don't Toss Your Turtle! Seizures and Fever in an Infant

61

Table 11.2 Differential diagnosis of a child with fever, seizures, and a subdural hematoma

Subdural empyema or infective subdural hematoma
- Gram-positive bacteria
  - Coagulase-negative *Staphylococcus*
  - *Staphylococcus aureus*
  - *Streptococcus* spp. (including *S. pneumoniae*)
- Gram-negative bacteria
  - *Haemophilus influenzae*
  - *Klebsiella* spp.
  - *Escherichia coli*
  - *Salmonella* spp.
- Mycobacteria
- Fungi (including *Candida* spp.)

Meningitis
- Bacterial
- Fungal
- Tuberculous (*Mycobacterium tuberculosis*)

Encephalitis
- Herpes simplex virus (HSV)
- Enteroviruses, including Coxsackievirus and echovirus
- Human herpes virus-6 (HHV-6)

Shigella infection with neurologic complications

Febrile seizure

Malignancy
- Brain tumors
- Infantile leukemia

Metabolic
- Glutaric aciduria type 1

Genetic epilepsies with febrile seizures

frank pus and blood. The fluid was sent for diagnostic studies. The cell count and other tests of the evacuated fluid analysis are shown in Table 11.3. The Gram stain showed Gram-negative bacilli (Fig. 11.2), and the bacterial culture grew *Salmonella* Sandiego (Table 11.3). The case was reported to the state Department of Public Health.

Further imaging was performed to rule out another focus of *Salmonella* infection, including chest X-ray, echocardiogram, and abdominal ultrasound, which were normal. Given that *Salmonella* superinfection of a subdural empyema is a rare extraintestinal manifestation of *Salmonella* infections, the presentation was concerning for a primary immunodeficiency.

11.1 Work-Up for Primary Immunodeficiency

The Immunology Service was consulted, and the assessment for an immunologic disorder in our patient was negative (Table 11.4). Measurement of immunoglobulin G (IgG) is useful in cases of suspected antibody deficiency. Measurement of immunoglobulin E (IgE) is useful in a patient with recurrent bacterial infections and dermatitis because if the level is greater than 2000 IU/mL, hyperimmunoglobulin E syndrome is suspected. Measurement of IgG antibody titers to tetanus, diphtheria, *Haemophilus influenzae* type B, and protein-conjugated pneumococcal vaccines is used to assess response to protein antigens, which is critical to assess the integrity of humoral immunity. The mitogen lymphocyte proliferation test is used to evaluate the integrity of T-cell responses to plant mitogens phytohemagglutinin (PHA) and pokeweed mitogen (PMW), which are powerful stimulants of T cells.

Lymphocyte subset analysis by flow cytometry is also an essential tool in the diagnosis of primary immunodeficiencies. Flow cytometry enables qualitative and quantitative enumeration of lymphocyte subsets, including CD4+ and CD8+ T cells, B cells, and natural killer (NK) cells. This test is important in determining if there are defects in T-cell numbers (as in severe combined immunodeficiency [SCID] or DiGeorge syndrome) or defects in T-cell function (as in common variable immunodeficiency [CVID]). The dihydrorhodamine (DHR) flow cytometry test is sent to evaluate for chronic granulomatous disease (CGD), primarily a defect in neutrophil function, with reduced ability to produce a respiratory burst for pathogen killing.

11.2 Salmonellosis

Our final diagnosis was *Salmonella enterica* serovar Sandiego superinfection of a left-sided subdural hematoma. The most likely source of the infection was enteritis, which presumably led to bacteremia with seeding of the hematoma. Blood cultures, interestingly, showed no growth. The

Table 11.3 Laboratory results on fluid drained from subdural space

Test (normal range for CSF)	Result
Total cell count (0–30/μL)	196,750 (H)
WBC (0–30/μL)	154,500 (H)
RBC (0/μL)	42,250 (H)
Neutrophils (0–6%)	98% (H)
Eosinophils (0%)	0%
Lymphocytes (40–80%)	1% (L)
Monocytes (15–45%)	1% (L)
Basophils (0%)	0%
Plasma cells (0%)	0%
Unclassified cells (0%)	0%
Protein (60–90 mg/dL)	2142
Glucose (50–70 mg/dL)	<20
Gram stain	Gram-negative bacilli
Culture result	*Salmonella* spp.
Serotype	*Salmonella* Sandiego
Antimicrobials: susceptible to	Ceftazidime, ceftriaxone, trimethoprim/sulfamethoxazole, and ampicillin

CSF cerebrospinal fluid

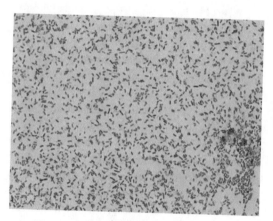

Fig. 11.2 Gram stain morphology from fluid drained from subdural space showing Gram-negative bacilli, speciated to *Salmonella*

patient was treated with intravenous (IV) ceftriaxone for 6 weeks. He defervesced a few days after the evacuation of the subdural empyema. He was discharged without neurologic complications.

Salmonella are Gram-negative bacilli that belong to the family *Enterobacteriaceae*. More than 2500 *Salmonella* serovars have been described; most serovars causing human disease are classified within O serogroups A through E. Species and subspecies are distinguished using biochemical reactions. There are only two recognized species, *Salmonella enterica* and *Salmonella bongori* [1].

Table 11.4 Immunology work-up

Lymphocyte subset 3 (quantifies T cells), blood	Normal
Quantitative immunoglobulins and Total IgE, serum	Normal
Mitogen proliferation test	Normal
Tetanus toxoid IgG, serum	Positive and appropriately responded to vaccination history
Diphtheria toxoid IgG, serum	Positive and appropriately responded to vaccination history
Pneumococcal IgG, serum	Partial immunity consistent with incomplete vaccination course; appropriate given patient's age and immunization history
Haemophilus influenzae type B IgG, serum	Normal
Isohemagglutinins Anti-A, Anti-B, serum	Normal
Dihydrorhodamine 123 test flow cytometry	Normal
Absolute CD4+ T cells, blood (normal range, 1400–4300/μL)	1544.78
Absolute CD3+ T cells, blood (normal range, 1900–5900/μL)	2688.54
Ratio CD4:CD8 (normal range, 1.3–4.7)	2.0

11 Don't Toss Your Turtle! Seizures and Fever in an Infant

63

Nontyphoidal *Salmonella* organisms are among the most common causes of laboratory-confirmed cases of enteric infection. The principal reservoirs for these organisms are birds, mammals, reptiles, and amphibians. However, some African serotypes that cause invasive human disease may have a human reservoir. In industrialized countries, the major food sources of transmission to humans are poultry, beef, eggs, and dairy products. Many other foods, such as fruits, vegetables, peanut butter, frozen pot pies, powdered infant formula, cereal, and bakery products, have been implicated in outbreaks in the United States (US) and Europe [1, 2]. Turtles with a shell length of <4 in. are a well-known carrier of *Salmonella* species that can cause human infections. *Salmonella* Sandiego was isolated from most ill patients in one case series of infections linked to small turtles [3].

Unlike nontyphoidal *Salmonella* serovars, the enteric fever serovars (*Salmonella* serovars Typhi, Paratyphi A and Paratyphi B) are uncommon in the USA. They can cause a protracted bacteremic illness known as typhoid (*Salmonella* Typhi) and paratyphoid (*Salmonella* Paratyphi A or B), and they are collectively called enteric fevers [1, 2]. They are restricted to human hosts and cause both clinical and subclinical infections. Chronic human carriers, usually involving infection of the gallbladder and occasionally the urinary tract, constitute the primary reservoir in areas with endemic infection, well known from the historical figure of Typhoid Mary.

The incidence of nontyphoidal *Salmonella* infection is highest in children <4 years of age. In the USA, rates of invasive infections and mortality are highest in infants, the elderly, people with hemoglobinopathies, and immunocompromised hosts. The incubation period for nontyphoidal *Salmonella* gastroenteritis usually is 12–36 h (range, 6–72 h). For enteric fever, the typical incubation period is 7–14 days (range, 3–60 days) [1, 2].

Nontyphoidal *Salmonella* organisms cause a spectrum of illness ranging from asymptomatic gastrointestinal tract carriage to gastroenteritis and bacteremia. Focal infections, such as meningitis, brain abscess, and osteomyelitis, may be diagnosed even in the absence of documented bacteremia. Gastroenteritis is the most common illness associated with nontyphoidal *Salmonella* infection, most often resulting in symptoms of diarrhea, fever, and abdominal cramps. Isolation of *Salmonella* from stool, blood, urine, bile, and/or cultured material from a focus of infection is diagnostic. Gastroenteritis is diagnosed by stool culture. Diagnostic tests to detect *Salmonella* antigens by enzyme immunoassay, latex agglutination, and monoclonal antibodies have been developed. Commercial immunoassays may also be used to detect antibodies to enteric fever serovars [1, 2], but the tests have limited sensitivity and specificity [4].

Antimicrobial therapy is not indicated for most patients with asymptomatic infection or uncomplicated gastroenteritis caused by nontyphoidal *Salmonella* serovars. Therapy does not shorten the duration of diarrheal disease and can even prolong the duration of fecal excretion of the pathogen. Although of unproven benefit, antimicrobial therapy is recommended for gastroenteritis caused by nontyphoidal *Salmonella* serovars in people at increased risk of invasive disease. This includes infants <3 months of age and people with chronic gastrointestinal tract disease, cancer, hemoglobinopathies, human immunodeficiency virus (HIV) infection, or other immunosuppressive illnesses or therapies [1, 2]. If antimicrobial therapy is initiated in patients with gastroenteritis, amoxicillin or trimethoprim-sulfamethoxazole (TMP-SMX) may be used for susceptible strains. Resistance to these agents is becoming increasingly common, especially in resource-limited countries. In cases of resistance, a fluoroquinolone or azithromycin is usually an effective substitute. For HIV-infected patients with localized invasive disease or bacteremia, empiric therapy with IV ceftriaxone is recommended. Once antimicrobial susceptibilities are available, ampicillin or ceftriaxone for susceptible strains is recommended.

Empiric treatment of enteric fever with ceftriaxone or a fluoroquinolone is recommended, and azithromycin may be an effective alternative. Once antimicrobial susceptibility results are known, therapy should be changed as necessary.

Corticosteroids may be beneficial in patients with severe enteric fever, which can lead to delirium, obtundation, coma, or shock [1, 2].

Typhoid vaccine is usually used in people at high risk of infection with *Salmonella* serovar Typhi. Two typhoid vaccines are licensed for use in the USA: a Vi capsular polysaccharide vaccine for parenteral use and an oral live-attenuated vaccine. Neither one provides complete protection. The vaccine efficacy appears high in US travelers [5]. However, the vaccines are not nearly as effective in populations where typhoid is endemic [6]. Efficacy at 1 and 2 years was 35% and 58% for the oral vaccine and 69% and 59% for the intramuscular vaccine, respectively [7]. Immunization is recommended only for specific populations, including travelers to areas where risk of exposure is recognized; people with intimate exposure to a documented typhoid fever carrier, as occurs with prolonged household contact; laboratory workers having frequent contact with *Salmonella* serovar Typhi; and people living outside the USA in areas with endemic typhoid infection [1, 2].

Key Points/Pearls

- Nontyphoidal *Salmonella* infections are far more common in the USA than typhoid fever.
- Populations at particular risk for invasive disease include infants <3 months of age and people with chronic gastrointestinal disease, cancer, hemoglobinopathies, HIV infection, or other immunosuppressive illnesses or therapies.
- The principal reservoirs for nontyphoidal *Salmonella* include birds, mammals, reptiles, small turtles, and amphibians; a thorough review of exposure history may reveal clues that can help to narrow the differential diagnosis.
- Nontyphoidal *Salmonella* cause asymptomatic gastrointestinal tract carriage, gastroenteritis, bacteremia, and focal infections including meningitis, brain abscess, and osteomyelitis.
- Superinfection of a subdural empyema should be considered in a child with chronic subdural hematoma and the clinical triad of prolonged fever, gastroenteritis, and neurological abnormalities.
- *Salmonella* Sandiego, a rare nontyphoidal *Salmonella* serotype, has been implicated in a number of US outbreaks linked to contact with small turtles.
- Antibiotics usually are not indicated for patients with either asymptomatic nontyphoidal *Salmonella* infection or uncomplicated gastroenteritis; they are usually recommended only in certain populations at high risk for invasive disease.
- Typhoid vaccines are recommended and considered highly effective in travelers to countries where typhoid is endemic.
- The live typhoid vaccine is contraindicated in immunocompromised patients.
- Prolonged nontyphoidal *Salmonella* bacteremia may be due to an aortic mycotic aneurism, a life-threatening condition that requires vascular surgery interventions.

References

1. American Academy of Pediatrics. *Salmonella* infections. In: Kimberlin DW, Brady MT, Jackson MA, Long SS, editors. Red book: 2015 Report of the Committee on Infectious Diseases. 30th ed. Elk Grove Village: American Academy of Pediatrics; 2015. p. 695.
2. Pegues DA, Miller SI. *Salmonella* species, including *Salmonella* Typhi. In: Mandell GL, Bennett JE, Dolin R, editors. Mandell, Douglas, and Bennett's principles and practice of infectious diseases, vol. 2. 7th ed. Philadelphia: Elsevier; 2010. p. 2887.
3. United States Centers for Disease Control and Prevention. National enteric disease surveillance: four multistate outbreaks of human *Salmonella* infections linked to small turtles. http://www.cdc.gov/salmonella/small-turtles-10-15/index.html. Posted May 18, 2016. Accessed 22 June 2017.
4. Siba V, Horwood P, Vanuga K, et al. Evaluation of serological diagnostic tests for typhoid fever in Papua New Guinea using a composite reference standard. Clin Vaccine Immunol. 2012;19(11):1833–7.
5. Mahon BE, Newton AE, Mintz ED. Effectiveness of typhoid vaccination in US travelers. Vaccine. 2014;32:3577–9.
6. Jackson B, Iqbal S, Mahon B. Updated recommendations for the use of typhoid vaccine—advisory committee on immunization practices, United States, 2015. MMWR. 2015;64(11):305–8.
7. Tabarani CM, Bennett NJ, Kiska DL, Riddell SW, Botash AS, Domachowske JB. Empyema of preexisting subdural hemorrhage caused by a rare *Salmonella* species after exposure to bearded dragons in a foster home. J Pediatr. 2010;156(2):322–3.

Kathleen Linder and Kevin Gregg

A 30-year-old female with past medical history of diabetes mellitus type 1 presented with 24 h of nausea and non-bloody, non-bilious vomiting accompanied by sharp right upper quadrant (RUQ) and epigastric pain that worsened after eating. She did not complain of abdominal cramping or diarrhea. The patient also reported decreased urinary output, fatigue, and malaise but reported no fevers or chills. Review of systems was notable for intermittent rhinorrhea and sinus congestion 2 weeks prior to presentation that had recently resolved.

The patient's past medical history was notable for a kidney/pancreas transplant 2 years earlier managed with an immunosuppressive regimen of mycophenolate mofetil, tacrolimus, and prednisone. She had no other notable surgical history. She reported no tobacco, alcohol, or illicit drug use. She lived with her mother in northern Illinois and they had no pets. She had no recent travel history or known sick contacts.

On admission examination, the patient was afebrile with a temperature 36.6 °C, tachycardic with a heart rate of 104 beats per minute, and tachypneic with a respiratory rate of 20 breaths per minute. Her blood pressure was 126/86 mmHg. Her cardiac examination demon-strated a regular rhythm with no rubs, murmurs, or gallops. Her lungs were clear to auscultation bilaterally. Abdominal exam demonstrated moderate epigastric, RUQ, and right lower quadrant tenderness on palpation; the abdomen was soft and non-distended without any guarding or rebound. The patient had no lower extremity edema, and her neurologic exam was normal.

The serum white blood cell (WBC) count was 12,000/μL (76% neutrophils, 15% lymphocytes), hemoglobin 16.5 g/dL, and platelet count 255,000/μL. The electrolytes were normal with an elevation of the blood urea nitrogen at 52 mg/dL (normal range, 8–20 mg/dL). The patient's serum creatinine was 5.7 mg/dL from a baseline of 1.0 (normal range, 0.5–1.0 mg/dL). A hepatic function panel showed elevated aspartate aminotransferase (AST) and alanine aminotransferase (ALT), at 231 U/L and 174 U/L, respectively (normal ranges, AST 8–30 U/dL and ALT <30 U/dL). Total bilirubin was 0.6 mg/dL. Serum lipase was 484 U/L (normal range, 0–160 U/L).

Given the patient's presenting symptoms and abnormal laboratory values, an abdominal ultrasound was obtained that demonstrated normal liver echogenicity with no evidence of cholelithiasis; the transplanted kidney was noted to be normal without hydronephrosis. A chest x-ray was normal.

The patient was given a diagnosis of pancreatitis (with an initial Ranson score of 0) and was admitted for intravenous hydration and pain

K. Linder, M.D. • K. Gregg, M.D. (✉)
University of Michigan Health System,
Ann Arbor, MI, USA
e-mail: kvngregg@med.umich.edu

© Springer International Publishing AG 2018
M. David, J.-L. Benoit (eds.), *The Infectious Disease Diagnosis*,
https://doi.org/10.1007/978-3-319-64906-1_12

Fig. 12.1 Transesophageal echocardiogram image of the mitral valve demonstrates an echodensity consistent with a vegetation (*white arrow*). *LA* left atrium, *LV* left ventricle

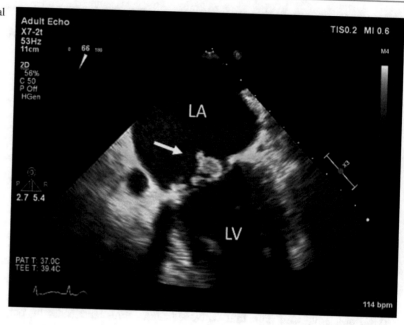

control. She was made NPO. She made gradual improvement over the subsequent 6 days; however, she had acute worsening of her pain on the sixth hospital day. The serum WBC count was 6800/μL. Lipase remained elevated at 1265 U/L. A computed tomography (CT) scan of the abdomen and pelvis was obtained and demonstrated a left adnexal, rounded fluid collection that measured 5.6 × 4.5 cm (Fig. 12.1). Blood and urine cultures were collected at this time and both had positive growth for *Escherichia coli*. The patient was started on intravenous (IV) piperacillin/tazobactam 3.375 g every 8 h (adjusted for renal function) for treatment of the bacteremia and the urinary tract infection. The patient subsequently developed fevers as high as 38.5 °C. Serial repeat blood cultures remained positive for *E. coli* for the next 4 days despite piperacillin/tazobactam therapy, to which the organism was found to be susceptible (minimum inhibitory concentration < 8 μg/mL). A transvaginal ultrasound was performed to characterize the adnexal collection and revealed a hemorrhagic cyst; this was thought to be unrelated to the patient's current presentation. A repeat ultrasound of the transplanted kidney now demonstrated trace fluid surrounding the allograft, consistent with hydronephrosis and possible pyelonephritis. A transthoracic echocar-

diogram (TTE) showed normal cardiac function and no vegetations; however, a transesophageal echocardiogram (TEE) showed an echodensity consistent with a vegetation on the mitral valve.

The patient met criteria for definite infective endocarditis by the modified Duke criteria (Table 12.1). However, she did not meet criteria for surgical intervention for endocarditis (Table 12.2) and was treated with a 6-week course of IV ceftriaxone 2 g every 24 h, to which the organism was susceptible (MIC < 0.12 μg/mL) [2]. She had an uneventful treatment course and made a full recovery with return to her baseline renal function.

12.1 Infective Endocarditis (IE)

IE is infection of one or more of the heart valves or endocardial tissue. Unfortunately, its incidence is increasing in the United States [3, 4]. The clinical presentation of this infection is widely variable, and presentation can range from an indolent, subacute illness to catastrophic acute cardiac failure. The most common clinical signs of IE include fever (90% of cases) and presence of a previously unrecognized cardiac murmur (85%) [5]. Metastatic foci of infection and

Table 12.1 Modified Duke criteria for diagnosis of infective endocarditis (IE) [1]

Major criteria	Minor criteria

1. Positive blood cultures
  • Typical IE organism (viridans streptococci, *S. aureus*, *Streptococcus gallolyticus* subsp. *gallolyticus* [previously named *S. bovis*], HACEK, enterococci) in two separate cultures
  • Atypical IE organism with ≥2 separate cultures ≥12 h apart or three or a majority of four separate cultures of blood (first and last sample drawn 1 h apart)
  • Positive *Coxiella* culture or phase 1 IgG titer >800
2. Evidence of endocardial involvement
  • Positive echocardiography: vegetation, abscess, or dehiscence of prosthetic valve
  • New valvular regurgitation
	1. Predisposing factor (known cardiac structural disease, IV drug use)
	2. Fever ≥38.0 °C
	3. Vascular phenomena (i.e., septic pulmonary emboli, mycotic aneurysm, conjunctival hemorrhages, or Janeway lesions)
	4. Immunologic phenomena (i.e., glomerulonephritis, Osler nodes, or positive rheumatoid factor)
	5. Positive blood cultures not meeting major criteria or serologic evidence of infection with organism consistent with IE

Definite IE requires the presence of two major criteria or the presence of one major and three minor criteria or the presence of all five minor criteria
Possible IE requires the presence of one major and one minor criterion or the presence of three minor criteria

Table 12.2 Indications for surgery in infective endocarditis [2]

Acute heart failure or cardiogenic shock due to valvular regurgitation or obstruction
Periannular extension of infection/perivalvular abscess
Systemic embolism and/or large vegetation >1.5 cm
Cerebrovascular complications
Persistent bacteremia after >5 days of appropriate antimicrobials
Difficult to treat organism (e.g., *Staphylococcus aureus*, *Pseudomonas aeruginosa*, *Coxiella burnetii*, or *Candida* spp.)
Prosthetic valve endocarditis

Table 12.3 Causative organisms of infective endocarditis and their relative frequency [8]

Streptococcus spp.	**48%**
Streptococci	36%
Enterococci	10%
Other *streptococci*	2%
Staphylococcus spp.	**36%**
S. aureus	27%
Coagulase-negative *staphylococci*	10%
Other microorganisms[a]	**9%**
≥2 microorganisms	**2%**
No microorganism identified	**5%**

[a]Other microorganisms include the HACEK group (*Haemophilus* spp., *Aggregatibacter actinomycetemcomitans*, *Aggregatibacter aphrophilus*, *Cardiobacterium hominis*, *Eikenella corrodens*, *Kingella kingae*), *Enterobacteriaceae*, *Pseudomonas aeruginosa*, *Candida* spp., and other organisms

embolic phenomena are common. Janeway lesions (nontender erythematous nodules on the palms and soles caused by embolic microaneurysms) and Osler nodes (acutely painful nodules on the pads of the fingers and toes caused by immune complex deposition) are rare but pathognomonic findings [6]. Laboratory testing results are nonspecific but may include leukocytosis, anemia, and elevated inflammatory markers. Urinalysis may show microscopic hematuria, red cell casts, or pyuria [5]. Electrocardiography (ECG) demonstrates cardiac conduction abnormalities in ~25% of patients, and abnormalities are more common in prosthetic valve endocarditis and in more invasive disease, such as development of paravalvular abscess [7].

The most common etiologic agents of IE are *Streptococcus* spp. and *Staphylococcus* spp., which cause nearly 70% of all cases, but many other pathogens are also known to cause endocardial infection (Table 12.3) [8]. One group of fastidious Gram-negative organisms, the HACEK group (*Haemophilus* spp., *Aggregatibacter actinomycetemcomitans*, *Aggregatibacter aphrophilus*, *Cardiobacterium hominis*, *Eikenella corrodens*, and *Kingella kingae*), causes 3–8% of cases of IE and typically present in a subacute fashion [5, 8].

IE due to other Gram-negative organisms, such as described in this case, is rare. Risk factors for Gram-negative IE include health-care exposure and implanted endovascular devices [9] as well as intravenous drug use [8–10].

A definite diagnosis of endocarditis can be made based on the presence of active tissue invasion on histologic exam of an intracardiac abscess or vegetation or by positive culture from valvular vegetation(s) [11]. Most often, however, pathologic specimens are not available, and diagnosis is made with a combination of clinical, radiographic, and microbiologic findings. The modified Duke criteria for IE can be applied to determine a likely diagnosis (Table 12.1) [1, 11].

Echocardiography is an essential tool in the diagnosis of IE. TTE is less invasive than TEE and is the recommended initial evaluation [3]. The sensitivity of TTE ranges from 32 to 75% with a specificity of >90% [12–14]. The sensitivity of echocardiography is improved to 85–90% with TEE, and this evaluation is recommended following negative TTE if there is a high pretest probability for IE, the patient is at increased risk for IE (prosthetic heart valves, congenital heart disease, previous endocarditis, new murmur, heart failure, or other stigmata of endocarditis), or the patient's TTE was of poor quality [3]. TEE is also recommended in cases of *Staphylococcus aureus* bacteremia, as it has been shown to diagnose IE in 20% of cases with a negative TTE [14].

Treatment of IE is targeted toward the pathogen isolated. At least 4 weeks of IV antimicrobials are recommended, and the majority of patients require a 6-week course [3]. Some patients require surgical intervention, particularly those with acute hemodynamic instability and disease that is not likely to clear with antibiotics alone (Table 12.2) [2]. Infectious diseases consultation should be obtained early in cases of suspected IE.

Key Points/Pearls

- Endocarditis should be suspected in patients who have a new murmur on cardiovascular exam and those with evidence of embolic phenomena.

- Gram-positive organisms are the most common etiologic agents of IE (particularly *Staphylococcus* and *Streptococcus* spp.), but Gram-negative organisms can cause IE and should be considered in the appropriate context (such as sustained bacteremia or consistent clinical findings).

- Definitive diagnosis of IE is made by histopathology consistent with valvular infection, but as this is not always available, the Duke criteria can be used to assist in making a diagnosis (Table 12.1).

- TEE is more sensitive than TTE to demonstrate valvular vegetations, but this superiority may be offset by the more invasive nature of the TEE; in patients with a high clinical suspicion of IE and a negative TTE, TEE should be pursued.

- Medical therapy is targeted toward the pathogen isolated; surgical intervention is sometimes required (Table 12.2).

- When multiple blood cultures are positive prior to starting antibiotics, an endovascular infection is likely; blood cultures may remain positive for days after starting antibiotics, especially when the pathogen is *Staphylococcus aureus*.

- When indicated, early surgical management of bacterial IE improves survival.

- Some pathogens causing IE do not grow on blood cultures and require specialized testing: *Bartonella* spp., *Coxiella burnetii* (Q fever), *Tropheryma whipplei* (Whipple's disease), *Chlamydia psittaci* (psittacosis), *Mycoplasma*, *Legionella*, and *Aspergillus*; *Brucella* spp. require prolonged incubation to grow.

- Due to improvements in automated blood culture systems, HACEK bacteria and nutritionally variant streptococci (*Abiotrophia defectiva* and *Granulicatella adiacens*) are routinely identified by culture within 5 days.

- Some valvular vegetations are not infectious, e.g., marantic endocarditis due to malignancy and Libman-Sacks endocarditis due to lupus erythematosus or antiphospholipid antibody syndrome.

References

1. Li JS, Sexton DJ, Mick N, et al. Proposed modifications to the Duke criteria for the diagnosis of infective endocarditis. Clin Infect Dis. 2000;30(4):633–8.

2. Prendergast BD, Tornos P. Surgery for infective endocarditis: who and when? Circulation. 2010;121:1141–52.

3. Baddour LM, Wilson WR, Bayer AS, et al. Infective endocarditis in adults: diagnosis, antimicrobial therapy, and management of complications. A scientific statement for healthcare professionals from the American Heart Association. Circulation. 2015;132:1–53.

4. Pant S, Patel NJ, Deshmukh A, et al. Trends in infective endocarditis incidence, microbiology, and valve replacement in the United States from 2000 to 2011. J Am Coll Cardiol. 2015;65(19):2070–6.

5. Cahill TJ, Prendergast BD. Infective endocarditis. Lancet. 2016;387(10021):882–93.

6. Farrior JB, Silverman ME. A consideration of the difference between a Janeway's lesion and an Osler's node in infectious endocarditis. Chest. 1976;70(2):239–43.

7. Meine TJ, Nettles RE, Anderson DJ, et al. Cardiac conduction abnormalities in endocarditis defined by the Duke criteria. Am Heart J. 2001;142(2):280–5.

8. Selton-Suty C, Celard M, Le Moing V, et al. Preeminence of Staphylococcus aureus in infective endocarditis: a 1-year population based survey. Clin Infect Dis. 2012;54(9):1230–9.

9. Morpeth S, Murdoch D, Cabell CH, et al. Non-HACEK gram-negative bacillus endocarditis. Ann Intern Med. 2007;147(12):829–35.

10. Reyes MP, Ali A, Mendes RE, Biedenbach DJ. Resurgence of Pseudomonas endocarditis in Detroit, 2006-2008. Medicine (Baltimore). 2009;88(5):294–301.

11. Durack DT, Lukes AS, Bright DK. New criteria for diagnosis of infective endocarditis: utilization of specific echocardiographic findings. Duke Endocarditis Service. Am J Med. 1994;96(3):200–9.

12. Habib G, Badano L, Tribouilloy C, et al. Recommendations for the practice of echocardiography in infective endocarditis. Eur J Echocardiogr. 2010;11(2):202–19.

13. Reynolds HR, Jagen MA, Tunick PA, Kronzon I. Sensitivity of transthoracic versus transesophageal echocardiography for the detection of native valve vegetations in the modern era. J Am Soc Echocardiogr. 2003;16(1):67–70.

14. Fowler VG Jr, Li J, Corey GR, et al. Role of echocardiography in evaluation of patients with Staphylococcus aureus bacteremia: experience in 103 patients. J Am Coll Cardiol. 1997;30(4):1072–8.

A Young Adult with Cough and Wheezing Since Infancy

13

M. Ellen Acree

A 20-year-old male presented to the Infectious Diseases clinic for evaluation of treatment options for recurrent respiratory papillomas. The patient was born with vocal cord paralysis and underwent tracheostomy at 4 weeks of life. At age 2 months, he was found to have a papilloma in his trachea, which was treated with intralesional steroids and laser excision. During his childhood years, his tracheostomy was closed, and he was found to have occasional, small papillomas in the trachea on airway inspection. However, when he reached puberty, the number and size of the papillomas increased dramatically. He required laryngoscopies for excision of the papillomas and intralesional cidofovir injections approximately every 3 months. Shortness of breath and hoarseness would develop periodically, indicating the need for a laryngoscopy in the near future.

At age 13 years, the patient was found on chest imaging to have pulmonary lesions, which was concerning for lower respiratory tract spread of the papillomas. He was begun on weekly α-interferon injections, which he continued for approximately 1 year. Unfortunately, the size and number of his papillomas did not improve, nor did the frequency of his laryngoscopies. He was

M.E. Acree, M.D.
Section of Infectious Diseases and Global Health, Department of Medicine, University of Chicago, Chicago, IL, USA
e-mail: Mary.Acree@uchospitals.edu

given a guarded prognosis, which prompted a second opinion at a tertiary medical center.

At age 16 years, the patient was admitted to our pediatric hospital for bronchoscopy and laryngoscopy. He was found to have diffuse circular papillomas throughout the trachea. A large sessile lesion was found almost completely occluding the entrance to the right upper lobe. The Pediatric Infectious Diseases service was consulted, who recommended addition of inhaled cidofovir therapy and sulindac, which is a nonsteroidal anti-inflammatory drug that had been shown in in vitro studies to induce apoptosis of human papillomavirus (HPV)-associated cervical carcinoma cells.

The patient continued with laryngoscopies approximately every 3 months for excision of papillomas. At age 20 years, he presented to the emergency department with hemoptysis. Repeat chest computed tomography (CT) scan demonstrated complete obstruction of the right upper lobe bronchus with a large endobronchial mass, which was presumably a papilloma (Fig. 13.1). The patient was also noted to have a postobstructive pneumonia and interval worsening of severe mediastinal lymphadenopathy. Bronchoscopy and endobronchial ultrasound and biopsy of the mass were performed. Pathology revealed squamous papilloma with focal, severe dysplasia. The patient completed a course of antibiotic therapy for pneumonia and was scheduled with the adult Infectious Diseases clinic for consideration of additional treatment options.

© Springer International Publishing AG 2018
M. David, J.-L. Benoit (eds.), *The Infectious Disease Diagnosis*,
https://doi.org/10.1007/978-3-319-64906-1_13

The patient was restarted on α-interferon. Tissue from a recent papilloma excision was sent for HPV genotyping, which was consistent with either HPV 6 or 11. Figure 13.2a shows positive nuclear staining for low-risk HPV DNA (serotypes 6 and 11) within a benign intra-airway papilloma using in situ hybridization. With the knowledge that his HPV type was included as a component of the commercially used recombinant HPV vaccine, the decision was made to administer the vaccine series in an effort to stimulate an HPV-directed immune response. Additionally, topical imiquimod was

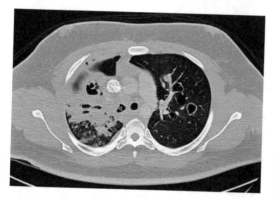

Fig. 13.1 Computed tomography of the chest with intravenous contrast showing obstruction of the right upper lobe bronchus (*arrow*), presumably due to an endobronchial papilloma. Severe postobstructive pneumonia is also demonstrated

applied to the vaccine injection site, which is currently being evaluated in clinical trials as a way to augment the HPV vaccine-associated immune response.

Unfortunately, the patient continued to have hemoptysis, and repeated laryngoscopies showed no regression of his papillomas. Intravenous cidofovir therapy was initiated, but shortly thereafter he required another admission for refractory hemoptysis, which was found to be stemming from the large, right-sided endobronchial lesion. After multiple failed bronchial artery embolizations, the patient underwent right pneumonectomy. He initially did well after surgery and was discharged to home on oxygen administered by nasal cannula. However, he presented approximately 1 week later with shortness of breath. He was found to have hypercarbic respiratory failure, which progressed to acute respiratory distress syndrome (ARDS), and this was the cause of his death at age 20 years. Of note, pathology from his pneumonectomy revealed squamous cell cancer with positive mediastinal lymph nodes. Figure 13.3 shows a cut section of the lung with multiple areas of squamous cell carcinoma invading the adjacent lung parenchyma. Figure 13.4 shows photomicrographs of four pathologic specimens obtained at the time of pneumonectomy.

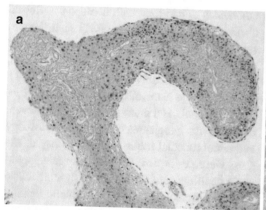
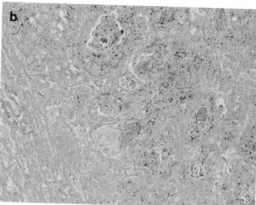
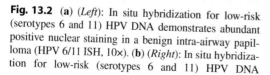

Fig. 13.2 (**a**) (*Left*): In situ hybridization for low-risk (serotypes 6 and 11) HPV DNA demonstrates abundant positive nuclear staining in a benign intra-airway papilloma (HPV 6/11 ISH, 10×). (**b**) (*Right*): In situ hybridization for low-risk (serotypes 6 and 11) HPV DNA demonstrates positive nuclear staining in an area of invasive squamous cell carcinoma (HPV 6/11 ISH, 10×) (Photos courtesy of Dr. David B. Chapel, University of Chicago, Department of Pathology)

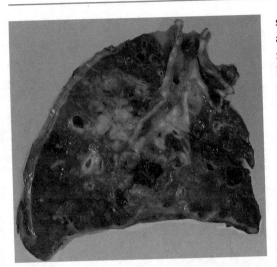

Fig. 13.3 Cut section of the lung showing multiple foci of white-tan squamous cell carcinoma, arising from an intermediate bronchus and invading the adjacent lung parenchyma. Hemorrhage and necrosis are grossly visible (Photo courtesy of Dr. David B. Chapel, University of Chicago, Department of Pathology)

13.1 Human Papillomavirus (HPV)

HPV is a DNA virus that causes common warts, anogenital warts, and a number of cancers in immunocompetent and immunocompromised hosts. It has more than 100 types. Several of the manifestations of HPV infection and their associated HPV types are presented in Table 13.1. Cutaneous warts include deep plantar warts, common warts, and plane or flat warts. Anogenital HPV infections, including condyloma acuminata, are the most commonly acquired viral sexually transmitted infections. Notably, there is a strong association between HPV and development of malignancy, including cancer of the cervix, vulva, vagina, penis, anus, and oropharynx, among other locations. Gardisil (Merck, West Point, PA) and Cervarix (GlaxoSmithKline, London, UK) are two recombinant HPV vaccines that have been developed to prevent HPV-associated anogenital warts, dysplasia, and cancers in males and females via the production of neutralizing antibodies. Gardisil is indicated for males and females between the ages of 9 and 26 years. Initially, Garidisil was a quadrivalent vaccine, protecting against HPV

serotypes 6, 11, 16, and 18. More recently, five additional serotypes have been added to the recombinant vaccine. Three randomized, double-blind, placebo-controlled clinical trials examined the efficacy of quadrivalent Gardisil for prevention of HPV-associated disease in females aged 16–26 years. Per-protocol data from these trials showed an efficacy against HPV 6-, 11-, 16- and 18-related cervical intraepithelial neoplasia 2 of 98.2% and vulvar intraepithelial neoplasia 2/3 of 100%. Efficacy against HPV 6- and 11-associated genital warts was 98.9%. Of note, in the trials assessing females with HPV vaccine type detected at study enrollment, there was no change in progression to disease with administration of the vaccine. In males aged 16–26 years, quadrivalent Gardisil was shown in one trial to have a per-protocol efficacy against HPV 6-, 11-, 16-, and 18-related genital warts of 89.4%.

13.2 Recurrent Respiratory Papillomatosis

Respiratory papillomas are the most common benign laryngeal tumor in children. Juvenile recurrent respiratory papillomatosis (RRP) is typically identified between the ages of 2 and 3 years and is related to acquisition of HPV during passage through the birth canal of an infected mother. Risk factors for development of RRP include being a firstborn child, which often implies longer labor, having a teenage mother with genital condylomata, and having a mother with a lower socioeconomic status. RRP is caused most commonly by HPV types 6 and 11 and less commonly by type 16. The estimated incidence of juvenile RRP is 4.3 per 100,000 children. RRP can cause obstruction of the larynx, which can lead to hoarseness and respiratory difficulty. Laryngoscopy will often reveal multiple verrucous growths along the true vocal cords, along the false vocal cords, in the subglottic region, and in the trachea.

Many children with RRP will require multiple procedures to excise the papillomas. Often, the lesions will diminish around puberty. Rarely, the papillomas can spread into the lower respiratory tract and undergo malignant

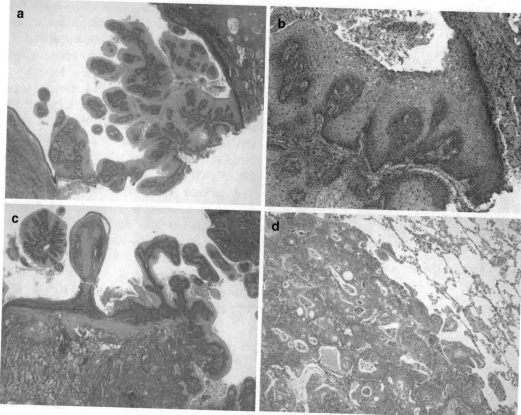

Fig. 13.4 (a) (*Left upper*): Benign squamous papillomas extend from an airway wall, resulting in airway occlusion. The airway beyond the obstructing papilloma was significantly dilated on gross examination (H&E, 2.5×). (b) (*Right upper*): A benign squamous papilloma (*left*) extends into an airway lumen, with no invasion into the airway wall (*right*). HPV-related changes are present in the squamous epithelium, but high-grade dysplasia is absent (H&E, 2.5×). (c) (*Left lower*): Benign squamous papillomas extend from the bronchiolar wall into the airway lumen (top half of photomicrograph). There is promi-

nent hyalinization of one papillary fibrovascular core. Squamous cell carcinoma arises from the benign papillary epithelium and invades the underlying lung parenchyma (*lower right*) (H&E, 2.5×). (d) (*Right lower*): Squamous cell carcinoma (*lower left*) invades and destroys the normal alveolar lung parenchyma (*upper right*). Note the pushing border of invasion, neutrophilic microabscesses, and tumor necrosis. Significant keratinization is absent (H&E, 10×) (Photos courtesy of Dr. David B. Chapel, University of Chicago, Department of Pathology)

transformation. Multiple therapies have been attempted for RRP, including interferon, photodynamic therapy, ribavirin, acyclovir, intralesional and intravenous cidofovir, intralesional mumps vaccine, bevacizumab, and others. Systemic therapy should be considered when the patient requires more than four surgical interventions per year, when there is evidence of spread to the lungs, when the papillomas are noted to regrow rapidly after excision, and when there is airway obstruction. Approximately 10% of patients with RRP will require systemic therapy. α-interferon is the most common sys-

temic therapy utilized in patients with RRP. It is believed to trigger a host immune response that inhibits viral protein synthesis. However, responses have been mixed in the literature and there are tolerability concerns. Some experts recommend a trial of α-interferon for 6 months followed by an assessment of disease response before deciding to continue.

Key Points/Pearls

- Recurrent respiratory papillomatosis (RRP) of childhood is a disease caused by human papillomavirus (HPV), most often type 6 or 11,

Table 13.1 Human papillomavirus (HPV) types and their disease association

Disease	HPV types with frequent association
Plantar warts	1, 2
Common warts	1, 2, 4
Common warts of meat, poultry, and fish handlers	2, 7
Flat and intermediate warts	3, 10
Condylomata acuminata	6, 11
Low-grade intraepithelial neoplasia	6, 11
High-grade intraepithelial neoplasia	16, 18
Cervical carcinoma	16, 18
Recurrent respiratory papillomatosis	6, 11
Conjunctival papillomas and carcinomas	6, 11, 16

Abbreviated from [3]

which is acquired during passage through the birth canal.

- RRP causes papilloma growth in the larynx and trachea and rarely can spread to the lower respiratory tract and undergo malignant transformation.
- RRP is often treated with local, intralesional therapy.
- Systemic therapy should be considered in patients who require multiple surgical interventions per year, when there is spread to the lungs, when the papillomas rapidly regrow after excision, and when there is airway obstruction.

- Although HPV 6 and 11 are considered low risk for malignancy, in RRP, they may cause squamous cell cancer of the lung as in this patient.
- Gardasil 9 includes HPV types 6 and 11 that are considered low risk for malignancy but cause genital warts and HPV types 16, 18, 31, 33, 45, 52, and 58 that associated with high risk for cervical, vaginal, vulvar, anal, penile, and oropharyngeal squamous cell cancer.
- HPV 16 and 18 cause approximately 70% of all cervical cancers, and HPV types 31, 33, 45, 52, and 58 cause about 15% of all cervical cancers.

Bibliography

1. Venkatesan N, Pine H, Underbrink M. Recurrent respiratory papillomatosis. Otolaryngol Clin North Am. 2012;45(3):671–94.
2. Derkay C. Recurrent respiratory papillomatosis. Laryngoscope. 2001;111(1):57–69.
3. Bonnez W. Papillomaviruses. In: Bennett JE, Dolin R, Blaser MJ, editors. Mandell, Douglas, and Bennett's principles and practice of infectious diseases. 8th ed. Philadelphia: Elsevier/Saunders; 2015. p. 1794–806.
4. Centers for Disease Control and Prevention (CDC). Human papillomavirus vaccination: recommendations of the Advisory Committee on Immunization Practices (ACIP). MMWR Morb Mortal Wkly Rep. 2014;63(RR05):1–30. http://www.cdc.gov/mmwr/preview/mmwrhtml/rr6305a1.htm. Accessed 22 June 2017.

Elevated Liver Enzymes in Pregnancy

14

Daniela Pellegrini

A 32-year-old female, G1P0, 32 weeks pregnant, with diet-controlled gestational diabetes, and a history of Crohn's disease requiring several bowel resections (partial colectomy and lysis of adhesions) and placement of an ileostomy was admitted to the hospital because of an illness associated with elevated serum transaminases. She had significant nausea and vomiting during the first and second trimesters of the pregnancy, but these symptoms subsided until 2 weeks prior to her presentation when nausea and vomiting recurred. Several days prior to admission, she developed a diffuse follicular-appearing pruritic rash that she attributed to a new soap she used in her bath. She was not immunosuppressed for Crohn's disease; years prior, she had been treated with adalimumab, an inhibitor of tumor necrosis factor-α, but she could not tolerate it. Routine labs obtained to monitor her inflammatory bowel disease (IBD) showed elevation of aspartate aminotransferase (AST) to 480 U/L (normal range, 8–37 U/L) and alanine aminotransferase (ALT) to 671 U/L (8–35 U/L), with alkaline phosphatase of 130 U/L (30–120 U/L) and normal total bilirubin of 0.5 mg/dL. The patient was admitted for an expedited workup.

At admission, she complained of abdominal pain and cramping associated with contractions from suspected blockage of her ostomy and ongoing nausea and vomiting. She denied fevers, chills, sick contacts, recent travel, or increased output from the ostomy. She had elevated blood pressure measurements throughout pregnancy but no other symptoms or signs of preeclampsia.

The patient had significant chronic abdominal pain related to her previous surgeries, which required chronic use of pain medications. Her past medical history also included depression, central venous catheter-associated deep venous thrombosis, and urinary tract infections.

She was a former smoker for 1 year but denied drug and alcohol use. She was married and lived with her husband. They had pets at home, but she reported no recent travel outside of the Midwest. She denied excessive use of Tylenol and she was not aware of any unusual food exposures. She was unemployed at the time of admission but had previously worked in an office. Current medications included docusate, methadone, ondansetron, and oxycodone. She had a documented allergy to sulfonamide antibiotics.

Her vital signs at the time of admission were: oral temperature 36.6 °C (97.9 °F), blood pressure 125/86 mmHg, pulse 85 beats per minute, respiratory rate 18 breaths per minute, and oxygen saturation 98%. The physical examination was remarkable for a diffuse, red, follicular-appearing, pruritic rash without ulcerations or

D. Pellegrini, M.D.
Section of Infectious Diseases and Global Health,
Department of Medicine, University of Chicago,
Chicago, IL, USA
e-mail: Daniela.Pellegrini@uchospitals.edu

© Springer International Publishing AG 2018
M. David, J.-L. Benoit (eds.), *The Infectious Disease Diagnosis*,
https://doi.org/10.1007/978-3-319-64906-1_14

discrete lesions, mucosal involvement, or desquamation. Head, ear, eye, nose, throat, cardiac, and pulmonary examinations were normal. No scleral icterus or jaundice was appreciated. The abdomen was gravid and diffusely tender to palpation with no focal areas of significant pain. The left-sided ileostomy had brown, non-bloody, soft stool. She had trace of lower extremity edema bilaterally.

The white blood cell count was 12,200/µL (normal range, 3500–11,000/µL), hemoglobin was 11.7 g/dL, and platelet count was 230,000/µL. A comprehensive metabolic panel showed an albumin of 2.9 g/dL (normal range, 3.5–5.0 g/dL) and elevated transaminases (AST 237 and ALT 363 U/L). Other liver function tests (LFTs) were normal.

The liver consultation service recommended viral hepatitis studies, including hepatitis A IgM, hepatitis B core IgM, hepatitis B surface antigen, hepatitis C antibody, and hepatitis E antibody. Other viral studies included herpes simplex virus (HSV) type 1- and type 2-specific IgG, cytomegalovirus (CMV) IgM and IgG, varicella zoster virus (VZV) serum IgG, serum polymerase chain reaction (PCR) for both CMV and Epstein-Barr virus (EBV), and urine PCR for CMV. Laboratory results are shown in Table 14.1. Viral hepatitis serologies were negative, HSV type 1 IgG was positive, VZV IgG was positive, and CMV IgM and IgG were positive. An abdominal ultrasound was suggestive of fatty liver and hepatic parenchymal dysfunction with no mass or ductal dilation. The Doppler showed patent hepatic vasculature.

Table 14.1 Laboratory results, blood

Test	Result
Herpes simplex virus (HSV) type 1 IgG	Positive
HSV type 2 IgG	Negative
Varicella zoster virus (VZV) IgG	Positive
Epstein-Barr virus (EBV) PCR	Negative
Cytomegalovirus (CMV) IgM and IgG	Positive
Acute hepatitis viral panel[a]	Negative
Hepatitis E antibody	Negative

[a]Assesses acute infection with hepatitis A, B, and C viruses

PCR polymerase chain reaction

The differential diagnosis of elevated transaminases during pregnancy is complex (Table 14.2). A group of disorders are triggered by the pregnant state, including hyperemesis gravidarum with onset in the first trimester, intrahepatic cholestasis of pregnancy (IHCP) with onset in the second trimester, and three disorders with onset in the third trimester that increase morbidity and mortality for both mother and fetus but resolve postdelivery: acute fatty liver disease of pregnancy (AFLP), preeclampsia/eclampsia, and the HELLP syndrome (hemolysis, elevated liver enzymes, low platelet count). Budd-Chiari syndrome may occur during pregnancy or more often postpartum due to the physiologic hypercoagulable state. Another group of disorders preexist the pregnancy but may flare either during pregnancy or postpartum (Wilson's disease, autoimmune hepatitis).

The differential diagnosis of elevated transaminases during pregnancy also includes viral hepatitis (i.e., hepatitis A, B, C, and E), HSV, VZV, and CMV [1–3]. Hepatitis due to HSV type 1 is severe, and hepatitis E virus can be severe

Table 14.2 Differential diagnosis of elevated transaminases during pregnancy

Noninfectious syndromes induced by pregnancy
First trimester onset: hyperemesis gravidarum
Second half of pregnancy: intrahepatic cholestasis of pregnancy
Third trimester onset:
Acute fatty liver disease of pregnancy
HELLP syndrome (hemolysis, elevated liver enzymes, and low platelets)
Preeclampsia and eclampsia
Other noninfectious syndromes
Wilson's disease (fulminant hepatitis during pregnancy)
Autoimmune hepatitis (flare during pregnancy or postpartum)
Budd-Chiari syndrome late pregnancy or postpartum (ascites, hepatomegaly, abdominal pain)
Infectious
Viral hepatitis (hepatitis A, B, C, or E)
Herpes simplex virus (HSV)
Varicella zoster virus (VZV)
Cytomegalovirus (CMV)

when acquired during the third trimester, especially outside the United States (USA). Hepatitis A, B, and C infections occur during pregnancy but are not greatly affected by the pregnancy. However, vertical transmission is a significant risk with both hepatitis B and hepatitis C.

The rash in our patient was consistent with an infectious etiology, and the pruritus might have been related to cholestasis. Acute fatty liver was considered given the abnormal ultrasound findings noted below. Hyperemesis gravidarum was not likely because it has an early onset in the pregnancy, and the emesis was neither severe nor persistent. HELLP syndrome was unlikely because the platelet count and hemoglobin were in the normal range. Hepatitis A, B, C, or E infection would usually be associated with higher ALT and AST levels.

The patient was diagnosed with CMV infection due to the positive IgM and IgG for the virus, although one could not be sure if this was primary infection or reactivation with end-organ involvement, and the Infectious Diseases Service was consulted. Intravenous (IV) ganciclovir was initiated, and LFTs were monitored. The patient was given a 10-gm dose of CMV IV immune globulin once. CMV serum and urine PCR assays were both negative.

The patient was discharged on ganciclovir to complete a 2-week course. The elevated liver enzymes (ALT and AST) steadily improved and eventually normalized shortly after she delivered a healthy baby via C-section performed because the fetus was in breech position.

cephaly, rash, low birth weight, splenomegaly, hepatomegaly, and retinitis. CMV is common in the USA, and upward of 80% of reproductive-age women have shown evidence of prior infection with this virus. Since 2016, there has been great concern for Zika virus infection during pregnancy with a risk of microcephaly and neurological abnormalities. With the exception of travelers to Zika endemic areas, CMV is a much more common threat to pregnant women who live in the continental USA, Hawaii and Alaska.

Pregnant women who are immunocompromised, either due to human immunodeficiency virus (HIV) infection or immunosuppressive medications, are at higher risk of developing an acute CMV infection and transmitting the infection to the fetus.

CMV reactivation is associated with a much lower risk to the fetus than primary infection during pregnancy [1]. In the setting of documented seroconversion (newly acquired CMV IgG antibody), primary infection is established. However in most cases there is no prior CMV serology. CMV IgM is considered reliable to diagnose primary CMV infection during pregnancy [4]. However, CMV IgM antibody can persist for months to years after primary infection and can also be found in the setting of reactivation, mostly in immunocompromised persons. The IgG avidity test may help in clarifying the significance of IgM antibody [4]. Viremia typically occurs in primary infection in the immunocompetent host and is undetectable or absent in recurrent infections [5].

14.1 Cytomegalovirus (CMV) in Pregnancy

CMV is a common cause of congenital infection, and primary maternal CMV infection carries a 35% risk of vertical transmission. Pregnant women who acquire primary CMV infection during the first trimester are much more likely to deliver babies with central nervous system (CNS) abnormalities, including seizures, than those who were infected before they became pregnant. Congenital CMV may cause jaundice, micro-

14.2 Cytomegalovirus (CMV) Hepatitis

Supporting the diagnosis of primary CMV infection in our patient is evidence of liver involvement demonstrated by her elevated ALT and AST. With primary CMV infection, the AST and ALT elevation typically is not higher than five times the normal range. Patients do not develop jaundice and are anicteric [5]. While primary CMV infection, reinfection, or reactivation can cause significant disease in immunocompromised patients, infection in those who are immunocompetent rarely leads to end-organ disease; only a few cases of CMV hepatitis have been reported [6].

Given the poor prognosis associated with vertical transmission of CMV to the fetus, it is appropriate to discuss with the pregnant mother the possible benefit of antivirals and CMV IV immune globulin, with the understanding that therapy is still investigational. CMV has been treated using ganciclovir in newborns who have symptomatic CMV infection, but little is known regarding the safety and efficacy of this medication during pregnancy. Animal studies suggest that CMV immune globulin may reduce fetal sequelae from CMV infection [1].

Key Points/Pearls

- The levels and kinetics of CMV IgM and IgG antibodies may not fully distinguish between primary CMV infection versus reactivation/reinfection in pregnancy; specialized testing may be useful.
- Acute CMV infection can cause a rise in liver enzymes although typically no more than five times the normal range.

- Acute CMV infection rarely causes end-organ disease in immunocompetent hosts but occasionally causes CMV hepatitis.
- Although investigational, antivirals and possibly CMV IV immune globulin may have benefit in pregnant women who have primary CMV infection.

References

1. Carlson A, Norwitz ER, Stiller RJ. Cytomegalovirus infection in pregnancy: should all women be screened? Rev Obstet Gynecol. 2010;3(4):172–9.
2. Tran TT, Ahn J, Reau NS. ACG clinical guideline: liver disease and pregnancy. Am J Gastroenterol. 2016;62(Suppl 4):S314–7.
3. Ch'ng CL, Morgan M, Hainsworth I, Kingham JG. Prospective study of liver dysfunction in pregnancy in Southwest Wales. Gut. 2002;51:876–80.
4. Revello MG, Gerna G. Diagnosis and management of human cytomegalovirus infection in the mother, fetus and newborn infant. Clin Microbiol Rev. 2002;15(4):680–715.
5. Taylor GH. Cytomegalovirus. Am Fam Physician. 2003;67(3):529–4.
6. Azad AK, Chowdhury AJ, et al. Cytomegalovirus induced hepatitis in an immunocompetent host. Mymensingh Med J. 2008;17(2 Suppl):S104–6.

Eye Pain and Visual Disturbance in an HIV/AIDS Patient

Fredy Chaparro-Rojas

A 49-year-old male with a history of human immunodeficiency virus (HIV) infection not on antiretroviral therapy due to non-compliance, presented to our tertiary care medical center reporting a 3-day history of right periorbital pain, ocular pain, edema, and decreased vision. He reported that the symptoms were first noted upon waking up and soon progressed to blurry vision, photophobia, and headaches. He denied neck pain or a stiff neck but reported subjective fevers. He denied trauma, surgery on his eyes, insect bites, or recent upper respiratory symptoms.

On examination, he was found to be febrile (102.3 °F) and tachycardic (pulse of 108 beats per minute) but alert and oriented. Significant right periorbital edema, erythema, tenderness to palpation, and purulent discharge were noted as well as conjunctival injection and lens opacity. His extraocular movements were intact but his visual acuity was decreased. His left eye examination was normal (Fig. 15.1). He had no lymphadenopathy, rash elsewhere on his body, or heart murmur. Also, no focal neurologic deficits or meningeal signs were noted.

The initial evaluation was notable for leukocytosis and neutrophilia (white blood cell [WBC] count 14,400/µL [normal range, 4600–9300/µL],

neutrophils 12,800/µL [1500–8000/µL]), CD4+ T-cell count of 1 cell/µL (359–1519 cells/µL), anemia (hemoglobin 10.2 g/dL [14.1–18.0 g/dL]), and transaminitis (aspartate aminotransferase [AST] 380 U/L [15–37 U/L] and alanine aminotransferase [ALT] 177 U/L [12–72 U/L]). An ophthalmologic examination demonstrated a hypopyon of the right eye and was consistent with panophthalmitis. Vitrectomy was performed, and intravitreal vancomycin and ceftazidime were administered by ocular injection.

A work-up was then undertaken to identify the etiology of panophthalmitis. His blood cultures grew methicillin-resistant *Staphylococcus aureus* (MRSA), without an evident primary source, and the patient was therefore started on intravenous (IV) vancomycin. The evaluation for a source of bacteremia included a transesophageal echocardiogram (TEE) that showed no findings suggestive of endocarditis and a computed tomography (CT) scan of the chest, abdomen, and pelvis that showed no evidence of pneumonia, intra-abdominal abscess, or pyelonephritis.

Cultures of the vitreous humor also grew MRSA, confirming the diagnosis. Therapy with intravitreal antibiotic injections and vitrectomy was performed every 48 h during the hospitalization.

Admission blood testing revealed that he had advanced acquired immune deficiency syndrome (AIDS), with a CD4+ T-cell count of 1 cell/µL, as noted above, and serum HIV viral load of 66,395 copies/mL. Initiation of antiretroviral therapy

F. Chaparro-Rojas, M.D.
Delaware Valley Infectious Diseases Associates, Wynnewood, PA, USA
e-mail: freddych6@yahoo.com

© Springer International Publishing AG 2018
M. David, J.-L. Benoit (eds.), *The Infectious Disease Diagnosis*,
https://doi.org/10.1007/978-3-319-64906-1_15

Fig. 15.1 Orbital cellulitis and presence of conjunctival hemorrhage, hypopyon, and lens opacity consistent with panophthalmitis

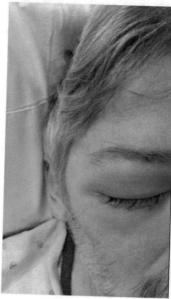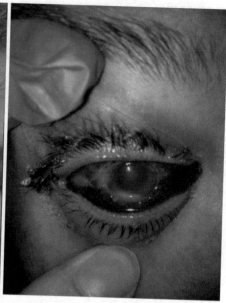

was deferred until his HIV genotype returned, given the risk of resistance due to the patient's history of prior treatment and his history of nonadherence.

After a prolonged course of IV vancomycin, the patient's blood cultures eventually cleared, turning negative after almost 2 weeks of positive results. IV antibiotic therapy was continued for complicated MRSA bacteremia for an additional 6 weeks. The patient progressed well with resolution of fevers and improvement in the periorbital edema and erythema. However while the treatment was successful in stopping the progression of the disease and preserving the eye, the patient's visual acuity remained seriously compromised.

15.1 Complicated MRSA Bacteremia and Secondary Panophthalmitis in HIV/AIDS

Patients with HIV infection may suffer from multiple conditions that can affect the eyes and surrounding structures. By direct inoculation of infectious agents or by dissemination of systemic processes, ocular infections are usually aggressive, and the prognosis depends on timely and accurate diagnosis and treatment. The differential diagnosis of rapidly progressive ophthalmologic conditions in patients with advanced HIV/AIDS includes retinitis, preseptal cellulitis, conjunctivitis, trauma, drug reactions (including rifabutin-associated uveitis with hypopyon), neoplastic infiltration, uveitis, and surgical complications (Table 15.1). A thorough ophthalmologic examination is necessary to identify the part of the eye involved and to narrow the differential diagnosis.

Orbital and periorbital cellulitis must be differentiated because the approach and treatment are different. Periorbital cellulitis, also known as preseptal cellulitis, is the inflammation and infection of the eyelid and skin surrounding the eye, anterior to the orbital and conjunctival septum. Orbital cellulitis is an inflammation of eye tissues posterior to the orbital and conjunctival septum and most commonly refers to extension of infection originating from acute sinusitis (usually ethmoidal sinusitis) or from bacteremia. Orbital cellulitis may cause proptosis and ophthalmoplegia and result in infectious cavernous sinus thrombosis with ptosis, mydriasis, and oculomotor nerve palsies. Orbital cellulitis requires emergent initiation of IV antibiotic therapy and may require a surgical procedure. In contrast to orbital cellulitis, patients with periorbital cellulitis do not have bulging of the eye (proptosis), limited eye movement (ophthalmoplegia), pain on eye movements, or loss of vision.

Table 15.1 Ophthalmic manifestations and complications of human immunodeficiency virus (HIV) infection

Anterior segment
• Kaposi's sarcoma

• Infections
  – Varicella zoster virus (VZV) ophthalmicus, common and potentially severe
  – Herpes simplex virus (HSV) keratitis with large ulcers rather than the typical dendritic ulcers seen in immunocompetent patients
  – Fungal infections (*Candida* spp., Microsporidia-associated keratitis)

• Uveitis
  – Syphilis (*Treponema pallidum*): syphilitic anterior uveitis is common and may be sight threatening
  – Reactive arthritis

Posterior segment

• Non-opportunistic conditions
  – HIV retinopathy (cotton wool retinal infiltrates, a benign condition) and optic nerve involvement
  – Syphilis can involve the posterior segment as well

• Opportunistic infections
  – Cytomegalovirus (CMV) retinitis is the most common, typically a vasculitis with hemorrhages and exudates, and can become sight threatening if not treated quickly
  – VZV-associated progressive outer retinal necrosis (VZV-PORN), the most severe
  – *Toxoplasma* chorioretinitis
  – *Candida* endophthalmitis
  – Bacterial retinitis and endophthalmitis including *Staphylococcus* spp.
  – *Cryptococcus* chorioretinitis
  – *Pneumocystis* choroiditis
  – Acute retinal necrosis due to HSV and VZV

Table 15.2 Categories and most common pathogens in endophthalmitis

Acute postcataract	Coagulase-negative staphylococcal species
Bleb related	Viridans streptococci, *Streptococcus pneumoniae*, *Haemophilus influenzae*
Chronic pseudophakic	*Propionibacterium acnes*
Fungal	*Candida* spp., *Aspergillus* spp., *Fusarium* spp.
Post-traumatic	*Bacillus cereus*
Endogenous	*Staphylococcus aureus*, *Streptococcus* spp., Gram-negative bacilli

In endophthalmitis, infection involves the vitreous humor, the aqueous humor, or both. In panophthalmitis, both orbital cellulitis and endophthalmitis are documented.

This patient presented with a clinical picture consistent with endogenous endophthalmitis/panophthalmitis. This entity constitutes an ophthalmologic emergency given its rapid progression and sight-threatening course. Endophthalmitis is broadly classified as endogenous or exogenous. Endogenous endophthalmitis is usually associated with a bacteremia, in which microorganisms seed the eye, and it is commonly associated with systemic symptoms of infection such as fever. Exogenous endophthalmitis, in contrast, is the most common presentation associated with surgery, trauma, or severe corneal infections. It usually lacks systemic manifestations.

The differential diagnosis of acute changes in vision in the HIV patient is broad, but certain findings may help to narrow the list (Table 15.1). Viral and parasitic infections commonly cause uveitis—for example, cytomegalovirus [CMV] retinitis or *toxoplasma* chorioretinitis—but rarely cause endophthalmitis. CMV retinitis is generally diagnosed on the basis of characteristic retinal changes, and indirect ophthalmoscopy usually reveals yellow-white, fluffy, or granular retinal lesions, often located close to retinal vessels and associated with hemorrhage. Testing for CMV viremia by DNA polymerase chain reaction (PCR), blood antigen, or blood culture is not diagnostically helpful. Patients with *Toxoplasma* chorioretinitis (a posterior uveitis) often have raised, yellow-white, cottony lesions in a nonvascular distribution (unlike the perivascular exudates of CMV retinitis) on ophthalmologic examination.

Endophthalmitis can be also classified by the mechanism of infection as shown in Table 15.2.

15.2 Community-Associated MRSA Infections in HIV/AIDS

In our case, several blood cultures were positive for MRSA, and MRSA was also isolated from the vitreous humor, confirming a case of endogenous endophthalmitis. However, no source of bacteremia was identified. The MRSA genotyping showed the typical characteristics of the USA300 strain type (i.e., it had MLST ST8, and it carried the SCC*mec* type IV element and the genes encoding the Panton-Valentine leukocidin [PVL]), which is the most common strain type of community-associated MRSA (CA-MRSA) in the United States.

Recent studies suggest that HIV-infected persons have a propensity for contracting CA-MRSA infections and colonization [1]. An HIV-infected patient is 18-fold more likely than an HIV-uninfected person to develop infections caused by CA-MRSA with twice the rate of recurrent disease [2]. Risk factors for CA-MRSA infection in an HIV-infected patient include higher HIV viral loads, lower nadir and current CD4+ T-cell counts, absence of antiretroviral therapy, same-sex intercourse among men, multiple sexual partners, recent sexually transmitted infections, close contact with MRSA-infected persons, and injection drug use [3]. However, CA-MRSA also affects HIV-infected patients with relatively high CD4+ T-cell counts, suggesting an antigen-specific immune defect. The higher incidence of CA-MRSA infection in the HIV-infected population may be related to the underproduction of cells producing the cytokine interferon-γ (IFN-γ). Researchers have demonstrated decreased function of IFN-γ-producing cells from HIV-infected patients in response to in vitro stimulation with MRSA [4].

Key Points/Pearls

- Endophthalmitis is an ophthalmologic emergency.
- Diagnosis of endophthalmitis must be suspected from a patient's history and physical examination and confirmed by cultures of the vitreous or aqueous humor.

- Treatment of endophthalmitis requires a combination of surgery (vitrectomy), intraocular antibiotics, and systemic antibiotics that achieve reasonably good intraocular levels.
- HIV-infected patients are at a higher risk of MRSA colonization and CA-MRSA infections likely due to immunological, behavioral, and social predisposing factors.
- HIV-infected patients with CD4 T-cell count below 50 are at high risk of CMV retinitis, which is treatable if diagnosed early, and treated with IV ganciclovir or oral valganciclovir.
- HIV-infected patients also may rarely develop VZV-PORN (progressive outer retinal necrosis), which leads to rapid and irreversible loss of vision.
- Syphilis frequently affects the eyes, and most often causes anterior uveitis, but may cause panuveitis, optic neuritis, and the Argyll-Robertson pupil.

References

1. Zervou FN, Zacharioudakis IM, Ziakas PD, Rich JD, Mylonakis E. Prevalence of and risk factors for methicillin-resistant *Staphylococcus aureus* colonization in HIV infection: a meta-analysis. Clin Infect Dis. 2014;59(9):1302–11.
2. Crum-Cianflone NF, Burgi AA, Hale BR. Increasing rates of community-acquired methicillin-resistant *Staphylococcus aureus* infections among HIV-infected persons. Int J STD AIDS. 2007;18(8):521–6.
3. Shadyab AH, Crum-Cianflone NF. Methicillin-resistant *Staphylococcus aureus* (MRSA) infections among HIV-infected persons in the era of highly active antiretroviral therapy: a review of the literature. HIV Med. 2012;13(6):319–32.
4. Utay NS, Roque A, Timmer JK, et al. MRSA infections in HIV-infected people are associated with decreased MRSA-specific Th1 immunity. PLoS Pathog. 2016;12(4):e1005580.

Undetected: When Medication Nonadherence Accompanies an Undetectable Viral Load

16

Matthew Richards and Connor Williams

A 19-year-old African-American male presented to the adolescent infectious disease clinic after being diagnosed with human immunodeficiency virus (HIV) infection 18 months before. Records from the patient's previous medical provider showed that the patient had initiated highly active antiretroviral therapy (HAART) (rilpivirine/tenofovir/emtricitabine) 4 months after diagnosis and had experienced side effects (drowsiness, dizziness, and nausea) with imperfect medication adherence for the next 5 months. These records indicated the patient received three blood tests during this 5-month period, and there was only one reported HIV viral load, which was undetectable 1 month after initiating HAART. After 5 months of treatment, he stopped taking HAART for the following 11 months and reported acute levels of psychosocial stress during this period related to alcohol consumption (4–5 drinks/day) and violent disputes with his partner, leading to high levels of stress and insomnia. During the time that he was not adherent, the patient had three HIV viral load measurements, which were 21,891/mL, 158/mL, and 331/mL, respectively. The patient's previous physician had noted the final two measurements

to be remarkably low despite the patient's reported medication nonadherence.

At the time of presentation to the clinic, the patient reported that he had restarted HAART (darunavir/ritonavir and tenofovir/emtricitabine) 1 month prior, and laboratory measurements indicated an undetectable HIV viral load. During the initial visit, screening revealed that the patient was infected with *Chlamydia*, which was treated. The patient was again prescribed darunavir/ritonavir and tenofovir/emtricitabine.

During his first visit to the clinic, the patient reported a severely depressed mood and a sense of hopelessness. He disclosed that he had endured many months of physical, verbal, and emotional abuse in his most recent relationship, and many other challenges were causing him great stress. After his partner permanently moved out of their shared apartment, the patient had become delinquent in his rent and unable to pay his bills without the financial support of his partner. The patient faced impending homelessness. He was unemployed, having recently lost his job after an incident with his supervisor in which his HIV infection was revealed to coworkers. The patient reported that his use of cigarettes, marijuana, and alcohol had increased significantly in the weeks prior to his presentation to the clinic. He identified his depressed mood and lack of motivation to find employment and alternative housing as driving factors for his increased frequency of substance abuse. Later in the same clinic visit, he

M. Richards, A.M., L.C.S.W., M.Div. (✉)
C. Williams, A.M., L.C.S.W.
Department of Pediatrics, University of Chicago, Chicago, IL, USA
e-mail: mrichards@peds.bsd.uchicago.edu

© Springer International Publishing AG 2018
M. David, J.-L. Benoit (eds.), *The Infectious Disease Diagnosis*,
https://doi.org/10.1007/978-3-319-64906-1_16

reported that he had attempted suicide few days before, and he agreed to speak with a licensed clinical social worker (LCSW). Together they contracted for the patient's immediate safety, detailing a plan for calling identified social supports and/or emergency services if he believed he would be a threat to his own life in the days following his appointment. The LCSW scheduled the patient for an intake appointment for the following week.

At his subsequent visit, the patient met with the LCSW for a comprehensive assessment that identified the core areas of concern. They discussed immediately available resources that would support his overall well-being and also developed a treatment plan that addressed adherence to HAART, psychiatric symptoms, and development of life skills related to attending community college and securing stable employment. The multidisciplinary team ensured his access to an infectious disease physician, a case manager, the LCSW, and a peer health navigator who were able to implement and support an integrative treatment plan. Early phases of the treatment focused on ensuring his safety and connection to basic resources. His case manager helped him to secure housing four times during 2.5 years of care. The patient first stayed at a youth shelter for 2–3 months before transitioning to living with friends for a brief period of time. He later obtained housing through an outside program for people living with HIV/AIDs (PLWH), but after only 18 months, he terminated his contract with the program because of a disagreement with his housing manager. Later, he moved into an apartment with a friend during a period of unemployment and financial instability. The volatility in his housing history paralleled the instability in other psychosocial domains.

Once his housing needs were met early in the treatment process, he and his case manager explored potential employment opportunities. After a prolonged process of applying to many different jobs in the service industry, the patient began working as a dishwasher for a fast food restaurant chain. A few months later, he reported feeling that his supervisor and coworkers were mistreating him, creating tension between him-

self and his manager that resulted in termination of his employment. Several months later he began part-time work for a medical office. This job provided him with minimal income, leaving him unable to meet his overall financial needs. He frequently reported that he was behind on his bills, and he was often unable to pay his monthly rent in full. After approximately 18 months of employment, he quit his second job following tension with his supervisor. He reported that he left his job because he felt that the staff at his work place showed him disrespect.

While his case manager addressed his social needs related to housing and employment, the patient was apprehensive about engaging in behavioral health services. In his previous encounters with mental health providers, he felt stigmatized. He had previously been prescribed a variety of psychotropic medications beginning when he was 15 years old. At that time, he was first hospitalized for suicidal ideation, substance use, and behavior that he described as "angry outbursts." He reported that he struggled with adherence to his psychotropic medication because he felt it was a mechanism of control over his mind and his general sense of freedom. He completed a series of brief assessments including the Generalized Anxiety Disorder 7 (GAD-7) anxiety screener, the Patient Health Questionnaire-9 (PHQ-9) depression screener, the Primary Care-Posttraumatic Stress Disorder screener (PC-PTSD), and a conjoint screener for alcohol and drug abuse (CAGE-AID). He was diagnosed with severe anxiety and moderately severe depression, and he was found to be using both drugs and alcohol at levels that suggested possible addiction.

He engaged intermittently with the LCSW for psychotherapy. The initial goals of this treatment were to reduce the immediate presenting mood symptoms, while also exploring a history of relational instability and identifying new areas of cognitive, emotional, and behavioral responses to inconsistencies in his relationships. His substance use was sporadic throughout treatment, and motivational interviewing techniques were used to highlight his ambivalence toward change, while also identifying and addressing areas in which substance use conflicted with treatment goals. His mood symptoms cycled through periods of stabilization, usually improving when psychosocial stressors were mitigated and/or when substance use was decreased. Through psychological treatment, he gained insight into personal triggers, allowing him to anticipate his own reactions to stressful circumstances and develop strategies for responding more adaptively—especially in the context of important relationships. As treatment progressed, he stayed more engaged with his providers by telephone and e-mail. He also began to rely on family members when he struggled with taking HAART or with attending appointments.

Despite the intensive approach taken to this patient's care, he experienced problems in service engagement and retention in care. His medical provider scheduled medical visits with him every 3–4 months. During the 2.5 years chronicled, the longest interval between clinical visits was 6 months. Notably, he had laboratory assessments on 16 occasions, all showing an undetectable HIV viral load and CD4+ T cell counts between 890 cells/mL and 1800 cells/mL. He reported that he would intermittently stop taking HAART for 1–2 months at a time, and yet the measured viral loads remained consistently undetectable.

As to nonmedical services, he cycled through 3- to 6-month periods of consistent presentation to psychotherapy appointments and case management meetings. These periods of engagement were followed by shorter episodes (typically for 1–3 months) of disconnection from one or both services. His care team worked collaboratively to retain him in services, often through case conferences to identify best practices to reengage him with the program. He maintained relationships with the allied health team, usually reaching out to his LCSW or case manager for assistance during times of stress. When the team was successful in bringing him into the clinic—most often through direct transportation assistance—each member of his care team was informed. Same-day appointments with other care providers were scheduled when possible. Text message and phone call reminders about appointments were used, and his case manager often visited him at home when he was unresponsive to other methods of contact. Home visits were almost always successful in reengaging him, especially when transportation was provided to his appointments.

During his most recent visit to the infectious disease clinic, he reported continued unemployment and financial concerns after being terminated from his job. His financial hardships had taken a toll on his important relationships—especially with his roommate—and he reported isolating himself in his room most days, drinking heavily. His most recent laboratory results reflected that he was virally suppressed with a CD4+ T cell count of 1214 cells/mL. Although his adherence to HAART appeared to have improved greatly, the care team was unsuccessful in engaging him in his quarterly medical visit. He was also less responsive to phone calls and other means of communication. Based on past experience, the clinical team expects that the current period of appointment nonadherence will follow past patterns and that the patient will be reengaged through intensive case management.

16.1 Treatment Conceptualization

Social-ecological approaches to human behavior examine the "complex associations between social and structural (access to care) factors, individual practices, the physical environment, and health" [1]. Social-ecological theory posits that variables at the individual, interpersonal, community, and macro levels shape complex human behaviors like engagement in the HIV care process. From this theoretical perspective, interventions that neglect the broad array of contextual factors that shape health behaviors are likely to fail.

The circumstances of this patient are characteristic of the manner in which social determinants of health and mental health can shape a person's capacity to remain engaged in HIV care. Despite significant progress in the medical management of HIV, a majority of patients in the United States remain disengaged from the HIV care process (see Fig. 16.1). Engagement in the HIV care process and achieving suppression of

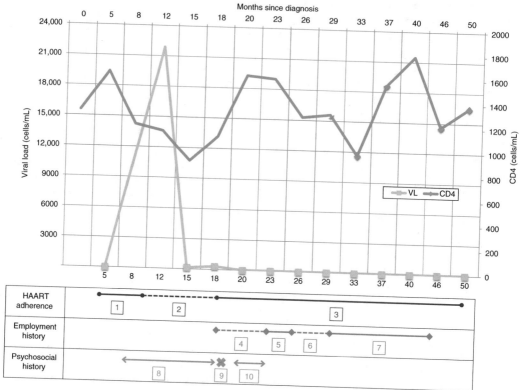

Fig. 16.1 Human immunodeficiency virus (VL) viral load, CD4+ T cell count, adherence with HAART, and indicators of psychosocial stressors during 50 months of care. (*1*) Four months after his diagnosis, the patient initiated highly active retroviral therapy (rilpivirine/tenofovir/emtricitabine). He reported moderate adherence for 5 months after being prescribed this regimen. (*2*) The patient reported nonadherence to the regimen for approximately 11 months (between 9 and 18 months after his diagnosis). (*3*) He presented to the clinic for the first time approximately 18 months after diagnosis. The patient indicated that he was moderately adherent to newly prescribed regimen (darunavir/tenofovir/emtricitabine). Moderate adherence was reported throughout the course of treatment at the clinic, with 1–2 month periods in which the patient reported complete nonadherence. (*4*) The patient reported losing employment at approximately 18 months after his diagnosis. He experienced unemploy-

ment for approximately 5 months. (*5*) He reported obtaining new full-time employment approximately 23 month after his diagnosis and maintained employment for approximately 3 months. (*6*) He reported losing employment approximately 26 months after his diagnosis and reported that he was unemployed for approximately 3 months. (*7*) The patient reported obtaining new part-time employment approximately 29 months after his diagnosis; he maintained employment for approximately 17 months. (*8*) The patient reported experiencing domestic violence (verbal, emotional, and physical) in his relationship for approximately 10 months (time period between 8 months and 18 months after his diagnosis). (*9*) He reported suicide attempt approximately 18 months after his diagnosis. (*10*) He reported living in a shelter for approximately 3 months (time period between 20 months and 23 months after his diagnosis)

the viral load improve long-term health outcomes for people living with HIV (PLWH) and are significantly correlated with reduced risk of onward HIV transmission [2]. The direct benefit to PLWH and the preventive value of viral suppression make it essential that providers of HIV care be aware of the factors that place an individual at risk of disengagement from the HIV care process

and develop a comprehensive treatment plan that attempts to address them (methods for improving engagement in care are shown in Table 16.1).

A variety of factors have been identified that shape vulnerability to disengagement from the care process, including lower-income status, diagnosed mental health or substance use disorder, incarceration, unstable housing, stigma,

Table 16.1 Evidence-based approaches for improving engagement in HIV medical care[a]

Intervention	Description
Intensive case management	Long-term interventions such as medical case management and brief interventions such as Antiretroviral Treatment and Access to Services (ATAS)
	Both interventions employ social workers who assess the complex array of variables inhibiting engagement in the HIV care process, and then develop and implement an "action plan" for engagement in care that facilitates linkage to and engagement at the HIV care site
Patient/health navigation and outreach service	Paraprofessionals or health outreach personnel provide HIV education and social support and increase access to resources that help neutralize barriers to entry into HIV care
	These brief interventions are often delivered in community-based settings with the goal of bridging the patient into a clinical environment
Technology-based interventions	Social workers, case managers, and health outreach personnel text message brief reminders affirming the importance of engagement in care to HIV-infected patients on an ongoing basis
	These interventions are best used in conjunction with medical case management once a client is connected to HIV care
Network interventions	Patients identify a member of their family or social network to provide appointment and medication adherence support

[a]Adapted from [3]

or a low level of social support [3]. These factors contribute to a dynamic pattern of patients cycling in and out of care that Michael Mugavero has described as "churn" [3]. As Mugavero notes, comprehensive models of health behavior—such as the social-ecological framework—are needed to describe the multiple factors that influence the considerable HIV-infected patient population experiencing churn. These models then need to be translated into multidisciplinary practice within the clinical environment. While factors and combinations of factors that shape vulnerability to disengagement are documented in the scientific literature, less has been written about the psychosocial interventions that should be implemented in clinical settings to neutralize these nonmedical barriers to engagement (see Fig. 16.2).

The research literature on HIV engagement in care interventions broadly supports the use of case management, patient navigation, and technology-based interventions [3]. Another area of current investigation relates to network-based engagement in care interventions. These could include interventions in which a patient identifies a member of his or her family or social network to provide appointment and medication adherence support [4]. Case management interventions include long-term interventions such as medical case management and brief interventions such as Anti-Retroviral Treatment and Access to Services (ARTAS) that both employ social workers who assess the complex array of variables inhibiting engagement in HIV care and then develop and implement an "action plan" for engagement in care that facilitates linkage to and engagement at the HIV care site [5]. Patient navigation and outreach interventions employ paraprofessionals or health outreach personnel to provide HIV education, social support, and increase access to resources that will neutralize barriers to entry into HIV care. These brief interventions are often delivered in community-based settings with the goal of bridging the patient into a clinical environment [6]. Technology-based interventions include using text messaging to send brief reminders affirming the importance of engagement in care to HIV-infected patients on an ongoing basis. One of the limitations of this intervention is that it focuses on appointment and medication adherence but fails to address the broad array of contextual factors (e.g., poverty, housing status, mental health conditions, and substance dependence) that may undermine engagement in HIV care. However, technology-based interventions may serve as a useful adjunct to case management once patients are linked to care.

Fig. 16.2 HIV stages of care. There is an urgent need to reach more people with testing and to make sure that those infected with the virus receive prompt, ongoing care and treatment. SOURCES: CDC National HIV Surveillance System and Medical Monitoring Project, 2011 and CDC Vital Signs, Nov. 2014, www.cdc.gov/vitalsigns. *Antiretroviral therapy

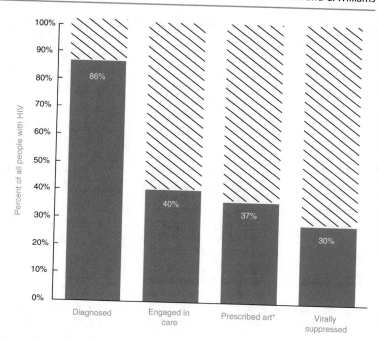

16.2 Social-Ecological Approaches as Applied to the Present Case Study

In this case study, we demonstrated how barriers to engagement should be assessed and addressed through the provision of psychosocial services within the context of a comprehensive treatment plan. The capacity for ongoing engagement in care is deeply interconnected with exposure to social determinants risk factors [3]. Therefore, these factors must be regularly assessed and addressed on an ongoing basis, including periods between medical appointments. In this case study, poor medication adherence and missed appointments appeared to be associated with psychosocial stressors. Missed appointments were highly predictive of medication nonadherence. This suggests that a patient's disengagement from nonmedical services during the course of treatment may be a risk factor for medication nonadherence; this may be an important area for future research. Because providers of nonmedical services are often in greater contact with patients between medical appointments, engagement patterns with these service providers might be used as a measure of risk for medication nonadherence between medical appointments.

An overreliance on biomedical measures of treatment engagement (HIV viral load and CD4+ T cell counts) may not always provide a reliable measurement of care engagement patterns. We propose that allied health services function both to mitigate exposure to psychosocial risk factors and provide a potentially reliable measure of care engagement patterns over time that can be used to give the medical provider a more accurate view of the patient's medication adherence. As demonstrated in this case study, the patient's HIV viral loads were consistently undetectable at clinic visits despite self-reported periods of extended nonadherence between appointments and inconsistencies in appointment adherence. This is not necessarily surprising because attendance at the medical appointment may itself suggest that a patient has higher capacity for medication adherence at that time. However, this suggests the possibility that data captured at medical visits may not be representative of a patient's medication adherence between appointments. Periods of extended nonadherence to HAART increase the risk of development of viral resistance and further HIV propagation, and therefore it is important to identify them.

Key Points/Pearls

- Exposure to psychosocial risk factors such as homelessness, poverty, HIV stigma/discrimination, untreated mental health and substance dependence, and lack of health insurance enhances vulnerability to disengagement from HIV care.
- Each patient's psychosocial assets and vulnerabilities must be assessed across the HIV treatment cascade to inform an interdisciplinary treatment plan that addresses psychosocial needs to neutralize risk factors for disengagement from HIV care.
- Assessment should be ongoing with the expectation that a patient's psychosocial vulnerabilities will change over time.
- Beyond biomedical measurements of HIV medication adherence (HIV viral load and CD4+ T cell count), information gained by providers of nonmedical services (e.g., mental health professionals, case managers, health educators, or navigators) can provide deeper insight into medication adherence behaviors between appointments that may not be reflected in laboratory measurements.

Acknowledgment The authors wish to thank Dr. Julia Rosebush, D.O. for her assistance with this report.

References

1. Baral S, Logie CH, Grosso A, Wirtz AL, Beyrer C. Modified social ecological model: a tool to guide the assessment of the risks and risk contexts of HIV epidemics. BMC Public Health. 2013;13:482.
2. Cohen MS, Chen YQ, McCauley M, et al. Prevention of HIV-1 infection with early antiretroviral therapy. N Engl J Med. 2011;365(6):493–505.
3. Mugavero MJ, Amico KR, Horn T, Thompson MA. The state of engagement in HIV care in the United States: from cascade to continuum to control. Clin Infect Dis. 2013;57(8):1164–71.
4. Bouris A, Voisin D, Pilloton M, et al. Project nGage: network supported HIV care engagement for younger black men who have sex with men and transgender persons. J AIDS Clin Res. 2013;4.
5. Craw JA, Gardner LI, Marks G, et al. Brief strengths-based case management promotes entry into HIV medical care: results of the antiretroviral treatment access study-II. J Acquir Immune Defic Syndr. 2008;47(5):597–606.
6. Hightow-Weidman LB, Jones K, Wohl AR, et al. Early linkage and retention in care: findings from the outreach, linkage, and retention in care initiative among young men of color who have sex with men. AIDS Patient Care STDs. 2011;25(Suppl 1):S31–8.

Danger in Paradise

17

Margaret Newman

A 31-year-old man became sick on the last day of his 3-week-long trip to Southeast Asia with sudden onset of fever, arthralgia, and headache. He attributed his symptoms to exhaustion and boarded a plane back to the United States (USA), but the symptoms persisted. The following day he also had several loose, non-bloody stools which were self-limited. Three days after departing Hong Kong, he presented to his Student Health Center for evaluation. Prior to his trip, he had not visited a travel clinic or received malaria prophylaxis.

The patient was originally from Colombia, but he had moved to the USA for his undergraduate and graduate education. He had not been to South America for more than 2 years. His trip to Southeast Asia included 10 days in Thailand, 4 days in Cambodia, 6 days in Laos, and 1 day in Hong Kong. His American girlfriend accompanied him on the trip and did not develop similar symptoms. While on vacation, they rode elephants, hiked through a jungle, and slept on a beach. They also swam in a waterfall and encountered local monkeys, though he did not recall any bites or scratches from a monkey. He drank mostly bottled water, but he ate local sushi and drank fruit juices purchased from street vendors. He denied any local sexual contacts. He used insect repellent intermittently during his trip but suffered many mosquito bites. He felt well throughout the majority of the trip.

The patient's past medical history was unremarkable. He was taking no prescribed medications, although he did take a few doses of acetaminophen and ibuprofen for the joint pains over the previous 3 days. He was enrolled in business school and lived in Chicago. He did not use drugs or smoke cigarettes. In addition to the fever, headache, and arthralgia, the patient also complained of appetite loss and fatigue. He was not having any abdominal pain or vomiting. He had no vision changes or neck pain.

On presentation, the patient was found to be febrile to 102 °F, mildly tachycardic at 99 beats per minute, normotensive at 115/75 mmHg, and had a respiratory rate of 16 breaths per minute. He had no enlarged joints and no findings of synovitis, but the provider incidentally noted a faintly erythematous, patchy rash over both anterior knees (see Fig. 17.1). The patient had not previously noted the rash as it was not tender or pruritic. His eyes were notable for mild scleral injection bilaterally. There was no appreciable lymphadenopathy, and the oropharynx was clear. The abdomen was soft and non-tender without enlargement of spleen or liver.

An infectious diseases consultation service was requested by the Student Health Clinic

M. Newman, M.D.
Section of Infectious Diseases and Global Health, Department of Medicine, University of Chicago Medicine, Chicago, IL, USA
e-mail: Margaret.Newman@uchospitals.edu

© Springer International Publishing AG 2018
M. David, J.-L. Benoit (eds.), *The Infectious Disease Diagnosis*,
https://doi.org/10.1007/978-3-319-64906-1_17

provider. The differential diagnosis for a returning traveler from Southeast Asia with a febrile illness of a relatively short incubation (maximum 21 days) is summarized in Table 17.1. It includes mosquito-borne infections (malaria, dengue fever, Zika virus, chikungunya virus, and Japanese encephalitis), mite-borne scrub typhus (*Orientia tsutsugamushi*), *Salmonella typhi* (typhoid fever), brucellosis, leptospirosis, acute viral hepatitis (especially A or E), and visceral leishmaniasis. Acute retroviral syndrome (human immunodeficiency virus [HIV]) and secondary syphilis would usually be in the differential diagnosis as they may cause similar symptoms, but these diagnoses were less likely in view of the patient's reported sexual history. More commonly encountered viral causes of fever and arthralgias, such as seasonal influenza, mononucleosis, and parvovirus, were also considered. Other rickettsial diseases (such as Flinders Island spotted fever in Southeast Asia) may present with similar symptoms, but a prominent diffuse rash would be expected. Tularemia and ehrlichiosis can also cause fever, arthralgia, and rash, but these diseases are not endemic in either Southeast Asia or Chicago.

Given the prolonged processing time required for serological studies for several of these infectious syndromes, it was recommended that the patient have basic electrolyte and hematologic laboratory studies, with hospital admission if they were abnormal. A malaria smear was negative, but the creatinine was significantly elevated to 2.1 mg/dL (normal range, 0.5–1.4 mg/dL) from a baseline value 0.9 mg/dL. The patient was admitted to the hospital for further evaluation. Liver function tests were slightly elevated, with alanine aminotransferase (ALT) of 49 U/L (8–35 U/L) and aspartate aminotransferase (AST) of 45 U/L (8–37 U/L). Antibody tests for dengue virus, chikungunya virus, Zika virus, and leptospirosis were sent to the US Centers for Disease Control and Prevention (CDC) for processing. A fourth-generation HIV screening test was nonreactive. A respiratory viral panel polymerase chain reaction (PCR) test was negative. Repeat malaria smears were also negative. Table 17.2 shows a complete list of the patient's laboratory test results. The acute kidney injury resolved after 12 hours of intravenous fluids, liver function tests normalized the following day, and the patient's symptoms improved. At this point he was discharged from the hospital with a 7-day course of empiric oral doxycycline while the infectious diseases serologies sent to the CDC were still pending. Several days later, the *Leptospira* IgM antibody test came back positive. Antibody tests for dengue, chikungunya, and Zika viruses were negative.

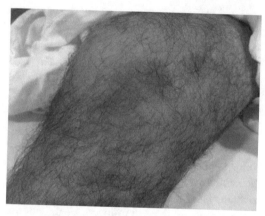

Fig. 17.1 Rash on the anterior right knee at presentation

Table 17.1 Differential diagnosis for a traveler returning from Southeast Asia with fever, myalgia, arthralgia, and rash with a relatively short incubation period (<21 days)

Dengue fever (flavivirus)
Zika virus (flavivirus)
Chikungunya virus and other uncommon alphaviruses
Scrub typhus (*Orientia tsutsugamushi*)
Leptospirosis (*Leptospira* spp.)
Salmonella typhi (typhoid fever)
Acute human immunodeficiency virus (HIV) infection
Influenza
Flinders Island spotted fever (*Rickettsia honei*)
Secondary syphilis (*Treponema pallidum*)
Mononucleosis (Epstein-Barr virus)
Parvovirus
Measles
Rubeola
Hepatitis A
Hepatitis E
Japanese encephalitis infection (flavivirus)
Malaria (usually no rash)

Table 17.2 Laboratory values

Test name	Patient value	Reference range
White blood cell count	8100/μL	3500–11,000/μL
Hemoglobin	14.6 g/dL	13.5–17.5 g/dL
Hematocrit	42%	41–53%
Mean corpuscular volume (MCV)	87.8 fL	81–99 fL
Platelet	126,000/μL	150,000–450,000/μL
Neutrophils	77%	39–75%
Lymphocytes	16%	16–47%
Monocytes	7%	4–12%
Eosinophils	0%	0–7%
Basophils	0%	0–2%
Sodium	138 mmol/L	134–149 mmol/L
Chloride	97 mmol/L	95–108 mmol/L
Blood urea nitrogen (BUN)	23 mg/dL	7–20 mg/dL
Glucose	110 mg/dL	60–109 mg/dL
Potassium	3.6 mmol/L	3.4–5.0 mmol/L
Carbon dioxide	21 mmol/L	23–30 mmol/L
Creatinine	2.1 mg/dL	0.4–1.4 mg/dL
Total bilirubin	0.4 mg/dL	0.1–1.0 mg/dL
Total protein	7.5 g/dL	6.0–8.3 g/dL
Albumin	4.2 g/dL	3.5–5.0 g/dL
Alkaline phosphatase	82 U/L	30–120 U/L
Aspartate aminotransferase	45 U/L	8–37 U/L
Alanine aminotransferase	49 U/L	8–35 U/L
Lactic acid	0.8 mmol/L	0.7–2.1 mmol/L
Urinalysis	Color yellow	Specific gravity 1.016–1.022
	Clarity turbid	pH 5.0–9.0
	Specific gravity 1.016	Urobilinogen 0.1–1.0 g/dL
	pH 5.0	
	Leukocyte esterase negative	
	Nitrites negative	
	Protein 2+	
	Blood 3+	
	Glucose 1+	
	Ketones negative	
	Bilirubin negative	
	Urobilinogen 0.2 g/dL	
Respiratory viral panel[a]	Negative	Negative
Malaria smear (Giemsa), thick and thin smears	Negative	Negative
Dengue fever Ab, IgG	Negative	Negative
Dengue fever Ab, IgM	Negative	Negative
Chikungunya Ab, IgG	Negative	Negative
Chikungunya Ab, IgM	Negative	Negative
Leptospira Ab, IgM	Positive	Negative
HIV 1/2 antibody/antigen screen	Nonreactive	Nonreactive
Blood cultures	Negative	Negative

[a]The respiratory viral panel tests by the polymerase chain reaction for the following pathogens: adenovirus, coronavirus 229E, coronavirus HKU, coronavirus NL63, coronavirus C43, human metapneumovirus, rhinovirus/enterovirus, H1 2009 subtype of influenza A, H1 subtype of influenza A, H3 subtype of influenza A, influenza A, influenza B, parainfluenza 1–4, respiratory syncytial virus (RSV), *Bordetella pertussis, Chamydophila pneumoniae, and Mycoplasma pneumoniae*

17.1 Leptospirosis

Leptospira is a zoonotic spirochete bacterial genus that frequently contaminates soil or surface water. It was first discovered in 1883 in sewer workers, as the pathogen is commonly spread by rodent urine in stagnant water. The clinical syndrome of renal failure, jaundice, and thrombocytopenia was described by Adolf Weil (1848–1916) in 1886 [1]. The *Leptospira* spirochete resides in the renal tubules of chronically infected animal hosts who do not display symptoms of illness, and bacteria are shed in the urine. They survive in surface fresh water for months to years. Rodents often spread disease in urban areas, but dogs and livestock can also be infected.

Humans may be infected via direct contact with animals or, more often, indirectly through contact with water or soil contaminated by the urine of infected animals, such as when skin abrasions or mucous membranes are exposed to contaminated water [2]. Leptospirosis is an occupational zoonosis more common in persons who handle animals (veterinarians, workers on dairy farms, abattoir workers, butchers, hunters, animal and dog handlers) or are exposed to contaminated wet soil or surface water (e.g., rice farming). Recreational- and sport-related exposures have become more prevalent.

Human disease is most prevalent in tropical regions, especially where precipitation is frequent, and large epidemics may occur after heavy rainfalls and floods. Leptospirosis is present in both tropical and temperate regions of the world including the USA. The World Health Organization (WHO) estimates the rate of leptospirosis at 0.1–0.2 cases per 100,000 people in temperate climates and 100/100,000 in tropical climates [3].

Leptospirosis in humans can present with a wide spectrum of severity, from a mild febrile illness to severe, life-threatening illness associated with multi-organ dysfunction.

Uncomplicated anicteric leptospirosis is by far the most common presentation. In the early septicemic phase, patients have acute onset of high fever, chills, headache, nausea, vomiting, and the very intense myalgias of the calf, paraspinal, and abdominal muscles that may often suggest the diagnosis. Conjunctival suffusions (erythema without discharge) are another diagnostic clue often identified on day 3 or 4. When seen, the rash is usually transient and may be urticarial, macular, maculopapular, erythematous, or purpuric. Labs may show leukocytosis or a normal white count with a left shift, thrombocytopenia, mild anemia, mild hyperbilirubinemia, and in some a mildly elevated creatinine.

Fever may recur after a remission of 3–4 days, producing a biphasic illness. In the immune phase, patients may develop recurrent fever and constitutional symptoms, such as aseptic meningitis, eye involvement, and peripheral neuropathy. Some patients may go on to develop chronic or recurrent uveitis.

Icteric leptospirosis (Weil disease) occurs in less than 10% of diagnosed cases. It may appear to be severe from the onset, or it may develop as a biphasic illness that initially appeared to be mild. Weil disease is a syndrome of high fever, jaundice with very high bilirubin but only moderately elevated transaminases (in the 100s), non-oliguric acute renal failure, and rarely thrombocytopenia and disseminated intravascular coagulation leading to cutaneous, gastrointestinal, and pulmonary hemorrhage. When bleeding is prominent, hemorrhagic fever with renal syndrome due to hantaviruses is in the differential diagnosis. Some patients with severe leptospirosis have isolated pulmonary involvement with hemorrhage and acute respiratory distress syndrome (ARDS).

It is estimated that about 50,000 cases of leptospirosis are fatal worldwide each year [4]. Patients with suspected leptospirosis should be monitored closely for renal or liver injury. Earlier treatment with appropriate antibiotics is associated with decreased risk of severe illness and complications. In a 2015 review of mortality trends of leptospirosis, there was a significant correlation between presence of jaundice and mortality [4].

Increased age and renal dysfunction were also associated with increased risk of death.

Diagnosis of leptospirosis is complicated by the lack of a cost-effective and simple diagnostic test. Of existing diagnostic tests, the microcapsule agglutination test (MAT) is considered to be the gold standard. However, the test requires the maintenance of live *Leptospira* cultures and technical expertise, and may take several days to result [5], which is often not practical in areas of the world most affected by leptospirosis. In addition, the MAT does not differentiate between past infection and active infection or between different serovars of *Leptospira*. The lateral flow test and latex agglutination test are older immunoassays routinely used to detect *Leptospira*-specific antibodies, but they are less specific than the MAT [5]. PCR-based tests have also been developed to help distinguish between different serovars of *Leptospira*, but they are similarly infeasible in countries with limited resources.

Prevention of leptospirosis with vaccination is limited by the genetic variations with a large number of species that cause human disease in the world, making it unlikely that a single vaccine will be effective. Vaccination for pets is available in the USA, but it does not prevent the spread of the pathogen to humans. Prophylactic medication for travelers was proven to be effective in a study of US soldiers stationed in Panama. Of the 940 soldiers enrolled in the blinded study, 0.2% of those who took 200 mg of doxycycline weekly developed leptospirosis, compared with 4.2% in the placebo group [6]. Similar studies have been attempted in endemic regions without a statistically significant difference between placebo and prophylaxis groups. The WHO officially recommends that travelers who are going to a region affected by natural disasters and likely contaminated fresh water receive doxycycline prophylaxis [1].

Treatment of leptospirosis is primarily doxycycline 200 mg daily for 7 days [7]. Studies of *Leptospira* isolates from several of the most commonly affected regions in the world identified no instances of doxycycline or tetracycline resistance, although higher MICs were noted with *Leptospira* strains from Egypt. *Leptospira* is susceptible in vitro to most penicillins, macrolides, cephalosporins, and fluoroquinolones. Severe leptospirosis often is treated with intravenous penicillin or a third-generation cephalosporin, but treatment may be complicated by the Jarisch-Herxheimer reaction, similar to that associated with other spirochete infections including syphilis and relapsing fever [7]. Studies of serologic biomarkers in leptospirosis patients have shown that cytokines such as TNFα, IL-6, IL-8, and PTX3 may be positively correlated with mortality from the infection [8], but the use of these prognostic tests is not yet validated.

Key Points/Pearls

- Consider leptospirosis as a potential diagnosis in a returning traveler with fever, myalgia (calf, spinal, and abdominal muscles), arthralgia, conjunctival suffusions, and sometimes a rash, diarrhea, and/or jaundice, the CBC may show leukocytosis or a left shift, thrombocytopenia; hyperbilirubinemia without significant transaminitis is present in most patients.

- Leptospirosis is a zoonotic pathogen that poses a significant health risk to native populations of and travelers to endemic regions and is contracted by exposure of mucous membranes or skin breaks indirectly to freshwater contaminated by animal urine or directly to infected animals (especially rodents, dogs, and cattle).

- Severe jaundice and acute renal injury are poor prognostic indicators of outcome in severe leptospirosis (Weil disease), and bleeding may be prominent (skin, GI, and lungs).

- Pulmonary hemorrhage and ARDS are seen in severe cases, sometimes without icterus.

- MAT is the reference standard test for diagnosis of leptospirosis; testing capabilities for leptospirosis are limited in endemic regions.

- Leptospirosis can be prevented in travelers by avoiding exposure to contaminated freshwater and taking doxycycline weekly when this is unavoidable (such as after flooding).

- Empiric treatment of mild leptospirosis is a course of oral doxycycline.
- Severe leptospirosis should be treated in hospital with intravenous penicillin or a cephalosporin.

References

1. Terpstra WJ. Human leptospirosis: guidance for diagnosis, surveillance, and control. World Health Organization. 2003. http://www.who.int/csr/don/en/WHO_CDS_CSR_EPH_2002.23.pdf. Accessed 22 June 2017.
2. Monahan AM, Miller IS, Nally JE. Leptospirosis: risks during recreational activities. J Appl Microbiol. 2009;107:707–16.
3. WHO | Leptospirosis Burden Epidemiology Reference Group (LERG). WHO. World Health Organization. 2016. http://www.who.int/zoonoses/diseases/lerg/en/. Accessed 22 June 2017.
4. Taylor AJ, Paris DH, Newton PN. Systematic review of the mortality from untreated leptospirosis. PLoS Negl Trop Dis. 2015;9(6):e0003866.
5. Suputtamongkol Y, Pongtavornpinyo W, Lubell Y, et al. Strategies for diagnosis and treatment of suspected leptospirosis: a cost-benefit analysis. PLoS Negl Trop Dis. 2010;4(2):e610.
6. Takafuji ET, Kirkpatrick JW, Miller RN, et al. An efficacy trial of doxycycline chemoprophylaxis against leptospirosis. N Engl J Med. 1984;310(8):497–500.
7. Londeree WA. Leptospirosis: the microscopic danger in paradise. Hawaii J Med Public Health. 2014;73(11 Suppl 2):21–3.
8. Chirathaworn C, Kongpan S. Immune responses to Leptospira infection: roles as biomarkers for disease severity. Braz J Infect Dis. 2014;18(1):77–81.

Man with AIDS Presents with a Headache

David Kopelman and Emily Landon

A 48-year-old man presented to the emergency department (ED) with a headache. His symptoms had begun 2 weeks prior and without any clear trauma or trigger. He did not have a history of chronic headaches or migraines. The headache was described as diffuse, aching in quality, and constant throughout the day. One week before he noted associated dizziness and myalgias. Two days prior to presentation, his dizziness progressed and resulted in nausea with vomiting. Review of systems was notable for subjective fevers with chills, neck stiffness, and decreased oral intake due to poor appetite.

The patient's medical history was notable for human immunodeficiency virus (HIV) infection diagnosed 10 years prior. He had previously been on antiretroviral therapy but self-discontinued his medications 3 years before due to side effects. His most recent CD4+ T cell count was 67 cells/μL 1 month prior to presentation; he took no prophylaxis and had no history of opportunistic infections. Other chronic medical conditions included hypertension and glaucoma. He took no medications and had an allergy to penicillin, which induced hives. Social history was notable for active tobacco abuse (total 20 pack-years exposure), moderate alcohol use (multiple beers

daily), and recreational marijuana use. He was sexually active with one male partner, with whom he lived. He worked in the food service industry and had no recent travel or known sick contacts.

On physical examination, the patient's temperature was 38.8 °C, heart rate was 109 beats per minute, blood pressure was 182/107 mmHg, respiratory rate was 18 breaths per minute, oxygen saturation was 98% breathing room air, and body mass index was 19 kg/m^2. In general the patient appeared cachectic and mildly toxic; he requested that the lights be turned off during the examination because they made his headache worse. His mucous membranes were dry, but there was no oropharyngeal exudate. Supraclavicular, cervical, submandibular, and posterior auricular lymphadenopathy were not appreciated. Cardiac exam demonstrated regular tachycardia without any murmurs. Lungs were clear to auscultation bilaterally. The abdomen was scaphoid without any surgical scars; bowel sounds were present, and there was no tenderness to palpation. Skin examination did not reveal any rashes, lesions, or signs of trauma. The patient was oriented to person, place, and time, although his memory was impaired as he occasionally corrected and contradicted himself when describing the symptoms and time course of his illness. Cranial nerves II–XII were intact, but neck stiffness was noted. Reflexes were normal.

Laboratory testing revealed a white blood cell count of 5800/μL (normal range 3500–11,000/μL),

D. Kopelman, M.D. • E. Landon, M.D. (✉)
Department of Medicine,
University of Chicago, Chicago, IL, USA
e-mail: Emily.Landon@uchospitals.edu

© Springer International Publishing AG 2018
M. David, J.-L. Benoit (eds.), *The Infectious Disease Diagnosis*,
https://doi.org/10.1007/978-3-319-64906-1_18

Table 18.1 Laboratory testing results

Laboratory test	Result
Blood cultures	Negative
Urine culture	Negative
Urine *Histoplasma* antigen	Negative
CSF VDRL	Negative
CSF cryptococcal antigen	Negative
CSF bacterial culture	Negative
CSF acid-fast, fungal, and viral cultures	Pending

CSF cerebrospinal fluid, *VDRL* venereal disease research laboratory test

Table 18.2 Differential diagnosis of headache with fever in a patient with AIDS

Bacterial meningitis
Tuberculous meningitis
Cryptococcal meningitis
Viral meningitis:
• Enterovirus
• Cytomegalovirus (CMV)
• Adenovirus
• Influenza
• Colorado tick fever virus
• Lymphocytic choriomeningitis virus (LCMV)
Aseptic meningitis
Herpes simplex virus (HSV) encephalitis
Varicella zoster virus (VZV) encephalitis
Arbovirus infection:
• West Nile virus (WNV) encephalitis
• La Crosse encephalitis virus
• St. Louis encephalitis (SLE) virus
• Eastern equine encephalitis (EEE) virus
• Western equine encephalitis (WEE) virus
• Tick-borne encephalitis viruses (Russian spring-summer, Siberian and Central European subtypes)
Toxoplasmosis
Tuberculoma
Measles
Rubella (also known as German measles)
Influenza
Brain abscess
Acute human immunodeficiency virus (HIV) infection
Secondary syphilis (*Treponema pallidum*)
Typhoid fever (due to *Salmonella typhi*)
Intracranial neoplasm (e.g., PCL)
Subdural empyema
Acute rhinosinusitis

AIDS acquired immune deficiency syndrome, *PCL* primary central nervous system lymphoma

hemoglobin 16.9 g/dL (11.5–15.5 g/dL), and platelet count 119,000/μL (150,000–450,000/μL). Complete metabolic panel was within normal limits. Chest X-ray was unremarkable. A lumbar puncture (LP) was performed in the ED; cerebrospinal fluid (CSF) studies revealed normal opening pressure, white blood cell count of 232 cells/μL (predominantly lymphocytes, normal range 0–5 cells/μL), glucose 74 mg/dL (50–70 mg/dL), and protein 825 mg/dL (15–45 mg/dL). Further work-up was performed, as shown in Table 18.1. The differential diagnosis is presented in Table 18.2.

The patient was admitted from the ED to the hospital and started on intravenous vancomycin, ceftriaxone, and acyclovir. He experienced clinical improvement during his first week of hospitalization with decreased severity of his headache and resolution of the fever. Magnetic resonance imaging (MRI) of the brain was notable for diffuse white matter enhancement, but it did not show any masses. On hospital day 10, however, the patient experienced new, acute onset bilateral lower extremity weakness, urinary retention, and loss of sensation at the sacrum and in the distal extremities. MRI of the spine showed diffuse enhancement of the meninges but no spinal cord abnormalities, mass, or bony lesions.

The patient was started on high-dose steroids for his radiculopathy. Over the next few days, his weakness and altered sensation improved to near baseline. Review of the patient's CSF viral culture demonstrated cytopathic effect consistent with varicella zoster virus (VZV). He never developed a rash typical of varicella or zoster, nor did his sexual partner. The patient's antimi-crobials were switched to oral acyclovir, and he was discharged home.

18.1 Encephalitis in an Immunocompromised Host

The patient presented with headache associated with nausea and vomiting and was found to be febrile with neck stiffness and photophobia concerning for central nervous system (CNS) infection, particularly either meningitis (infection of the subarachnoid space and cerebral ventricles) or encephalitis (infection of the brain parenchyma). His history of HIV infection, progression to acquired immune deficiency syndrome (AIDS, in his case defined as having CD4+ T cell count <200 cells/μL), and lack of opportunistic infection prophylaxis broaden the differential diagnosis for the etiology of his symptoms. Fever and headache are the most common symptoms of both meningitis and encephalitis, and therefore, initial steps to narrow this differential begin with the physical examination. His neurological exam was non-focal with normal reflexes, but his memory was impaired. There was no suggestion of seizure activity or a post-ictal period. Meningismus and photophobia are more common in meningitis, but abnormal cognition (such as impaired memory) is more characteristic of encephalitis. Additionally, focal neurologic deficits are more common in encephalitis. Seizure activity can be seen in both [1].

CSF analysis is essential to the diagnosis of CNS infection and involves measurement of opening pressure, cell count, protein, glucose, and pathogen-specific antibody and polymerase chain reaction (PCR) assays based on clinical suspicion. The method of diagnosis of VZV encephalitis in this patient by positive CSF viral culture was unusual; he presented prior to the widespread adoption of CSF VZV PCR assays. In one review of 22,394 viral cultures of CSF samples from 33 states over the course of 11 years, virus was isolated in only 1270 (5.7%) cases, of which only a single case was VZV [2]. PCR is now widely available for many herpesviruses (herpes simplex virus [HSV]-1 and -2, cytomegalovirus, Epstein-Barr virus [EBV], and human herpes virus [HHV]-6). Because PCR enables viruses to be detected more quickly and with greater sensitivity than CSF culture, the latter is no longer routinely recommended by the Infectious Diseases Society of America (IDSA) unless there is clinical concern for non-viral causes of encephalitis [3]. The most common false-positive herpesvirus detected by PCR is HHV-6; the most common associated with a dual-positive result is EBV [4]. Additionally, detection of VZV-specific IgM antibodies in the CSF is diagnostic of acute infection because IgM antibodies do not generally cross the blood-brain barrier [3]. Routine measurement or serial monitoring of serum antibodies during acute illness or convalescence to demonstrate seroconversion has no value in determining whether to institute specific therapy for viral infections of the brain—though it may help clarify the precise infectious etiology in retrospect [1].

Neuroimaging rarely identifies a specific infectious etiology of a patient's symptoms, though there are suggestive findings (e.g., bilateral temporal lobe edema in the case of HSV). In cases of suspected meningitis or encephalitis, MRI is preferred over computerized tomography (CT) because it has greater sensitivity. Clarifying whether an intracranial mass lesion (tumor or abscess) is present in a patient with HIV/AIDS is also important. Similarly, an electroencephalogram (EEG) may help suggest particular pathogens based on the area of the brain involved. Brain biopsy is rarely used today given advancements in imaging and in molecular and serologic testing [3].

Regarding the timing of neuroimaging prior to performing LP, in multiple studies, researchers have attempted to identify risk factors and signs associated with abnormal imaging findings and risk of brainstem herniation. In one retrospective study of 301 patients diagnosed with bacterial meningitis, immunocompromise was predictive of abnormal CT imaging of the head in greater than one third of patients (24 out of 70, 34%) [5]. Given the overlap in clinical syndromes of encephalitis and meningitis described above, it is recommended to follow meningitis guidelines and obtain neuroimaging prior to performing LP [6].

18.2 Varicella Zoster Virus (VZV) Encephalitis

Encephalitis complicates 1–2 out of every 10,000 varicella cases. Neurologic symptoms tend to occur approximately 1 week after the onset of generalized vesicular varicella rash (chickenpox) and include headache, fever, vomiting, and altered mental status. CSF findings usually include elevated opening pressure, lymphocytic pleocytosis, mildly elevated protein, and normal glucose. Imaging is usually unrevealing, although it can show areas of edema or low attenuation consistent with demyelination [7].

This patient's lack of any vesicular rash was unusual. Cutaneous manifestations of VZV in the form of varicella in children with HIV infection and zoster in adults with AIDS are usually similar to those in immunocompetent hosts. However, unusual presentations of zoster in immunocompromised hosts have been described, including atypical generalized zoster (diffuse varicella-like skin lesions outside an isolated dermatome), zoster sine herpete (zoster-like neuropathic pain in the absence of any rash), multiple hyperkeratotic papules without dermatomal distribution, and ecthymatous VZV lesions that present with large punched-out ulcerations with a central black eschar and a peripheral rim of vesicles [7].

Precise diagnosis of VZV encephalitis was previously hindered by difficulty culturing the virus from CSF. This patient's CSF underwent viral culture. The light microscopy image of this patient's viral culture shown in Fig. 18.1 demonstrates classic findings of the VZV cytopathic effect resulting from mammalian cell viral infection. These findings, coupled together with his clinical syndrome, confirmed the diagnosis.

Neurologic complications associated with VZV can be seen in both varicella and zoster,

which are distinct clinical syndromes. While VZV encephalitis is considered the most serious CNS complication of varicella, cerebellar ataxia is slightly more common, with an incidence of approximately 1 in 4000 cases, and is usually seen in children. Ataxia can develop days before and up to weeks after onset of varicella rash, is usually self-limiting, and resolves without major deficits. Other syndromes that have been described include transverse myelitis, aseptic meningitis, and Guillain-Barré syndrome. Zoster can be complicated by myelitis, featuring paraparesis with a sensory-level and sphincter impairment (as in this patient). Vasculopathies have been described as well. Large-vessel or granulomatous arteritis is seen primarily in immunocompetent patients, whereas small-vessel or multifocal arteritis is more common in the immunocompromised [8]. These complications are altogether rare and expected to become even less common with the widespread use of the varicella vaccine in childhood [7].

The IDSA recommends that in patients for whom the clinician suspects viral encephalitis, acyclovir should be given empirically (in addition to any antibiotics warranted for bacterial meningitis). Once the diagnosis of VZV encephalitis is made, acyclovir is the preferred treatment, although ganciclovir can be considered as an alternative. Corticosteroids are used in cases of VZV encephalitis and vasculopathy, but there are no data to support this practice [3]. In one study of 514 consecutive patients with HIV presenting with neurological symptoms, VZV DNA was detected by PCR in CSF samples from 13 (2.5%). Four of these thirteen patients had clinical syndromes of VZV encephalitis or meningoencephalomyelitis, and their clinical outcomes correlated with clearance of VZV from the CSF following intravenous acyclovir therapy. The two patients whose CSF VZV became undetectable survived, whereas the two patients whose CSF did not clear ultimately expired [9].

Fig. 18.1 Cerebrospinal viral fluid culture in rhesus monkey kidney cells

Key Points/Pearls

- There is significant overlap in the clinical presentations of meningitis and encephalitis; however, seizures, altered mental status, cortical function deficit, and focal neurological findings are more common in encephalitis than in meningitis.

- The practice of CSF viral culture has been largely supplanted by virus-specific PCR testing.
- Imaging and EEG rarely point to a specific viral cause of encephalitis.
- In immunocompromised hosts, neuroimaging is recommended before performing a LP to detect mass lesions (tumor or abscess) that may increase the risk of herniation.
- In patients with AIDS, the syndrome of fever, headache, memory deficit, and photophobia is highly suggestive of opportunistic infection or primary CNS lymphoma associated with EBV reactivation; such patients should undergo brain imaging with both infused CT and MRI to detect mass lesions (most often toxoplasmosis or primary CNS lymphoma) and demyelination (progressive multifocal leukoencephalopathy due to John Cunningham virus [JCV]); LP should be performed to obtain opening pressure, cell count, glucose, protein, *Cryptococcus* antigen, VDRL, West Nile virus serology, and PCR for *M. tuberculosis*, enterovirus, HSV, VZV, EBV, and JCV; the most common etiologies of meningitis in this population are cryptococcosis, neurosyphilis, and tuberculosis.
- VZV encephalitis is one of many neurologic complications (both central and peripheral) of either primary varicella infection or zoster reactivation.
- Atypical presentations of rash in VZV are possible, especially in the immunocompromised host.
- For VZV encephalitis, acyclovir is the preferred treatment although ganciclovir can be considered as an alternative.

References

1. Whitley RJ. Viral encephalitis. N Engl J Med. 1990;323(4):242–50.
2. Polage CR, Petti CA. Assessment of the utility of viral culture of cerebrospinal fluid. Clin Infect Dis. 2006;43(12):1578–9.
3. Tunkel AR, Glaser CA, Bloch KC, Sejvar JJ, Marra CM, Roos KL, et al. The management of encephalitis: clinical practice guidelines by the Infectious Diseases Society of America. Clin Infect Dis. 2008;47(3):303–27.
4. DeBiasi RL, Kleinschmidt-Demasters BK, Weignberg A, Tyler KL. Use of PCR for the diagnosis of herpesvirus infections of the central nervous system. J Clin Virol. 2002;25(Suppl 1):S5–11.
5. Hasburn R, Abrahams J, Jekel J, Quagliarello VJ. Computed tomography of the head before lumbar puncture in adults with suspected meningitis. N Engl J Med. 2001;345(24):1727–33.
6. Tunkel AR, Hartman BJ, Kaplan SL, Kaufman BA, Roos KL, Scheld WM, et al. Practice guidelines for the management of bacterial meningitis. Clin Infect Dis. 2004;39(9):1267–84.
7. Gnann JW Jr. Varicella-zoster virus: atypical presentations and unusual complications. J Infect Dis. 2002;186(Suppl 1):S91–8.
8. Gilden DH, Kleinschmidt-DeMasters BK, Laguardia JJ, Mahalingam R, Cohrs RJ. Neurologic complications of the reactivation of varicella-zoster virus. N Engl J Med. 2000;342(9):635–45.
9. Cinque P, Bossolasco S, Vago L, Fornara C, Lipari S, Lazzarin A, et al. Varicella-zoster virus (VZV) DNA in cerebrospinal fluid of patients infected with human immunodeficiency virus: VZV disease of the central nervous system or subclinical reactivation of VZV infection? Clin Infect Dis. 1997;25(3):634–9.

Shirley Stephenson

A 50-year-old female presented to the Urgent Care Clinic with myalgias, lymphadenopathy, and rash 3 days after returning from a medical volunteer trip to the KwaZulu-Natal province of South Africa, where she worked as a healthcare provider and participated in home visits to patients with human immunodeficiency virus (HIV) infection and tuberculosis. One month prior to departure, she visited a travel clinic and received hepatitis A, hepatitis B, and typhoid fever vaccines. Although the volunteer group would not be headquartered in a region with malaria transmission, she was uncertain how far they might travel outside the town and thus received a prescription for atovaquone/proguanil (Malarone) for prophylaxis. She was counseled on insect precautions. In case of traveler's diarrhea, she had a 3-day supply of ciprofloxacin, which she did not self-administer during her trip. Prior to her travels she was up to date on measles, mumps, and rubella (MMR); tetanus, diphtheria, and acellular pertussis (Tdap); and influenza vaccines. She had a history of chickenpox. For her employment as a health care worker, she underwent annual tuberculosis testing, which had recently resulted negative. Her past medical history included anemia.

She felt well throughout the 2-week trip and enjoyed the home visits, where she had prolonged, close contact with the local population. She did not travel independently or leave the Southeastern region of the country. She sustained no accidental needle sticks or body fluid exposures in the clinic. The volunteers ate mostly the same foods and drank only bottled water. She did not have any new sexual partners, had no known exposure to bats, and was not bitten by any animals. The volunteers dedicated their last days in South Africa to leisure, venturing out for a boat trip, horseback riding, hiking, and a 1-day safari. The patient took her malaria prophylaxis throughout the trip, used insect repellant containing N,N-diethyl-meta-toluamide (DEET), and did not notice any mosquitos or bug bites during the trip.

During the patient's return flight, however, her right leg and left shoulder began itching. She developed a headache and mild neck stiffness. Upon arriving home, she found three raised, red lesions behind her right knee and two on her left shoulder. Over the next 2 days, scattered vesiculopapular lesions appeared on her trunk and limbs, some pruritic. Her right thigh became warm and tender. Myalgias, cervical and axillary tenderness, and a moderate headache persisted. Her measured temperature was 99–100 °F. She felt fatigued but attributed it to jet lag. She experienced no photophobia, nasal congestion, sore throat, shortness of breath, cough, chest pain, nausea, vomiting, diarrhea, bruising,

S. Stephenson, R.N., F.N.P.-B.C.
Department of Medicine, University of Chicago
Medicine, Chicago, IL, USA
e-mail: sstephenson@medicine.bsd.uchicago.edu

© Springer International Publishing AG 2018
M. David, J.-L. Benoit (eds.), *The Infectious Disease Diagnosis*,
https://doi.org/10.1007/978-3-319-64906-1_19

or confusion. As far as she knew, her fellow travelers had no similar symptoms.

On day 3 after symptom onset, she presented to the Urgent Care Clinic, and the provider consulted the infectious diseases service. The differential diagnosis for rash and flulike symptoms in a traveler returning from South Africa is summarized in Table 19.1. The patient's travel and contact with ill patients raised the possibility of numerous diagnoses. However, a careful history seemed to eliminate several. The medical volunteers on this trip never entered a malaria zone, and there is a relatively low risk of contracting Chikungunya virus in the area. Another more dangerous, tick-borne illness to consider was Crimean-Congo hemorrhagic fever (CCHF), but this viral disease tends to cause more severe symptoms such as high fever, intense headache, and vomiting before progressing to bruising, epistaxis, and petechiae. By contrast, Rift Valley fever (RVF), which is transmitted by insects and RVF-infected animal products, presents with milder symptoms, and if it evolves to a hemorrhagic fever, it does so within days. Treatment for both CCHF and RVF is supportive.

Table 19.1 Differential diagnosis of a fever, myalgias, vesiculopapular rash, and headache in a returning traveler from Southern Africa

African tick bite fever (*Rickettsia africae*)
Chikungunya virus
Crimean-Congo hemorrhagic fever
Disseminated gonococcal disease
Drug reaction
Enterovirus
Fungal infections
Leptospirosis
Malaria
Malignancy
Measles
Mediterranean spotted fever (*Rickettsia conorii*)
Meningococcal rash
Rift Valley fever
Rubella
Schistosomiasis (Katayama fever)
Syphilis
Typhoid fever

The patient's social history excluded sexually transmitted causes of rash such as syphilis and disseminated gonococcal infection. A recorded history of reactive titers for measles and rubella, a history of varicella infection, and typhoid fever vaccination further narrowed the list. Acute schistosomiasis infection (Katayama fever) can cause a pruritic rash, but the parasites are found only in freshwater, and the patient did not report swimming in any lakes or streams. Also of note, the fever and myalgias associated with schistosomiasis typically manifest 3–8 weeks after infection. Finally, the group traveled in late August, which is subtropical spring and a time of fewer mosquitos [1]. The patient did not visit any regions with malaria transmission, and she took prophylaxis, which decreased the likelihood that she contracted malaria.

The finding of multiple skin lesions and lymphadenopathy and a history of visits to rural homesteads and proximity to large game and cattle suggested a diagnosis of the highly prevalent African tick bite fever (ATBF). The patient was treated with 100 mg doxycycline twice daily for 10 days. She was instructed to seek emergency attention if her symptoms changed or worsened. She attended a follow-up appointment in the Infectious Diseases Clinic 2 days later, on day 5 after symptom onset. She complained of continued right leg warmth and tenderness. However, she had no new lesions, and her headache, neck stiffness, and myalgias had diminished. She denied other complaints and was hoping to return to work the next day.

On physical examination, her temperature was 97.3 °F, blood pressure 127/72 mmHg, and heart rate 81 beats per minute. She appeared fatigued and pale but exhibited no acute distress. Her legs were peppered with 2–3 mm vesiculopapular lesions. A 5 mm papule on her forehead remained, as did multiple similarly sized papules behind her left knee, left shoulder, and across her right upper abdomen. All of the lesions had an erythematous base, and some were scabbed. There was no apparent eschar, drainage, or petechiae. Her right thigh was mildly erythematous and warm. Her oropharynx was clear and conjunctivae normal. Her neck was supple, with mild lymphadenopathy.

She had normal abdominal, cardiovascular, and pulmonary examinations.

The complete blood count was notable for a hemoglobin of 7.0 g/dL (normal range, 13.5–17.5 g/dL), which was consistent with labs collected 2 months prior to travel. Total bilirubin was elevated at 1.5 mg/dL (0.1–1.0 mg/dL), and the rest of the complete metabolic panel was normal. Serum spotted fever group (SFG) antibodies, IgG and IgM, were both <1:64, which suggested the absence of acute rickettsial infection. However, antibodies for spotted fever, which show cross reactivity to any infection in the group, are typically not detectable until 7–10 days after symptom onset. Furthermore, SFG rickettsiae exhibit high sensitivity to doxycycline, and early treatment likely reduces antibody response, thus impairing detection [2].

19.1 African Tick Bite Fever (ATBF)

ATBF is caused by *Rickettsia africae*, a small, Gram-negative bacillus. It is a leading cause of illness among travelers to South Africa, with an estimated incidence of 4–5% among visitors from Europe, exceeding the incidence of malaria and typhoid fever [3, 4]. Awareness of ATBF outside endemic areas is relatively limited, but it has become better known with increasing travel to Southern Africa and safari tourism [4]. A comprehensive, 12-year GeoSentinel analysis found that among travelers seeking medical care after visiting Africa, as many as 13% were ultimately diagnosed with SFG rickettsioses [5]. Although other SFG rickettsiae have been identified in sub-Saharan Africa, studies using polymerase chain reaction (PCR) and Western blot to identify the rickettsial pathogens from ill travelers to the region found that more than 90% were caused by *Rickettsia africae* [6].

The vectors for ATBF in Africa are two species of hard ticks, *Amblyomma variegatum* (the tropical bont tick) and *Amblyomma hebraeum* (the South African bont tick). The latter is widespread in South Africa. *A. variegatum* is present in the Caribbean where ATBF is endemic

as well. By sensing odors and heat, ticks find their source for a blood meal. In Kenya, 92% of sampled *Amblyomma* ticks collected from cattle, goats, and sheep carried *Rickettsia africae* [7]. *Amblyomma* ticks readily feed on humans, inserting their hypostome through a small incision made in the host's skin, and are able to introduce *R. africae* [4]. *Amblyomma* ticks often select multiple feeding sites on the same host, resulting in one or more eschars at the sites of inoculation [2]. Ticks in the larval and nymph stages often go unnoticed by their host, and once attached may remain so for days until full, at which point they detach. Symptoms of ATBF typically appear 5–7 days after inoculation and are classically mild with sudden onset of fever, myalgia, one or more eschars, and a vesiculopapular rash. ATBF is in general much less severe than Rocky Mountain spotted fever (which is only endemic in the Americas) or Mediterranean spotted fever (endemic in Europe, Africa, and Asia) but is more common [1]. Although the majority of humans infected with *Rickettsia africae* develop fever, an eschar is not always present or may be obstructed by hair or skin folds [3]. Lymphadenopathy, aphthous stomatitis, and a maculopapular or vesicular rash may also be seen with ATBF [6], but the full spectrum of symptoms is not present in the majority of cases [4]. Although ATBF is usually self-limited, some patients do have a severe illness, and treatment should not be delayed.

SFG rickettsial infections are challenging to confirm with laboratory testing, and treatment should not be delayed [1, 5]. The first-line treatment for ATBF is doxycycline, 100 mg every 12 h for 7–14 days. Alternative antibiotics are not as effective (chloramphenicol, quinolones). If initial serology testing is negative, it should be repeated 1 month after symptom onset to assess for seroconversion of IgG and IgM. Testing can also be performed using a PCR assay, immunohistochemistry, and cultures from a swab or biopsy from eschar or rash. In the USA, these specimens must be submitted to state health departments, which forward them to the US Centers for Disease Control and Prevention (CDC). These diagnostic techniques are most sensitive during the first week of illness and within 24 h of initiation of treatment with antibiotics. Diagnosed cases can be reported using online forms to the CDC's Rickettsial Zoonoses Branch.

In the present case, the traveler completed her course of doxycycline and recovered within 1 week of treatment. Repeat testing was not performed, as she had received a blood transfusion and was undergoing a workup for anemia, which turned out to be due to an unrelated etiology. Had baseline labs not established that her anemia preceded travel, the clinical picture likely would have been more puzzling. Given the increasing number of global travelers, healthcare providers must recognize the risks specific to patient demographics and destinations. Risk factors for ATBF among visitors to Southern Africa include safaris, game hunting, and rural visits (e.g., cattle farms). Travelers should be counseled to wear long pants and sleeves, use insect repellant that contains extended-release DEET or permethrin-treated clothing, shower after outdoor activities, check themselves for ticks, remove ticks properly, and seek medical attention immediately if fever, rash or other signs of systemic illness develop. There is insufficient evidence to recommend doxycycline for chemoprophylaxis [1].

Key Points/Pearls

- ATBF, transmitted by *Amblyomma variegatum* (the tropical bont tick) and *A. hebraeum* (the South African bont tick), is relatively common in travelers to sub-Saharan Africa, particularly those visiting rural areas, game parks, and cattle farms.
- Travelers should be counseled on tick exposure prevention.
- Acute onset of fever, myalgia, headache, often with one or more eschars, a vesiculopapular rash, and lymphadenopathy are hallmarks of ATBF; one or more eschars may be present but

not be apparent on a casual examination; some patients do not have all the findings above.
- Early serologic testing may be negative in rickettsioses and should be repeated approximately 1 month after symptom onset if confirmation is necessary.
- If less than 1 month after onset of symptoms, the diagnosis relies on the clinical presentation and history of exposure to ticks, and sometimes advanced techniques, including PCR or immunohistochemistry of a skin biopsy.
- If ATBF is suspected, treatment should not be delayed, regardless of laboratory results; doxycycline is the treatment of choice.

References

1. McQuiston J. Rickettsial (spotted & typhus fevers) & related infections (anaplasmosis & ehrlichiosis). Centers for Disease Control and Prevention. CDC Health Information for International Travel 2016. New York: Oxford University Press; 2016.
2. Fournier PE, Jensenius M, Laferl H, Vene S, Raoult D. Kinetics of antibody responses in Rickettsia africae and Rickettsia conorii infections. Clin Diagn Lab Immunol. 2002;9(2):324–8.
3. Frean J, Blumberg L, Ogunbanjo GA. Tick bite fever in South Africa. S Afr Fam Pract. 2008;50(2):33–5.
4. Jensenius M, Fournier PE, Vene S, Hoel T, Hasle G, Henriksen AZ. African tick bite fever in travelers to rural sub-equatorial Africa. Clin Infect Dis. 2003;36(11):1411–7.
5. Jensenius M, Davis X, von Sonnenburg F, Schwartz E, Keystone J, Leder K, et al. Multicenter geosentinel analysis of rickettsial diseases in international travelers, 1996–2008. Emerg Infect Dis. 2009;15(11):1791–8.
6. Raoult D, Fournier PE, Fenollar F, Jensenius M, Prioe T, Pina JJ, et al. *Rickettsia africae*, a tick-borne pathogen in travelers to Sub-Saharan Africa. N Engl J Med. 2001;344:1504–151.
7. Maina AN, Jiang J, Omulo SA, et al. High prevalence of *Rickettsia africae* variants in *Amblyomma variegatum* ticks from domestic mammals in rural Western Kenya: implications for human health. Vector Borne Zoonotic Dis. 2014;14(10):693–702.

A Toddler with Pica

M. Ellen Acree

A 2-year-old female presented to the emergency department with daily fevers for approximately 1 month. Her temperatures ranged from 102 to 104 °F orally. She had been given ibuprofen two to three times daily with rapid return of fevers after the ibuprofen wore off. When febrile, the child wanted to remain in bed and refused to eat, but shortly after taking ibuprofen she would begin to behave almost normally. Her parents had taken her to a local emergency room approximately 1 week prior to the current presentation. The parents were told that she likely had a viral illness and advised to continue supportive measures. The child had no upper respiratory symptoms, cough, vomiting, diarrhea, joint swelling, mouth sores, or rash.

The child was born in Chicago and had never left the city. She lived at home with her parents, her maternal grandmother, and nine siblings. Her parents were born in Mexico. She did not attend daycare and was cared for by her maternal grandmother during the day. She was up to date on immunizations. She had no significant past medical or surgical history, had no allergies, and was on no medications. Her family history was notable for diabetes mellitus and hypertension in her maternal grandmother.

On physical examination, the patient was very tired-appearing and barely cried with peripheral IV placement. Her weight was at the 68th percentile, and she was afebrile but had been given ibuprofen shortly before arrival. She had hepatosplenomegaly, but otherwise her examination was unremarkable. Laboratory studies revealed a white blood cell count of 9600/μL (normal range 4000–13,800/μL) with 17% eosinophils (0–5%). The hemoglobin was 7.7 g/dL (11.3–13.2 g/dL) with a mean corpuscular volume of 56.3 fL (74–86 fL) and a reticulocyte percentage of 1.5 (0.5–1.0%). Iron studies were consistent with iron deficiency. Iron was low at 22 mcg/dL (40–160 mcg/dL), and percent saturation was low at 4.7% (14–50%). Ferritin was normal at 129 ng/mL (10–220 ng/mL), although this is notably an acute phase reactant. The renal and hepatic functions were normal. Inflammatory markers were elevated; the erythrocyte sedimentation rate was 78 mm/h (0–20 mm/h), and the C-reactive protein was 75 mg/L (<5 mg/L). IgE was elevated at 1131 IU/mL (<100 IU/mL). Human immunodeficiency virus (HIV) screening was negative. A chest X-ray was unrevealing, and an abdominal ultrasound confirmed hepatosplenomegaly.

The Pediatric Infectious Diseases consultation team obtained additional history from the patient's family. Over the previous few months, the child had been found eating dirt, sand from the sandbox, and cat litter. The Pediatric Infectious Diseases team recommended additional studies,

M.E. Acree, M.D.
Section of Infectious Diseases and Global Health, Department of Medicine, University of Chicago Medicine, Chicago, IL, USA
e-mail: Mary.Acree@uchospitals.edu

© Springer International Publishing AG 2018
M. David, J.-L. Benoit (eds.), *The Infectious Disease Diagnosis*,
https://doi.org/10.1007/978-3-319-64906-1_20

including serologies for Epstein-Barr virus (EBV), cytomegalovirus (CMV), *Toxoplasma*, *Bartonella*, *Toxocara*, and parvovirus. A PPD was placed. Three stool ova and parasite examinations were performed. The differential diagnosis for eosinophilia is presented in Table 20.1.

Table 20.1 Differential diagnosis for eosinophilia

Allergic reaction to medications including drug related eosinophilia systemic syndrome (DRESS)

- Iodides
- Aspirin
- Sulfonamides
- Dapsone
- Tetracyclines
- Nitrofurantoin
- β-lactam antibiotics
- Anticonvulsant drugs
- Allopurinol
- Colchicine

Atopy and allergy

- Hay fever
- Asthma
- Eczema

Serum sickness

Vasculitis

- Eosinophilic granulomatosis with polyangiitis (Churg-Strauss)
- Necrotizing granulomatosis with polyangiitis
- Polyarteritis nodosa

Immunobullous disorders

- Pemphigus
- Dermatitis herpetiformis
- Pemphigoid

Loeffler's endocarditis

Collagen vascular disease

- Rheumatoid arthritis
- Eosinophilic fasciitis
- Sarcoidosis

Malignancies

- Lymphoma (Hodgkin's disease and non-Hodgkin's T-cell lymphoma)
- Mycosis fungoides
- Chronic myeloid leukemia
- Adenocarcinoma (stomach, pancreas, ovary, uterus)
- Eosinophilic leukemia

Table 20.1 (continued)

Primary immune deficiency syndromes

- Hyper-immunoglobulin E Syndrome (Job's syndrome)
- DOCK8 deficiency
- Chronic granulomatous disease

Helminthic infections

- Acute infection with nematodes (Loeffler syndrome by *Ascaris*, hookworms, *Trichuris*, and *Strongyloides*), *Toxocara* (visceral larva migrans), flukes (blood flukes *Schistosoma*, lung fluke *Paragonimus*, and liver flukes *Fasciola*, *Clonorchis*, and *Opisthorchis*)
- Chronic infection with *Strongyloides*, filariasis (lymphatic filariasis including tropical pulmonary eosinophilia, onchocerciasis, loiasis), and gnathostomiasis

Echinococcosis when a cyst ruptures

Cutaneous larva migrans (dog hookworms)

Eosinophilic meningitis (*Angiostrongylus cantonensis*, *Baylisascaris procyonis*, and gnathostomiasis)

Other infections

- Coccidioidomycosis
- Allergic bronchopulmonary aspergillosis (ABPA)
- Human immunodeficiency virus (HIV)
- Human T-cell lymphotropic virus-1 (HTLV-1)

Therapeutic administration of cytokines IL-2 or granulocyte macrophage colony-stimulating factor (GM-CSF)

Idiopathic hypereosinophilic syndromes (HES)

Other than antipyretics, the patient was not on any medications, making drug allergy an unlikely cause of eosinophilia. She had no arthritis, arthralgia, or rash suggestive of collagen vascular disease. While malignancy was possible, her imaging did not reveal any suspicious masses, nor was her peripheral blood smear consistent with an oncologic process. She had no history of asthma, eczema, or seasonal allergies. Additionally, the patient had no significant infectious history, such as pneumonia, skin and soft tissue infections, or bone and joint infections to suggest a primary immunodeficiency, such as hyperimmunoglobulin E syndrome (Job's syndrome), DOCK8 deficiency, or chronic granulomatous disease.

The patient was discharged prior to many of her laboratory tests returning. A follow-up appointment at the Pediatric Infectious Diseases clinic was scheduled. Her serologies for EBV and CMV indicated past exposure, but IgM antibodies were negative. The *Toxoplasma*, *Bartonella*, and parvovirus serologies were negative. PPD was negative, when assessed prior to hospital discharge, and stool ova and parasite examination were negative. However, the *Toxocara* IgG was positive. This laboratory result was consistent with the child's presentation and supported a diagnosis of visceral larva migrans due to *Toxocara*. She was treated with albendazole 400 mg by mouth twice daily for 5 days. It was likely that the child's iron deficiency led to pica and consequent ingestion of *Toxocara* eggs.

20.1   Toxocariasis

The larvae of two species of *Toxocara* nematodes cause the larva migrans syndrome known as toxocariasis. These roundworms are found in the intestines of dogs and cats. *Toxocara canis* is the dog roundworm and is the more common cause of toxocariasis. *Toxocara cati* is the feline roundworm. *Toxocara* eggs are shed in the dog or cat feces, which contaminate the soil or sandboxes left uncovered. The eggs mature in the soil for 2–4 weeks before becoming infectious. When ingested by humans or other animals, the eggs hatch, and larvae penetrate the intestinal wall and migrate in the bloodstream, enabling them to spread to various locations (see Fig. 20.1). Figure 20.2 shows the hatching of a *Toxocara canis* larva. While most humans do not develop symptoms, certain people will go on to develop visceral larva migrans and/or ocular larva migrans, pathologic processes that are caused by organ or muscle damage from the migrating larvae. According to the United States (US) Centers for Disease Control and Prevention, almost 14% of the US population has been infected with *Toxocara*. Risk factors for *Toxocara* infection include greater animal exposures, age under 20 years, children with pica, lower socioeconomic status, and living in a hot, humid climate.

Signs and symptoms of toxocariasis vary from mild isolated eosinophilia to fevers, respiratory symptoms such as cough and wheezing, and abdominal pain with hepatomegaly. Rarely, symptomatic myocardial or central nervous system infection can develop. Ocular toxocariasis is caused by larval migration to the eye leading to granulomatous inflammation in the form of endophthalmitis, chorioretinitis, and/or uveitis. Symptoms of toxocariasis are related to the burden of larvae and their path of migration. Laboratory abnormalities include anemia, leukocytosis, hypergammaglobulinemia, and eosinophilia. Patients with ocular toxocariasis often present with decreased vision in one eye, which can be irreversible, and may demonstrate leukocoria (white pupil) on physical examination, which raises concern for retinoblastoma.

The diagnosis of toxocariasis is made by serologic testing in a patient with a history of likely exposure to *Toxocara* eggs and compatible signs, symptoms, and laboratory studies. An enzyme-linked immunosorbent assay (ELISA) using *Toxocara* larva antigens is the currently recommended test. While identifying the organism in a liver biopsy is diagnostic, this procedure is rarely performed. The antibody level in the serum may be absent or low in patients with ocular toxocariasis. Importantly, serologic testing may be positive in patients with past or asymptomatic infections. Paired serum samples demonstrating a rise in antibody titer over time can confirm a recent infection.

Toxocariasis is treated with albendazole or mebendazole. Steroids can be considered in certain situations, such as central nervous system or myocardial involvement, or in patients with ocular toxocariasis. Children should be prevented from ingesting substances that may contain *Toxocara* eggs, and pica secondary to iron deficiency should be addressed.

Key Points/Pearls
- Toxocariasis should be considered in children with a history of pica and eosinophilia.
- *Toxocara canis* and *T. cati* are the roundworms of dogs and cats, respectively, whose eggs when ingested after maturation in the environment can lead to visceral and ocular larva migrans.
- Toxocariasis can be asymptomatic or lead to organ damage that manifests as cough, wheezing, abdominal pain, fever, and hepatomegaly.

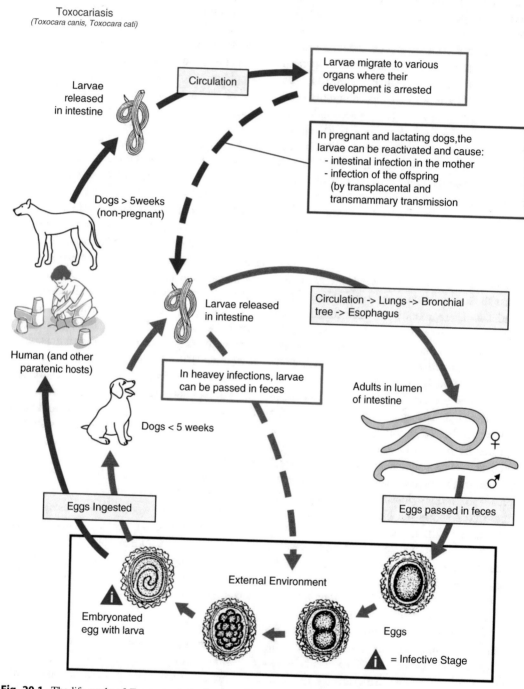

Fig. 20.1 The life cycle of *Toxocara canis*. Source: CDC/Alexander J. da Silva, PhD/Melanie Moser, available at https://stacks.cdc.gov/view/cdc/25578/Share. (Accessed on June 22, 2017)

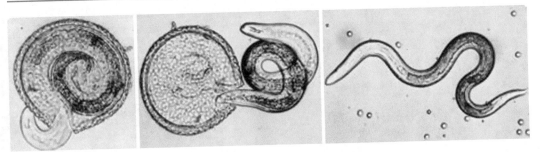

Fig. 20.2 Hatching of *Toxocara canis* larva. Source: CDC, available at https://www.cdc.gov/dpdx/toxocariasis/index. html. (Accessed on June 22, 2017)

- Ocular toxocariasis leads to leukocoria, which is in the differential diagnosis of retinoblastoma.
- Although the differential diagnosis of eosinophilia is broad, the patient had acute hypereosinophilia defined as an absolute eosinophil count above 1500, which points to a more limited list of diagnoses.
- Some helminthic infections mostly cause marked eosinophilia during the acute infection when helminths migrate through tissues: nematodes including geohelminths (*Ascaris*, hookworms, and *Trichuris*), trichinosis, and toxocariasis; flukes including acute schistosomiasis or Katayama syndrome, paragonimiasis, and liver flukes (*Fasciola*, *Clonorchis*, and *Opisthorchis*).
- Other helminthic infections cause pronounced, chronic eosinophilia, most commonly *Strongyloidiasis*, filariasis (lymphatic filariasis including tropical pulmonary eosinophilia, onchocerciasis, and loiasis), and gnathostomiasis.
- Cysticercosis and echinococcosis do not typically cause eosinophilia unless there is rupture of a cyst.

Bibliography

1. Centers for Disease Control and Prevention. Parasite – Toxocariasis (also known as Roundworm Infection). https://www.cdc.gov/parasites/toxocariasis. Accessed 22 June 2017.
2. Holland SM, Gallin JI. Disorders of granulocytes and monocytes. In: Kasper D, Fauci A, Hauser S, Longo D, Jameson JL, Loscalzo J, editors. Harrison's principles of internal medicine. New York: McGraw-Hill, Medical Pub. Division; 2015.
3. Ellison RT III, Donowitz GR. Acute pneumonia. In: Bennett JE, Dolin R, Blaser MJ, editors. Mandell, Douglas, and Bennett's principles and practice of infectious diseases. 8th ed. Philadelphia: Elsevier/ Saunders; 2015. p. 823–46.

Hidden Sphere

Jessica Ridgway

A 69-year-old man who had a heart transplant presented with 2 days of left-sided, sharp, pleuritic chest pain. The pain was associated with subjective fevers and chills as well as a cough productive of white sputum. He denied sore throat or sinus congestion. He had no sick contacts and no recent travel. The rest of his review of systems was negative.

His past medical history included a heart transplant 6 months prior for ischemic cardiomyopathy. He also had a history of hyperlipidemia and benign prostatic hyperplasia. Medications included tacrolimus, mycophenalate, prednisone, trimethoprim-sulfamethoxazole for *Pneumocystis jirovecii* pneumonia (PJP) prophylaxis, pravastatin, tamsulosin, as well as antihypertensive medications.

On physical examination, his temperature was 37.4 °C, blood pressure 128/70 mmHg, heart rate 120 beats per minute, respiratory rate 20 breaths per minute, and oxygen saturation 98% on room air. In general, he was in no acute distress. The head and neck exam was unremarkable. The pulmonary exam revealed decreased breath sounds and dullness to percussion at the left base. The car-diac exam showed tachycardia but no murmurs. The abdominal exam was benign. He had no rash.

His white blood cell (WBC) count was elevated at 20,300/µL (normal range, 4500–11,000/µL), and he was anemic with a hemoglobin of 9.4 g/dL (13.5–17.5 g/dL). His basic metabolic panel showed a creatinine of 1.4 mg/dL (0.8–1.3 mg/dL) but was otherwise unremarkable. Liver function tests and urinalysis were normal. Levels of tacrolimus and mycophenalate were within the therapeutic range.

A chest X-ray showed a patchy airspace opacity in the left lower lobe with an associated moderate pleural effusion. A thoracentesis was performed. Pleural fluid analysis revealed a pH of 7.39, lactate dehydrogenase (LDH) 161 U/L, and protein 3.7 mg/dL (normal range, <3 mg/dL). By comparison, the serum LDH was 323 U/L (140–280 U/L) and serum protein was 5.7 mg/dL. Gram stain of the pleural fluid showed no organisms but moderate WBCs. His computed tomography (CT) scan of the chest is shown in Fig. 21.1.

Microbiologic tests included a respiratory viral panel that was positive for rhinovirus, negative urinary *Legionella* antigen, negative urinary *Streptococcus pneumoniae* antigen, and negative urinary *Histoplasma* antigen. The Quantiferon gold interferon-γ release assay result was indeterminate. Initial blood cultures were negative. A bronchoscopy was performed, and broncho-alveolar lavage cultures for bacteria, fungi, and viruses were sent. An assay for PJP was also negative.

J. Ridgway, M.D., M.S.
Section of Infectious Diseases and Global Health, Department of Medicine, University of Chicago, Chicago, IL, USA
e-mail: Jessica.Ridgway@uchospitals.edu

© Springer International Publishing AG 2018
M. David, J.-L. Benoit (eds.), *The Infectious Disease Diagnosis*,
https://doi.org/10.1007/978-3-319-64906-1_21

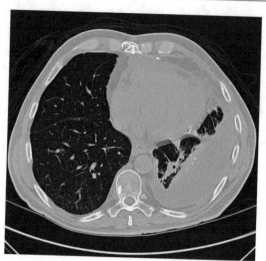

Fig. 21.1 Chest CT showing moderate left pleural effusion, left lower lobe consolidation, and pleural thickening

positive at 1:128. Although his initial admission blood cultures were negative, a blood culture drawn on hospital day 4 also became positive for *Cryptococcus neoformans*. A lumbar puncture was performed and showed normal opening pressure, 0 WBC/µL, glucose of 62 mg/dL, and protein of 27 mg/dL. The cerebrospinal fluid (CSF) cryptococcal antigen was negative.

The patient was treated with intravenous (IV) liposomal amphotericin and flucytosine. He also underwent decortication of the left lung and drainage of the pleural effusion. He developed acute kidney injury secondary to amphotericin and was subsequently changed to oral fluconazole 400 mg daily. His symptoms improved, and he was discharged in stable condition on fluconazole.

The patient received empiric antibiotics with vancomycin, piperacillin-tazobactam, and azithromycin to cover for potential healthcare-associated and community-acquired pneumonia. In solid organ transplant recipients, the risk for different infections varies based on time from transplant [1]. In the first month after transplant, infections are typically either derived from the donor organ or arise as a complication of the transplant surgery or hospitalization. From 1 to 6 months after transplant, patients are at highest risk for developing opportunistic infections, such as PJP, endemic fungal infections, and others. More than 6 months after transplant, patients are on reduced levels of immunosuppression and are subject to more common pathogens, such as causes of community-acquired pneumonia and respiratory viruses. The differential diagnosis for pulmonary infection in a solid organ transplant recipient is shown in Table 21.1 [2].

Although he had initially been afebrile on admission, on hospital day 3, the patient began spiking fevers as high as 38.9 °C and had no improvement in his symptoms. On hospital day 4, the pleural fluid culture turned positive for *Cryptococcus neoformans*. The patient's serum cryptococcal antigen was then sent and returned

21.1 Cryptoccocosis in Solid Organ Transplant Recipients

There are two species of *Cryptococcus* associated with human disease, *Cryptococcus neoformans* and *Cryptococcus gattii*. *Cryptococcus neoformans* is an encapsulated yeast that is ubiquitous in the environment (Fig. 21.2). It typically causes disease in immunocompromised individuals, particularly those with acquired immunodeficiency syndrome (AIDS) or after organ transplant. The incidence of cryptococcosis in solid organ transplant recipients is 2.8% in their lifetime [3]. The median time to onset of cryptococcosis in solid organ transplant recipients is 16–21 months posttransplant. While the vast majority of individuals with AIDS who suffer from an active cryptococcal infection present with cryptococcal meningitis, solid organ transplant recipients often show other manifestations. In solid organ transplant recipients with cryptococcosis, 61% present with disseminated or central nervous system (CNS) disease, 54% with pulmonary disease, and 8% with skin and soft tissue infection. Mortality among solid organ transplant recipients with CNS cryptococcal disease ranges from 14 to 42%.

Table 21.1 Differential diagnosis for pulmonary infection in solid organ transplant recipients

Gram positive bacteria	Gram negative bacteria	Fungi	Viruses	Other
Streptococcus pneumoniae	Legionella pneumophila	Pneumocystis jirovecii	Cytomegalovirus	Mycobacterium tuberculosis
Streptococcus spp.	Pseudomonas aeruginosa	Aspergillus spp.	Influenza	Nontuberculous mycobacteria
Staphylococcus aureus	Escherichia coli	Histoplasma capsulatum	Parainfluenza	Nocardia asteroides and other Nocardia species
	Klebsiella spp.	Blastomyces dermatitidis	Respiratory syncytial virus	Rhodococcus equi
	Enterobacter spp.	Cryptococcus neoformans		Actinomyces spp.
	Serratia spp.			
	Acinetobacter spp.			
	Proteus spp.			
	Citrobacter spp.			
	Haemophilus influenzae			

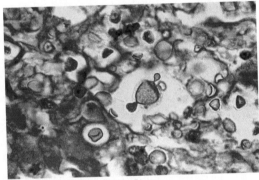

Source: https://phil.cdc.gov/phil/details.asp
Public Health Image Library. Centers for Disease Control and Prevention. Accessed September 5, 2017.

Fig. 21.2 *Cryptococcus neoformans* in a pulmonary specimen stained using hemotoxylin and eosin (https://phil.cdc.gov/phil/details.asp Public Health Image Library. Centers for Disease Control and Prevention. Accessed September 5, 2017)

Patients' risk of cryptococcosis varies with different immunosuppressive regimens. Steroids confer an increased risk, whereas patients on calcineurin inhibitors are less likely to have disseminated or CNS disease [4]. Incidence also varies by region, with higher incidence in the Eastern than Western United States. Men are more likely than women to develop cryptococcal disease [5].

Treatment for CNS, disseminated disease or severe pulmonary cryptococcal disease consists of induction therapy with liposomal amphoteri-cin B and flucytosine for at least 2 weeks. This is followed by consolidation with fluconazole 400–800 mg daily for 8 weeks, then maintenance with fluconazole 200–400 mg daily for 6–12 months [6]. For mild to moderate non-CNS disease, treatment consists of fluconazole 400 mg daily for 6–12 months.

Key Points/Pearls

- Solid organ transplant recipients are at risk for different infections based on time since their transplant: donor-derived and hospital-acquired infections in the first month, opportunistic infections from months 1 to 6, and community-acquired pathogens after 6 months.
- The most common manifestations of cryptococcal disease in solid organ transplant recipients are disseminated disease, CNS disease, and pulmonary disease.
- Treatment of disseminated or severe cryptococcal disease in transplant recipients includes induction with amphotericin and flucytosine followed by consolidation and maintenance with fluconazole.
- Rare cases of donor organ transplant-associated cryptococcosis have been reported, usually within a month of transplantation.
- Patients who receive calcineurin inhibitors are less likely to have disseminated cryptococcosis and more likely to have limited pulmonary

cryptococcosis; calcineurin inhibitors inhibit the growth of *Cryptococcus*.

- Although *Cryptococcus* is an opportunistic pathogen, it can also cause severe disease in apparently immunocompetent patients.
- *Cryptococcus gattii* frequently causes aggressive pulmonary or central nervous system infection in immunocompetent persons, often with extensive inflammation and large lung or brain cryptococcomas; this infection is slow to respond to antifungal therapy and may require surgical drainage of large cryptococcomas and/or prolonged antifungal therapy.
- An outbreak of *Cryptococcus gattii* has been identified in British Columbia and Washington state.
- The *Cryptococcus* antigen is a highly sensitive diagnostic test in AIDS patients with cryptococcal meningitis or disseminated infection, but has a lower sensitivity in transplant patients with cryptococcosis, or in any patient with only localized pulmonary or skin cryptococcosis.

References

1. Fishman JA, Rubin RH. Infection in organ-transplant recipients. N Engl J Med. 1998;338(24):1741–51.
2. Kupeli E, Eyuboglu FO, Haberal M. Pulmonary infections in transplant recipients. Curr Opin Pulm Med. 2012;18(3):202–12.
3. Singh N, Forrest G. Cryptococcosis in solid organ transplant recipients. Am J Transplant. 2009;9(Suppl 4):S192–8.
4. Vilchez RA, Fung J, Kusne S. Cryptococcosis in organ transplant recipients: an overview. Am J Transplant. 2002;2(7):575–80.
5. Husain S, Wagener MM, Singh N. *Cryptococcus neoformans* infection in organ transplant recipients: variables influencing clinical characteristics and outcome. Emerg Infect Dis. 2001;7(3):375–81.
6. Perfect JR, Dismukes WE, Dromer F, et al. Clinical practice guidelines for the management of cryptococcal disease: 2010 update by the Infectious Diseases Society of America. Clin Infect Dis. 2010;50(3):291–322.

The Importance of a Complete Social History

Lindsay A. Petty and Kenneth Pursell

A 48-year-old male with a history of well-controlled human immunodeficiency virus (HIV) infection treated with efavirenz/tenofovir/emtricitabine with a CD4+ T lymphocyte count of 368 cells/mm³ and HIV viral load <20 copies/mL and squamous cell cancer at the base of the tongue in remission after radiation therapy presented to Infectious Diseases Clinic with a lesion on his left hand.

The patient reported noticing the lesion approximately 2 months prior to presentation. It began as a small nodule that slowly increased in size and later developed a central area of skin breakdown. He did not recall any trauma from around the time he first noticed the lesion. He denied any pain or drainage. More recently he noticed a second, small, painless bump on his left forearm. He denied fevers, chills, nausea, vomiting, or other rashes or lesions. At the time of presentation, he worked as an administrative assistant. He denied alcohol or drug use, travel or pets. His HIV infection had been well controlled for approximately 11 years since starting on antiretroviral therapy.

On physical examination, the patient had a heart rate of 80 beats per minute, blood pressure 118/65 mmHg, temperature 37.2 °C, and respiratory rate of 10 breaths per minute. There was no cervical adenopathy, and mucous membranes were moist. His pulmonary, cardiovascular, and abdominal examination was normal. The pulses were equal. His skin exam was remarkable for a 1.5-cm, hard, non-tender, and mobile nodule on the side of his left hand (Fig. 22.1) that was erythematous with an area of central ulceration. There was no warmth. Proximal to this lesion on the left forearm (Fig. 22.2), there was also a 0.5-cm nodule that was firm, non-tender and mobile, and without any overlying skin changes.

The differential diagnosis for nodular lymphangitis, a skin lesion with lymphangitic spread proximally with associated lymphadenopathy, is

L.A. Petty, M.D. (✉)
University of Michigan, Ann Arbor, MI, USA
e-mail: lindsay.a.petty@gmail.com

K. Pursell, M.D.
Section of Infectious Diseases and Global Health,
Department of Medicine, University of Chicago,
Chicago, IL, USA

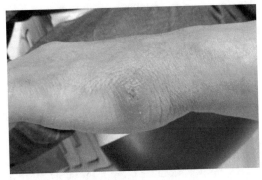

Fig. 22.1 Medial aspect of the left hand: 1.5-cm, hard, non-tender, and mobile nodule

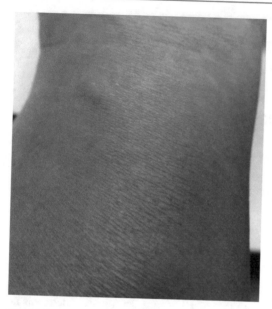

Fig. 22.2 Distal forearm, near the wrist: 0.5-cm nodule with no overlying skin changes that was firm, non-tender, and mobile

Table 22.1 Differential diagnosis for nodular lymphangitis

Sporothrix schenckii
Leishmania braziliensis
Nocardia brasiliensis
Mycobacterium marinum

presented in Table 22.1. *Sporothrix schenckii*, a dimorphic fungus, is the most common cause of nodular lymphangitis in the United States (USA) [1]. It occurs after exposure to wood or soil, and, therefore, farmers, gardeners, and forestry workers are at risk. *Leishmania braziliensis*, a protozoan infection, is acquired through the bite of an infected female sand fly in Brazil, Peru, and Central America. The lesions are often pruritic and not as painful as they appear; histological examination with Giemsa stain may reveal amastigotes. *Nocardia brasiliensis* are filamentous, Gram positive, branching, aerobic, often acid-fast bacilli. *N. brasiliensis* only accounts for about 7% of US cases of nodular lymphangitis, and it is a more frequent finding in immunocompetent hosts. Gardeners, farmers, and nursery employees are at an elevated risk for *N. brasiliensis* infection because this species can be recovered from soil.

Table 22.2 Laboratory results

Test	Result
Biopsy pathology	Epidermal acanthosis and hypergranulosis, with superficial and deep perivascular inflammatory infiltrate consisting of lymphocytes and histiocytes
Bacterial culture	Aerobic Gram-positive bacillus
Fungal culture	Negative
Acid-fast bacilli culture	Negative; incubation for 8 weeks

Table 22.3 Differential diagnosis for aquatic injuries: A list of pathogenic species

Vibrio spp.
Aeromonas hydrophila
Erysipelothrix rhusiopathiae
Mycobacterium marinum

Mycobacterium marinum is a slow-growing, non-tuberculous acid-fast mycobacterium, and disease is the result of trauma in an aquatic environment.

The patient was referred to Dermatology Clinic for a biopsy of the lesion. Pathology studies showed epidermal acanthosis and hypergranulosis, with superficial and deep perivascular inflammatory infiltrate consisting of lymphocytes and histiocytes. The fungal and acid-fast stains were negative, as were preliminary cultures (Table 22.2). The bacterial culture grew an aerobic Gram-positive bacillus that was sent to a reference laboratory for further testing to attempt to identify it.

When the patient was called with the results, he offered more information about his social history. He owned a saltwater aquarium with many exotic fish and occasionally had noted small scrapes while on his hands when cleaning the tank. He thought when asked about pets initially that his physician referred only to dogs or cats, but later he realized that other types of pets may have been important as well. The differential diagnosis of skin infections caused by aquatic injury can be found in Table 22.3 and include *Vibrio* spp., *Aeromonas hydrophila*, *Erysipelothrix rhusiopathiae*, and *Mycobacterium marinum* [2]. The first three develop more rapidly and cause painful lesions often associated with a cellulitis. Only *M. marinum* fits the clinical history and physical examination in this patient.

The patient started on therapy with oral minocycline and clarithromycin. He had resolution of the lesions after 2 months.

22.1 *Mycobacterium marinum*

M. marinum, an aerobic acid-fast bacillus, is a slow-grower non-tuberculous mycobacterial species that produces yellow pigment when exposed to light (photochromogen) and grows poorly at 37 °C but much better at 32 °C. It was first discovered as the cause of fish tuberculosis in 1926 at the Philadelphia Aquarium [3] and was determined to be a cause of skin disease in humans in 1951 [4]. Human infection can be caused by exposure to water housing both freshwater and saltwater fish, as well as shellfish, and it can cause fish illness or death as well. Lesions that *M. marinum* causes have been given the nickname "fish tank granuloma" given the exposure source [5]. Human infection is caused by even minor trauma in an aquatic environment, acquired by direct inoculation with the bacterium through broken skin, and there is no human-to-human transmission.

Disease caused by *M. marinum* is typically localized to the skin and subcutaneous tissue in an otherwise healthy host. Deeper infection in the bone or tenosynovitis is caused by direct extension. Systemic infection is rare and limited to immunocompromised hosts. Skin lesions are usually painless and can present as a papule, nodule, or plaque. Many cases result in sporotrichoid spread [5, 6], a lymphangitic spread from the primary lesion, with chains of granulomatous, inflamed, pustular skin lesions along that chain. In one study, 95% of lesions were found on the upper extremities, most likely because high-risk exposures often involve the use of these extremities in cleaning tanks and because the preferred temperature for growth of the organism is 30–32 °C [7]. Systemic symptoms such as fever and malaise are rare. Occupations or hobbies that put one at risk for disease include chefs, fish mongers, oyster shuckers, fish tank owners, and water sports enthusiasts.

M. marinum skin disease is diagnosed based on clinical history, physical exam and biopsy, and culture. However, the smear and culture are often negative and thus, a high degree of clinical suspicion based on history and physical examination are typically necessary [8]. There are no controlled trials for treatment, but two-drug therapy is recommended for 1–2 months after resolution of skin lesions. Therefore, treatment regimens are typically a 3–4 month course of clarithromycin in addition to rifampin, ethambutol, tetracyclines, or linezolid [5, 9, 10].

Key Points/Pearls

- In nodular lymphangitis, a papule forms at the site of pathogen inoculation through the skin, then ulcerates and suppurates; spread occurs along the draining lymphatics, with formation of new nodules along the lymphatics over time.
- Nodular lymphangitis has a short differential; the most important pathogens in the USA are *Sporothrix schenckii*, *Nocardia brasiliensis*, and *Mycobacterium marinum*.
- In travellers with nodular lymphagitis, one should also consider cutaneous leishmaniasis (especially *Leishmania braziliensis* complex and *L. tropica*), cutaneous nocardiosis due to *Nocardia asteroides*, skin infection due to rapidly growing *Mycobacteria* (especially *Mycobacterium chelonae*), and tularemia (*Francisella tularensis*) in persons exposed to game (rabbits) and ticks [11].
- It is critical to obtain a thorough social history to identify exposures that could suggest the diagnosis (jobs, hobbies, pets, or travel).
- Sporotrichosis, due to the soil dimorphic fungus *Sporothrix schenckii*, is the most common etiology of nodular lymphagitis and is present worldwide.
- The initial lesion of sporotrichosis ulcerates and suppurates, but remains painless, and neither lymphadenitis nor systemic symptoms develop; clues to this diagnosis include a history of gardening, working with roses and other flowers, and manipulation of sphagnum moss.
- Immunocompromised patients rarely get disseminated sporotrichosis; uncomplicated cases are treated with itraconazole.
- *Nocardia brasiliensis* causes a usually tender inoculation lesion that suppurates, and associated lymphadenitis is common, but the patient

usually has no or minimal systemic symptoms; clues to this diagnosis include gardening or soil exposure; immunocompromised patients may get disseminated disease; treatment includes trimethoprim/sulfamethoxazole and minocycline.

- *Mycobacterium marinum* causes a mildly tender inoculation lesion that suppurates, but associated lymphadenitis is rare and there are no systemic symptoms; clues to this diagnosis include exposure to fresh or salt water, including fish tanks and swimming pools.
- *M. marinum* infection is often called "fish tank granuloma;" treatment is not standardized, but a combination of two drugs is often used: clarithromycin, trimethoprim/sulfamethoxazole, rifampin, ethambutol, linezolid, and amikacin are active drugs.
- *M. marinum* is slow-growing and grows best at 32 °C; PCR may be useful for diagnosis, as the cultures are often negative.
- *M. marinum*, like *M. kansasii*, is photochromogenic, i.e., it produces a yellow pigment when exposed to light and both may cause a positive quantiferon gold interferon-γ release assay.

References

1. Giordano CN, Kalb RE, Brass C, Lin L, Helm TN. Nodular lymphangitis: report of a case with presentation of a diagnostic paradigm. Dermatol Online J. 2010;16(9):1.
2. Finkelstein R, Oren I. Soft tissue infections caused by marine bacterial pathogens: epidemiology, diagnosis, and management. Curr Infect Dis Rep. 2011;13(5):470–7.
3. Aronson JD. Spontaneous tuberculosis in saltwater fish. J Infect Dis. 1926;39(4):315–20.
4. Costanzo MR, Dipchand A, Starling R, et al. The International Society of Heart and Lung Transplantation Guidelines for the care of heart transplant recipients. J Heart Lung Transplant. 2010;29(8):914–56.
5. Lewis FM, Marsh BJ, von Reyn CF. Fish tank exposure and cutaneous infections due to *Mycobacterium marinum*: tuberculin skin testing, treatment, and prevention. Clin Infect Dis. 2003;37(3):390–7.
6. Gluckman SJ. Mycobacterium marinum. Clin Dermatol. 1995;13(3):273–6.
7. Aubry A, Chosidow O, Caumes E, Robert J, Cambau E. Sixty-three cases of *Mycobacterium marinum* infection: clinical features, treatment, and antibiotic susceptibility of causative isolates. Arch Intern Med. 2002;162(15):1746–52.
8. Elston D. Nontuberculous mycobacterial skin infections: recognition and management. Am J Clin Dermatol. 2009;10(5):281–5.
9. Rallis E, Koumantaki-Mathioudaki E. Treatment of *Mycobacterium marinum* cutaneous infections. Expert Opin Pharmacother. 2007;8(17):2965–78.
10. Griffith DE, Aksamit T, Brown-Elliott BA, et al. An official ATS/IDSA statement: diagnosis, treatment, and prevention of nontuberculous mycobacterial diseases. Am J Respir Crit Care Med. 2007;175(4):367–416.
11. Kostman JR, DiNubile MJ. Nodular lymphangitis: a distinctive but often unrecognized syndrome. Ann Intern Med. 1993;118(11):883–8.

Myalgias and Joint Pain in a Traveler to India

Oana Denisa Majorant and Sara Hurtado Bares

A 54-year-old Indian female with no significant past medical history presented with fever, headache, myalgias, and joint pain which began while she was vacationing in India.

The patient had returned from a 2-week trip to Delhi to visit family just 3 days prior to presenting for evaluation. She was well until 1 week into her stay in Delhi when she developed fevers up to 101 °F, headache, myalgias, and severe joint pain accompanied by swelling and erythema of the bilateral wrists, knees, ankles, and feet. Two days after the initial symptoms began, she developed a pruritic rash that started on the legs and later spread to her trunk and arms. The rash resolved spontaneously after approximately 5 days. She denied vision changes, conjunctivitis, cough, shortness of breath, abdominal pain, nausea, or vomiting. The patient had sought medical care while in India; however, no diagnosis was made and she was advised to take acetaminophen and ibuprofen as needed.

Interestingly, the patient's father and brother-in-law reported similar symptoms. The patient did not receive any vaccinations before traveling to India and did not take malaria prophylaxis. She consumed local vegetarian dishes and ate in the homes of numerous family members. She did not hike or swim and denied any tick bites but did recall some mosquito bites.

The patient had no significant past medical or surgical history. She was not taking regular medication aside from the acetaminophen and ibuprofen that she had started taking for the pain a few days prior to presenting for care. She was born in India but had moved to the United States (USA) more than 20 years before and at the time of her presentation was working as a college professor. She was in a monogamous relationship with her husband. There was no history of tobacco, ethanol abuse, or recreational drug abuse. She reported experiencing a rash while on sulfa drugs in the past.

On physical examination, the temperature was 37.2 °C, the blood pressure was 122/69 mmHg, the heart rate was 72 beats per minute, the respiratory rate was 18 times per minute, and the oxygen saturation was 99% while breathing room air. She was in no acute distress and breathing comfortably. She had no rash at the time of the presentation. She did not have any conjunctival pallor or scleral icterus, and her oropharynx was clear. She did not have any lymphadenopathy. The heart demonstrated a normal rate and a regular rhythm, and the lungs were clear to auscultation bilaterally. She had mild soft tissue swelling and tenderness to palpation of her knees, ankles, and metacarpal joints bilaterally (see Figs. 23.1 and 23.2).

O.D. Majorant, M.D. • S.H. Bares, M.D. (✉)
University of Nebraska Medical Center,
Omaha, NE, USA
e-mail: sara.bares@unmc.edu

© Springer International Publishing AG 2018
M. David, J.-L. Benoit (eds.), *The Infectious Disease Diagnosis*,
https://doi.org/10.1007/978-3-319-64906-1_23

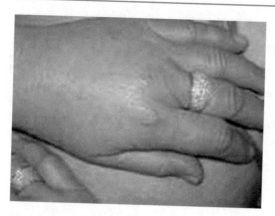

Fig. 23.1 Edematous polyarthritis of the hands [1]

Table 23.1 Differential diagnosis for traveler with fever, rash, arthritis, thrombocytopenia, and elevated transaminases

Chikungunya virus
Dengue fever
Zika virus
Malaria
Epstein-Barr virus (EBV)
Cytomegalovirus (CMV)
Parvovirus B19
Hepatitis A
Hepatitis B
Hepatitis C
Human immunodeficiency virus (HIV)
Seronegative rheumatoid arthritis

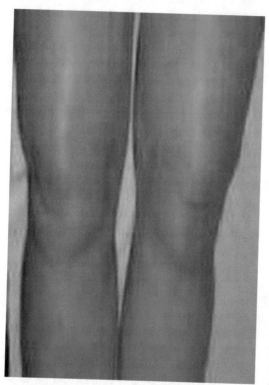

Fig. 23.2 Periarticular swelling and joint effusion in the knees [1]

The complete blood count was normal aside from a platelet count of 86,000/μL (normal range 150,000–400,000/μL). The comprehensive metabolic panel was normal aside from an aspartate transaminase of 81 U/L (15–41 U/L) and an alanine transaminase of 132 U/L (7–52 U/L). The erythrocyte sedimentation rate and C-reactive protein were elevated at 81 mm/h (0–20 mm/h) and 8.9 mg/dL (<1 mg/dL), respectively.

The differential diagnosis is presented in Table 23.1. Factors considered when developing the differential diagnosis included the symptoms and laboratory abnormalities described above, the timing and location of symptom onset, the exposure to mosquitoes, and the fact that the patient had family members with similar symptoms. Highest on the differential were dengue virus and chikungunya virus which are both associated with travel and are known to cause a febrile illness that can begin 1 to 2 weeks after exposure within an endemic area. Zika virus activity had not been reported in the year that this patient presented, but had she been in an endemic area, it could certainly have been on the differential diagnosis as well. Malaria can present in a similar fashion and was also included in the initial differential. Mononucleosis related to Epstein-Barr virus (EBV) or cytomegalovirus (CMV) can present with similar findings and occur independently of travel. Parvovirus can present with an acute polyarthritis syndrome so this diagnosis was also entertained. Finally, acute hepatitis due to hepatitis A, B, C, and E viruses were also considered, but the very short incubation period in this patient who was only 7 days into her trip when her symptoms started would

Table 23.2 Laboratory test results on the blood

Test	Result
Dengue IgM	Positive
Dengue IgG	Positive
Chikungunya IgM	Positive
Chikungunya IgG	Positive
Thick and thin blood smear	Negative
Parvovirus B19, IgM, and IgG	Negative
Hepatitis A IgM	Negative
Hepatitis B surface antigen	Negative
Hepatitis B core antibody, IgM	Negative
Hepatitis C antibody	Negative

make viral hepatitis unlikely. Because her father and brother-in-law reported similar symptoms, a mosquito-borne infection was much more likely (chikungunya, dengue, or malaria), although respiratory viral illnesses (e.g., influenza), food-borne illnesses, and even leptospirosis can also occur in clusters.

Further work-up was performed, as shown in Table 23.2, and the patient was ultimately diagnosed with dengue and chikungunya virus coinfection. It is important to note that although serum antibody and polymerase chain reaction (PCR) testing are both useful tests for the diagnosis of dengue and chikungunya, the ELISA IgM antibody tests are preferred if symptoms have been present for more than 8 days. PCR testing is preferred during the first 7 days of symptoms when antibodies may not yet be present.

23.1 Chikungunya–Dengue Fever Coinfection

Dengue fever is one of the most common mosquito-borne viral infections, with over 96 million symptomatic cases per year worldwide [2]. It is caused by the four dengue flavivirus serotypes transmitted by primarily day-biting *Aedes* mosquitoes, especially the peri-domestic *Ae. aegypti* which infests the cities of the developing world. Well-known for centuries, dengue was first recorded in the 1780s when

it was coined "break-bone fever" in reference to the acute febrile illness accompanied by the bone and muscle pain. In the last 70 years, dengue has become global, with urbanization and international travel as key factors in facilitating its spread from Asia to Africa, Latin America, and the Caribbean islands. Dengue is a major public health problem because it may result in severe and life-threatening disease with hemo-concentration, shock, and sometimes bleeding in a minority of infected persons, especially children.

Chikungunya fever is another important mosquito-borne viral infection, due to the chikungunya alphavirus, transmitted by the same *Aedes* mosquito vector as dengue. It was first described in the 1950s in Africa after an outbreak on the Makonde Plateau, on the border of Mozambique and Tanzania. It bears its name from a Makonde word meaning "that which bends up," a fitting description of the stooped posture that often develops as a result of the incapacitatingly painful arthralgias induced by the virus [3]. Chikungunya has more recently emerged as a true global pathogen affecting millions of people in more than 50 countries. In 2005, chikungunya reemerged in India and spread to Southeast Asia, and it took less than 10 years for the virus to enter the Western Hemisphere. By 2014, chikungunya had caused disease in more than 20 countries in the Caribbean and Central and South America [4], and the first domestically acquired case of chikungunya was reported in the USA in 2014 [5]. International travel and globalization have played an important role in the rapid geographical expansion of the virus.

Although rare, there have been reports of coinfection with chikungunya and dengue, as both are transmitted by the same mosquito vector, especially *Ae. aegypti* and *Ae. albopictus*. These mosquitoes are well adapted to urban environments, and they bite primarily during the day indoors and outdoors, although they may bite at night in well-lit areas. They are nervous feeders; if the meal is interrupted they may resume feeding on another household member, and this explains the frequent clustering of infections among family members. Studies have indicated that mosquitoes may be coinfected with both viruses, and they are able to deliver particles of both dengue and chikungunya virus through their saliva during a blood meal [6]. The first reported case of coinfection was documented in 1982 in Puerto Rico [7]. Since then, there have been multiple reports of coinfections, most of which have occurred during outbreaks [8].

23.2 Similarities and Differences: Chikungunya and Dengue

The two viruses share many clinical and epidemiological features, especially in regions where both viruses are endemic such as in parts of Asia as well as South America. There is significant overlap between the clinical presentations of uncomplicated dengue fever and early chikungunya fever, and the two infections may be indistinguishable based on clinical symptoms alone [9]. Both viruses have short incubation periods (always <2 weeks) and may cause fever, headache, rash, myalgias, arthralgias, and arthritis. Also, in both chikungunya and dengue, the initial work-up may reveal lymphopenia, thrombocytopenia, or neutropenia. Chikungunya is often distinguished from dengue clinically by the intense and sometimes prolonged arthralgia/arthritis that persists beyond the initial febrile episode and that may linger for weeks. Classic, uncomplicated dengue, on the other hand, is frequently characterized by an intense retro-orbital headache as well as more profound hematologic

abnormalities including neutropenia and thrombocytopenia (see Table 23.3).

It is important to differentiate between dengue and chikungunya, and, when this is not immediately possible initially, to be on the lookout for the World Health Organization (WHO) defined warning signs that identify patients at risk of developing severe dengue. An older WHO classification defined classic dengue, dengue hemorrhagic fever, and dengue shock syndrome but has been replaced by a more accurate classification of dengue without warning signs, dengue with warning signs, and severe dengue (Table 23.4). Death from severe dengue is prevented when patients with warning signs are managed carefully to avoid shock due to hemoconcentration as well as excessive edema. The WHO has published detailed guidelines for management of dengue applicable in resource-limited settings.

Arthritis from chikungunya virus is symmetrical, peripheral, nondestructive, severe, and persists from weeks to months in most patients, which is not seen with dengue. Because of the large number of infected patients when chikungunya enters a new geographic area where the whole population is susceptible, disabling arthritis affects many people for months and results in a high economic cost. Such prolonged arthritis is also seen with parvovirus B19, rubella, and the arthritogenic alphaviruses (chikungunya virus which has been spreading globally, *O'nyong nyong virus* in East Africa, *Sinbis virus* especially in northern Europe and Scandinavia, Mayaro virus in northern South America, and both Ross River and Barmah Forest viruses in Australia) [10].

Table 23.3 Similarities and differences between chikungunya and dengue [1]

	Patient in present case	Chikungunya	Dengue
Fever	High grade (101 °F)	High grade	Moderate – high grade
Headache	+	++	+++
Rash	+	+	++
Myalgia	+	+	++
Arthralgia	+++	+++	+
Neutropenia	–	+	+++
Thrombocytopenia	+	+	+++
Hemorrhage	–	+/–	++

Table 23.4 World Health Organization dengue case definitions

Dengue without warning signs	Fever and two of the following: • Nausea, vomiting • Rash • Aches and pains • Leukopenia • Positive tourniquet test
Dengue with warning signs	Dengue with any of the following: • Abdominal pain or tenderness • Persistent vomiting • Clinical fluid accumulation (ascites, pleural effusion) • Mucosal bleeding • Lethargy, restlessness • Liver enlargement >2 cm • Laboratory: increase in hematocrit with rapid decrease in platelet count

Severe dengue	Dengue with at least one of the following criteria:
	• Severe plasma leakage leading to shock (DSS) or fluid accumulation with respiratory distress
	• Severe bleeding as evaluated by a clinician
	• Severe organ involvement
	  – Liver: AST or ALT ≥1000
	  – CNS: impaired consciousness
	  – Failure of the heart and other organs

AST aspartate transaminase, *ALT* alanine transaminase, *CNS* central nervous system, *DSS* dengue shock syndrome

23.3 Second Infection Can Increase the Risk of Severe Dengue

Dengue fever occurs after exposure to any of the four distinct serotypes: DEN-1, DEN-2, DEN-3, and DEN-4. The disease presentation can range from a mild, nonspecific viral syndrome to classic dengue fever to severe dengue. Initial infection induces lifelong immunity to the serotype originally acquired, but the cross-immunity to the other serotypes only lasts for a few months. Moreover, a heterologous dengue infection (i.e., an infection with a different serotype) that occurs more than 1 year after the initial infection may lead to severe dengue. Antibody-dependent enhancement is one of the proposed mechanisms underlying the relationship between secondary infection and more severe disease. The hypothesis is that the preformed dengue antibodies link to the virus but do not destroy it and actually facilitate its entry into cells where it replicates [11]. This results in a higher viral burden, a strong immune response, and a subsequent increase in inflammatory mediators, which eventually results in capillary leakage and severe dengue disease. Of note, it is possible to get severe dengue with the first infection, such as when infants still have cross-reacting maternal antibody or with certain genotypes.

23.4 Treatment and Prevention

The mainstay of management for both viruses is supportive care as there is no effective antiviral therapy. Aspirin and nonsteroidal anti-inflammatory drugs are generally avoided in dengue fever due to the risk of bleeding.

For dengue, early recognition of the warning signs for severe disease is critically important for the appropriate triage and monitoring of the patient. Warning signs, which are outlined in Table 23.4, include abdominal pain, persistent vomiting, clinical fluid accumulation, lethargy, liver enlargement, and laboratory evidence of an elevated hematocrit (from hemoconcentration) with concurrent thrombocytopenia.

Severe dengue is much more common in children and can be managed according to WHO guidelines with careful fluid management as soon as warning signs are identified, which reduces mortality remarkably in hospitalized patients.

A special consideration is given to the persistent arthritis/tenosynovitis that can occur after chikungunya infection and may be severe enough to interfere with daily activities. The clinical symptoms vary from persistent polyarthralgias to synovitis, bursitis and enthesitis, and can evolve into a chronic inflammatory arthritis. In these cases, the management often requires a multidisciplinary team that involves rheumatologists, physical therapists, and medications such as meloxicam, chloroquine, corticosteroids, or even methotrexate [12].

Prevention is fundamental. Recommended measures include avoiding mosquito exposure as well as the use of a mosquito repellant containing *N,N*-diethyl-meta-toluamide (DEET), and protective clothing when outdoors, and air conditioning, DEET, or mosquito nets when indoors. Secondary prevention measures such as avoiding mosquito exposure during the first week of illness in order to reduce the risk of local transmission are also important. To date, there is no licensed vaccine for either dengue or chikungunya.

Key Points/Pearls

- Arboviruses represent an important cause of febrile illnesses in returning travelers and should be considered in the differential of fever occurring in the first 2 weeks after travel.
- *Aedes aegypti* and *Aedes albopictus* transmit the chikungunya alphavirus as well as the dengue and Zika flaviviruses.
- Chikungunya and dengue have similar epidemiological and overlapping clinical features that often make them indistinguishable; serology may be the only way to differentiate them.
- Zika virus infection can present similarly to chikungunya and dengue, although infection is often asymptomatic or associated with a mild illness.
- Only chikungunya causes a severe, disabling, painful, symmetric, peripheral, nondestructive arthritis that persists for weeks to months in a majority of infected persons; this is also seen with the other arthritogenic alphaviruses, which are restricted to limited geographic areas in Latin America (Mayaro), Africa (O'nyong-nyong), Northern Europe (Sinbis), and Australia (Ross River and Barmah Forest).
- Other important arthritogenic viruses include Parvovirus B19 and rubella.
- Only dengue causes a severe disease with hemoconcentration due to extravasation of fluid with shock and edema, as well as bleeding from severe thrombocytopenia.
- Severe dengue disease occurs in a minority of patients and is more common in those infected with a second serotype; it is essential to identify warning signs early and manage these patients' fluid balance carefully to prevent both shock and excessive edema as detailed in the WHO guideline applicable to resource-limited settings.
- Given the similar geographical distribution and the fact that they share a common vector, coinfection with these dengue and chikungunya viruses is possible.
- There is no specific vaccine for either of these viruses, and the treatment is supportive.
- Prevention is critical, and travelers to the affected areas should be advised to avoid mosquito exposure or use protective clothes and DEET when outside, although biting also occurs indoors.

References

1. Centers for Disease Control. Chikungunya: clinical management in dengue-endemic areas. http://www.cdc.gov/chikungunya/pdfs/CHIKV_DengueEndemic.pdf. Accessed 22 June 2017.
2. Bhatt S, Gething PW, Brady OJ, Messina JP, Farlow AW, Moyes CL, et al. The global distribution and burden of dengue. Nature. 2013;496(7446):504–7.
3. Halstead SB. Reappearance of chikungunya, formerly called dengue, in the Americas. Emerg Infect Dis. 2015;21(4):557–61.
4. Morrison TE. Reemergence of chikungunya virus. J Virol. 2014;88(20):11644–7.
5. Centers for Disease Control Newsroom Release (July 17, 2014). First Chikungunya case acquired in the United States reported in Florida [Press release]. http://www.cdc.gov/media/releases/2014/p0717-chikungunya.html. Accessed 30 Apr 2017.
6. Vazeille M, Mousson L, Martin E, Failloux AB. Orally co-Infected Aedes albopictus from La Reunion Island, Indian Ocean, can deliver both dengue and chikungunya infectious viral particles in their saliva. PLoS Negl Trop Dis. 2010;4(6):e706.
7. Gubler DJ, Kuno G, Sather GE, Waterman SH. A case of natural concurrent human infection with two dengue viruses. Am J Trop Med Hyg. 1985;34(1):170–3.
8. Ramachandran VG, Das S, Roy P, Hada V, Mogha NS. Chikungunya: a reemerging infection spreading during 2010 dengue fever outbreak in National Capital Region of India. Virusdisease. 2016;27(2):183–6.
9. Furuya-Kanamori L, Liang S, Milinovich G, Soares Magalhaes RJ, Clements AC, Hu W, et al. Co-distribution and co-infection of chikungunya and dengue viruses. BMC Infect Dis. 2016;16:84.

10. Suhrbier A, Jaffar-Bandjee MC, Gasque P. Arthritogenic alphaviruses—an overview. Nat Rev Rheumatol. 2012;8(7):420–9.

11. Halstead SB, Heinz FX, Barrett AD, Roehrig JT. Dengue virus: molecular basis of cell entry and pathogenesis, 25-27 June 2003, Vienna, Austria. Vaccine. 2005;23(7):849–56.

12. Blettery M, Brunier L, Polomat K, Moinet F, Deligny C, Arfi S, et al. Management of chronic post-chikungunya rheumatic disease: the Martinican experience. Arthritis Rheumatol. 2016;68(11): 2816–24.

A Marathon Runner with a Change in Mental Status

Michael Z. David

A 45-year-old, previously healthy African-American man presented in the late spring to the emergency department with complaints of 2 months of weight loss (47 lb) leading to a 25% weight reduction, fevers, night sweats, chills, a dry cough, and confusion for 3 days. Seven weeks earlier, he had noted the onset of a rash starting on the palms and soles and later on the dorsal surfaces of his hands and feet, transiently on his back and most recently, within the previous 3 weeks, on the nose and surrounding his mouth. Two of the lesions bled slightly. For 5 weeks, he had diarrhea that improved transiently with an over-the-counter antidiarrheal medication. Three months prior to presentation, he traveled to New Orleans and he had also been to Sacramento, California for work-related meetings.

As an outpatient prior to his presentation, he had an extensive workup for these symptoms. This included a normal computed tomography (CT) scan of the brain, and a negative esophogastroduodenoscopy and colonoscopy 3 weeks prior to admission. He also had a negative bacterial stool culture, negative human immunodeficiency virus (HIV) antibody test, negative rapid plasma reagin (RPR), and normal serum levels of angiotensin-converting enzyme and lactate dehydrogenase. However, a CT scan of the chest, abdomen, and pelvis showed diffuse retroperitoneal, hilar, and mediastinal lymphadenopathy. The erythrocyte sedimentation rate (ESR) was elevated, at 115 mm/h (normal range, 0–22 mm/h), several days prior to admission.

The patient worked as a lawyer, lived alone, denied the use of alcohol, tobacco, or illegal drugs, had no pets or recent known animal contact, denied foreign travel, had no known recent insect bites, homelessness, incarceration or known tuberculosis contacts, and denied any history of sexually transmitted infections. He had not been camping, hunting, or spelunking in recent years. He had run many marathons in the previous several years in various cities of the United States (USA) and was an active, avid runner.

On physical examination, the patient had a fever of 38.5 °C, hypotension of 82/50 mmHg, heart rate of 76 beats per minute, respiratory rate of 14 breaths per minute, and oxygen saturation of 99% on room air. He was tired appearing. He had a 2/6 holosystolic heart murmur audible throughout the precordium. He was forgetful and demonstrated confabulation, with a slow and sometimes changing response to questions during the examination and history. He had a flat affect, which was not his baseline according to

M.Z. David, M.D., Ph.D.
Section of Infectious Diseases and Global Health, Department of Medicine, University of Chicago Medicine, Chicago, IL, USA
e-mail: michdav@upenn.edu

© Springer International Publishing AG 2018
M. David, J.-L. Benoit (eds.), *The Infectious Disease Diagnosis*,
https://doi.org/10.1007/978-3-319-64906-1_24

family members. Skin examination revealed scattered firm papules on the palms, soles, dorsal surfaces of the hands and feet, the distal margin of the nares, and the perioral skin (see Fig. 24.1).

His laboratory studies are summarized in Table 24.1. They were most notable for an elevated serum white blood cell (WBC) count, eosinophilia (10% on the differential), anemia, thrombocytosis, a slightly elevated alkaline phosphatase, and an elevated gamma-glutamyl transferase (GGT). A lumbar puncture was performed, and the results are shown in Table 24.2. These demonstrated a lymphocytic pleocytosis, a markedly elevated cerebrospinal fluid (CSF) protein, and decreased CSF glucose. A chest X-ray showed right hilar fullness. Blood and CSF cultures were both negative for growth of fungi, bacteria, and acid fact bacilli. The quantiferon gold test, the serum and CSF cryptococcal antigen,

and the viral load for the human immunodeficiency virus (HIV) were all negative. The urine *Histoplasma* antigen and the serum *Blastomyces* antibody were negative.

A skin biopsy was obtained from a skin lesion on the posterior hand. The histologic images from this biopsy are shown in Fig. 24.2, demonstrating low- and high-power images of round structures in the skin consistent with spherules of *Coccidioides* spp. The serum *Coccidioides* antibody by enzyme immunoassay (EIA) was negative. On further specific questioning, the family reported that the patient had run in the Phoenix, Arizona, marathon for the past 3 years in January, the last time about 3 months prior to his presentation. This may have been the critical exposure to the region endemic for *Coccidioides* spp.

The differential diagnosis of palmar skin lesions with or without fever is presented in

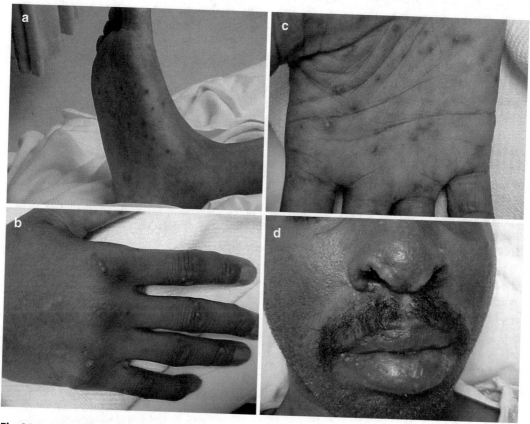

Fig. 24.1 Skin findings of physical examination, showing papular lesions on the soles (**a**), dorsal surface of the hand (**b**), palms (**c**), and perioral and nasal areas (**d**)

Table 24.1 Laboratory results in the present case

Laboratory test (blood)	Result	Normal range
White blood cell count	12,900/μL	3500–11,000/μL
Neutrophils	59%	39–75%
Lymphocytes	15%	16–47%
Eosinophils	10%	0–7%
Basophils	5%	0–2%
Hemoglobin	9.1 g/dL	13.5–17.5 g/dL
Hematocrit	28.1%	41–53%
Platelet count	536,000/μL	150,000–450,000/μL
Sodium	133 mmol/L	134–149 mmol/L
Potassium	3.7 mmol/L	3.5–5.0 mmol/L
Chloride	101 mmol/L	95–108 mmol/L
Bicarbonate	27 mmol/L	23–30 mmol/L
Blood urea nitrogen	9 mg/dL	7–20 mg/dL
Creatinine	0.5 mg/dL	0.5–1.4 mg/dL
Glucose	93 mg/dL	60–99 mg/dL
Alanine aminotransferase	15 U/L	8–35 U/L
Aspartate aminotransferase	24 U/L	8–37 U/L
Alkaline phosphatase	155 U/L	30–120 U/L
Total bilirubin	0.3 mg/dL	0.1–1.0 mg/dL
Gamma-glutamyl transferase	126 U/L	0–45 U/L
Total Protein	7.2 g/dL	6.0–8.3 g/dL
Albumin	4.1 g/dL	3.5–5.0 g/dL
Iron	128 μg/dL	40–160 μg/dL
Total iron-binding capacity	356 μg/dL	230–430 μg/dL
Ferritin	460 ng/mL	20–300 ng/mL

Table 24.2 Results of lumbar puncture (all values on cerebrospinal fluid)

Laboratory test	Result	Normal range
Total cell count	494/μL	0–30/μL
White blood cells	210/μL	0–30/μL
Red blood cells	284/μL	0/μL
Neutrophils	27%	
Lymphocytes	73%	
Eosinophils	0%	
Protein	210 mg/dL	60–90 mg/dL
Glucose	42 mg/dL	50–70 mg/dL

Table 24.3. The differential for our patient was quite broad initially although it could be narrowed on the basis of signs, symptoms, and history. Although another fungal infection was possible, the skin lesions of *Blastomyces* tend to have purulent drainage, unlike his dry, papular lesions. The skin lesions, with symptoms of central nervous system (CNS) involvement, made most other fungal pathogens unlikely. Tuberculosis or non-tubercular *Mycobacteria* was possible, but would be unlikely in an immunocompetent host, and eosinophilia would not be common. Cryptococcal meningitis and skin lesions would also be unlikely in this host although *Cryptococcus gattii* has been reported to cause meningitis in immunocompetent patients in the US Pacific northwest and the region around Vancouver Island in Canada. Viral pathogens can cause aseptic meningitis and a rash, but the observed papular skin lesions would have been quite unusual for a viral infection. Lesions on the palms and soles should always raise the question of Rocky Mountain spotted fever, meningococcemia, or syphilis. However, there were no

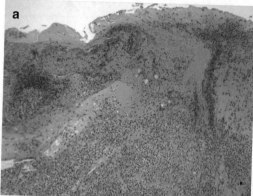

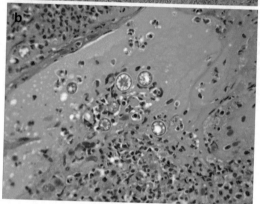

Fig. 24.2 Spherules of *Coccidioides* visible in the dermis of skin biopsy. (**a**) Low power, (**b**) high power

tick exposures, and the morphology of the skin lesions was not at all typical of a rickettsial infection. There were no known recent sexual exposures, and testing for syphilis was negative, making secondary syphilis very unlikely. Meningococcemia usually has a much more fulminant presentation with sepsis, and the lesions are often petechial or purpuric, unlike the papular lesions in our patient.

With the finding of the distinctive, and often pathognomonic, organisms in the skin biopsy (Fig. 24.2) along with the abnormal CSF findings (Table 24.2), a diagnosis of *Coccidioides* disseminated to the skin and meninges was made. Our patient was thus treated initially with high-dose fluconazole and then was indefinitely treated with 400-mg daily fluconazole orally. His fever abated within a week, and gradually the skin lesions and confusion resolved completely. He was able to return to work.

Table 24.3 Differential diagnosis for palm and sole skin lesions with or without fever (etiologies in bold text are more common)

Infectious
Blastomyces dermatitidis
Histoplasma capsulatum
Coccidioides immitis or *C. posadasii*
Cryptococcus spp.
Tinea
Viral exanthem
Hand, foot and mouth disease (coxsackieviruses, enteroviruses, echoviruses, polioviruses)
Measles
Tuberculosis (*Mycobacterium tuberculosis*)
Nontuberculous mycobacterial infections (e.g., fish-handler's disease, by direct inoculation)
Leprosy (*Mycobacterium leprae*)
Rocky Mountain spotted fever (*Rickettsia rickettsii*)
Secondary syphilis or congenital syphilis (*Treponema pallidum*)
Typhus (*Rickettsia prowazekii*)
Endocarditis (Janeway lesions, Osler's nodes)
Q fever (*Coxiella burnetii*)
Reactive arthritis due to a gastrointestinal pathogen or *Chlamydia*
Noninfectious
Miliaria rubra
Tylosis
Drug eruption
Sweet's syndrome
Stevens Johnson syndrome
Contact dermatitis, atopic dermatitis
Eczema
Scabies
Psoriasis
Insect bites
Skin cancer
Allergy
Seborrheic dermatitis
Erythema nodosum
Erythema multiforme

24.1 Coccidioidomycosis

Coccidioides immitis and *C. posadasii* are dimorphic fungal pathogens that cause respiratory and, less commonly, disseminated human infections known as coccidioidomycosis. Along with *Blastomyces, Histoplasma, Sporothrix,*

Paracoccidioides, and *Penicillium marneffei*, *Coccidioides* spp. are often referred to as an "endemic mycosis." This term refers to the limited geographic distributions of the dimorphic fungi. Coccidioidomycosis was first described in 1892 by Alejandro Posadas, a physician in Argentina who diagnosed the disease from skin lesions [1]. *Coccidioides* spp. cause a syndrome known as San Joaquin Valley fever that is sometimes called "valley fever." The distribution of the disease in the USA is limited to southern California, Nevada, and Utah, most of Arizona and New Mexico, and western Texas [2]. It was been estimated that the incidence of hospitalization for disseminated coccidioidomycosis was 4.8/100,000 per year in 2000–2009 in Arizona and 0.89/100,000 per year in 2003–2008 in California. The incidence was found to be much higher among African-Americans [3]. The disease also occurs in parts of Mexico and Central and South America. History of travel to an endemic area provides an important clue to the diagnosis for patients who present in other regions [2].

Infection occurs when fungal forms called arthroconidia (or spores, 3–5 μm in size) are inhaled from the soil, usually in dry, desert environments. The life cycle of these dimorphic species is complex. At human body temperature after seeding the respiratory tract of an infected patient, the *Coccidioides* spp. arthroconidia grow, enlarging into a rounded structure known as a "spherule." Within the spherule, cleavage planes appear and develop into many endospores that fill the mature spherule, which can reach up to 100 μm in diameter. The mature spherule eventually ruptures and releases endospores that can either go on to form new spherules in the host tissues or be disseminated back into the environment from the infected host. The rupture of spherules may be associated with an enhanced immune reaction and development of a focal lesion in the skin or other tissues. In the environment, the endospores germinate during the mycelial stage of their life cycle to become morphologically very distinct mold-form structures with septate hyphae which ultimately release free arthroconidia [2].

Clinical manifestations of coccidioidomycosis may vary from asymptomatic infection to severe, life-threatening involvement of the central nervous system. The incubation period is generally 1–4 weeks after exposure. It has been estimated that 60% of infections are asymptomatic and result in durable immunity. Typical symptoms of pulmonary infection by *Coccidioides* spp. include cough, chest pain, shortness of breath, fever, fatigue, weight loss, and headache. Many patients experience only a mild, flu-like illness. Approximately 10–50% of patients with pulmonary disease develop a hypersensitivity rash, often an erythematous or macular rash, but sometimes erythema nodosum or erythema multiforme. Hematogenous spread from the lungs occurs in only approximately 0.5–8% of clinically diagnosed cases, and when there is dissemination beyond the respiratory tract, the skin is the most common secondary site [2]. In addition to skin, many sites of infection have been reported, including cases of pericarditis, empyema, peritonitis, retropharyngeal infections, osteomyelitis, and myositis [4]. Laboratory abnormalities often include elevation of the ESR, peripheral eosinophilia, and chest X-ray abnormalities, which can vary [2].

Diagnosis of coccidioidomycosis is usually by biopsy and serology and less commonly by culture. EIA testing can give a false positive, whereas immunodiffusion-based assays for tube precipitin and complement-fixing antibody tests are less sensitive. Testing for the organism by polymerase-chain reaction (PCR)-based assays or tests aimed at antigen detection are not used frequently but may be useful in the future [5].

Meningitis is a rare complication of coccidioidomycosis, first described in 1905 [1]. The diagnosis is life-threatening; without treatment, mortality is almost 100%. Meningitis is suggested if there is evidence of *Coccidioides* infection and there is an elevated CSF WBC and protein (sometimes very highly elevated), along with a low CSF glucose. Meningitis may progress to vasculitis, hydrocephalus requiring placement of a shunt, or brain abscess [1].

24.2 Treatment of Coccidioidomycosis

The Infectious Diseases Society of America updated its treatment guidelines for coccidioidomycosis in 2016 [5]. For mild pulmonary infections in immunocompetent, previously healthy hosts, no therapy is needed, even in those with an asymptomatic, single pulmonary nodule or cavitary lesion proven to be caused by *Coccidioides* spp. However, if a patient has a serious comorbid condition even with asymptomatic infection or if there is a symptomatic cavitary lung lesion in any person, therapy with an azole drug, such as fluconazole at a dose of at least 400 mg daily, is recommended. For any extrapulmonary coccidioidal disease, treatment is recommended. Lumbar puncture is only advocated in those cases where persistent headache, nausea, and vomiting, or a new focal neurologic deficit is present in the setting of *Coccidioides* spp. infection; it is not necessary if there is no specific concern for CNS involvement [5].

Meningitis in coccidioidomycosis is a life-threatening condition that usually responds to therapy. Guidelines recommend 400–1200 mg of fluconazole daily for treatment. Lifelong suppressive therapy is recommended for *Coccidioides* meningitis. If fluconazole therapy fails in cases of meningitis, another effective azole antifungal or intrathecal amphotericin should be used. Special considerations must be taken for immunocompromised hosts, including HIV-infected patients, and pregnant women [5].

Key Points

- Coccidioidomycosis is an endemic dimorphic fungus with a complex life cycle.
- *Coccidioides* spp. have a distinctive geographic distribution in the Southwestern USA, Mexico, and Central and South America.
- Many infections occur in endemic regions of the USA every year, and the incidence increases when heavy rains are followed by drought and dust storms.
- Aerosolized arthrospores are inhaled into the lungs.
- The majority of infections are asymptomatic, and many mild infections in immunocompetent, healthy hosts require no therapy.
- African-Americans and Filipinos are at higher risk of severe coccidioidomycosis.
- Patients with AIDS are at high risk of dissemination and meningitis.
- Transplanted organs may transmit coccidioidomycosis to the transplant recipient.
- For immunocompromised hosts and in the case of extrapulmonary or disseminated disease in all patients, therapy is warranted.
- *Coccidioides* spp. can disseminate to nearly any organ in the body.
- Meningitis is nearly uniformly fatal if not treated and requires lifelong suppressive therapy, and fluconazole is the preferred agent; intrathecal amphotericin B is used in refractory cases.
- Diagnosis is definitive by pathology or culture while serological testing is often useful.
- Eosinophils are often increased within the infected tissues (skin lesion or lung biopsy), infected fluids (CSF, and pleural, pericardial, or joint effusion), and sometimes in the blood of patients with coccidioidomycosis.

References

1. Mathisen G, Shelub A, Truong J, Wigen C. Coccidioidal meningitis: clinical presentation and management in the fluconazole era. Medicine (Baltimore). 2010;89(5):251–84.
2. Nguyen C, Barker BM, Hoover S, et al. Recent advances in our understanding of the environmental, epidemiological, immunological, and clinical dimensions of coccidioidomycosis. Clin Microbiol Rev. 2013;26(3):505–25.
3. Seitz AE, Prevots DR, Holland SM. Hospitalizations associated with disseminated coccidioidomycosis, Arizona and California, USA. Emerg Infect Dis. 2012;18(9):1476–9.
4. Crum-Cianflone NF, Truett AA, Teneza-Mora N, et al. Unusual presentations of coccidioidomycosis: a case series and review of the literature. Medicine (Baltimore). 2006;85(5):263–77.
5. Galgiani JN, Ampel NM, Blair JE, et al. Infectious Diseases Society of America (IDSA) clinical practice guideline for the treatment of coccidioidomycosis. Clin Infect Dis. 2016;63(6):e112–46.

Unmasking One of the Great Masqueraders

Ralph Villaran

A 59-year-old female with a past medical history of hypertension, diabetes mellitus, hypothyroidism, toxic multinodular goiter, and hepatitis C was hospitalized. She had hepatitis C genotype 1b diagnosed 3 years prior to her admission with a liver biopsy showing moderate fibrosis, treated with pegylated interferon α-2a and ribavirin that was stopped 4 weeks prior to her hospitalization. She presented to the hospital with a high-grade fever for 4 weeks, a 15-lb weight loss, fatigue, abdominal discomfort, intermittent chills, sweats, and chronic dry cough. She had no complaints of nausea, vomiting, diarrhea, urinary symptoms, or mental status changes.

The patient was born in Pakistan and emigrated to the United States (US) 30 years prior. Her last visit to Pakistan was 3 years prior. She previously worked as a nurse. She did not have any history of smoking and alcohol or drug consumption and had no pets at home. Her family history was significant for diabetes, thyroid disease, and coronary artery disease, but no history of cancer. She had three successful pregnancies. She was known to be purified protein derivative (PPD) positive but had no history of active tuberculosis.

Her physical examination on admission revealed a temperature of 39.5 °C, heart rate of 126 beats per minute, blood pressure of 161/71 mmHg, and respiratory rate of 20 breaths per minute. She was fully awake, alert, and oriented in no acute distress. She appeared chronically ill, had pale conjunctivae, had no jaundice or rashes, and her lungs were clear. She was tachycardic and her cardiac rhythm was regular. She had no audible murmurs. Her bowel sounds were normal, but her abdomen was distended with mild diffuse tenderness on palpation. She had a possible fluid wave, but no palpable organomegaly or abdominal masses. Her neurological exam was normal.

The patient's laboratory results are shown in Table 25.1. Her initial chest x-ray showed diffuse interstitial opacities suggestive of edema with likely small bilateral pleural effusions. A computed tomography (CT) scan of the chest, abdomen, and pelvis showed small to borderline diffuse lymphadenopathy (mediastinal, axillary, diaphragmatic, mesenteric, retroperitoneal, and iliac) and no pulmonary infiltrates or nodules. There was a small amount of ascites with infiltrative changes of the omentum and pelvic fat suggestive of possible peritoneal carcinomatosis. There were large, bilateral ovarian cystic lesions (Figs. 25.1 and 25.2), splenomegaly with multiple small nonspecific hypodense lesions, an enlarged pancreatic head and thyromegaly with

R. Villaran, M.D.
Infectious Disease Specialists, Highland, IN, USA
e-mail: rvillaranmd@gmail.com

Table 25.1 Laboratory findings on blood, except for urinalysis

Test name (normal range)	Value
White blood cell count (4000–10,000/uL)	5100/μL
Hemoglobin (12–15 g/dL)	8.6 g/dL
Hematocrit (36–47%)	25.6%
Platelets (150,000–400,000/uL)	139,000/μL
Neutrophils (35–80%)	49%
Bands (0–10%)	18%
Lymphocytes (18–44%)	14%
Monocytes (4.7–12.5%)	14%
Sodium (135–145 meq/L)	129 meq/L
Potassium (3.5–5 meq/L)	3.8 meq/L
Chloride (95–105 meq/L)	93 meq/L
Carbon dioxide (18–22 meq/L)	24 meq/L
Blood urea nitrogen (BUN) (8–21 mg/dL)	11 mg/dL
Creatinine (0.8–1.3 mg/dL)	0.5 mg/dL
Glucose (65–110 mg/dL)	167 mg/dL
Protein (6–8 g/dL)	7.2 g/dL
Albumin (3.5–5 g/dL)	3.0 g/dL
Total bilirubin (0.3–1.2 mg/dL)	0.6 mg/dL
Alkaline phosphatase (50–100 U/L)	280 U/L
Aspartate aminotransferase (AST) (5–30 U/L)	102 U/L
Alanine aminotransferase (ALT) (5–30 U/L)	61 U/L
Prothrombin time (PT) (11–14 s)	14.5 s
International normalized ratio (INR) (0.9–1.2)	1.1
Partial thromboplastin time (PTT) (20–40 s)	33.2 s
Erythrocyte sedimentation rate (ESR) (0–20 mm/h)	135 mm/h
C-reactive protein (CRP) (<5 mg/dL)	41 mg/dL
Lactate dehydrogenase (LDH) (50–150 IU/L)	288 IU/L
Ferritin (15–200 ng/mL)	2963 ng/mL
Haptoglobin (30–200 mg/dL)	368 mg/dL
Thyroid-stimulating hormone (TSH) (0.5–5.0 μIU/mL)	1.0 μIU/mL
Rheumatoid factor (<25 IU/mL)	16 IU/mL
Antinuclear antibodies (ANA) (negative)	1:160
anti-dsDNA (<10)	<10
CA125 (<35 U/mL)	340 U/mL
CEA (<4 μg/L)	1.6 μg/L
Cryoglobulin (negative)	Negative
Blood cultures	Negative
Urinalysis	Unremarkable

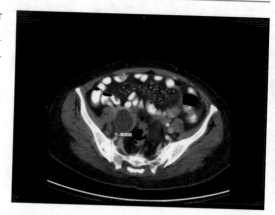

Fig. 25.1 CT scan of the abdomen and pelvis showing right ovarian cystic lesion with infiltrative changes of the omentum

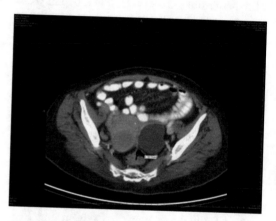

Fig. 25.2 CT scan of the abdomen and pelvis showing a left ovarian cystic lesion

multiple nodules. The diagnosis of a malignancy was strongly entertained.

Because there was only a small amount of ascites noted on the CT scan, no paracentesis was performed, and the patient underwent a diagnostic laparoscopy. This showed severe studding of the abdominal organs and abdominal peritoneal surface with small whitish lesions, dense pelvic adhesions, omental adhesions to the anterior abdominal wall, and a liver with a fibrotic appearance (Fig. 25.3).

A biopsy was obtained from visualized intraabdominal lesions. The pathology showed granulomatous disease consistent with tuberculous peritonitis with no evidence of malignancy. The acid-fast bacillus (AFB) stain was negative. The differential diagnosis is shown in Table 25.2.

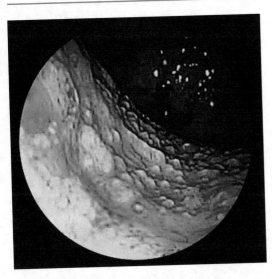

Fig. 25.3 Laparoscopic image showing studded appearance of the omentum

Table 25.2 Differential diagnosis of adnexal masses with peritoneal thickening and ascites

Intraabdominal abscess
Atypical mycobacterial infections
Intraabdominal actinomycosis may cause adnexal mass with extension to the peritoneum
Peritoneal tuberculosis
Ovarian carcinoma
Peritoneal carcinomatosis
Intestinal lymphoma
Ulcerative colitis

25.1 Peritoneal Tuberculosis

Tuberculosis (TB) is a leading global killer. In 2015, 10.4 million people worldwide developed TB and 1.4 million people died from it [1]. In the United States, 9421 active TB cases were reported in the same year, and 66% of the reported cases were in foreign-born individuals. From 1992 to 2014, the number of reported cases of TB in the United States declined each year [2].

Mycobacterium tuberculosis is the etiologic agent of TB. It is an aerobic, non-spore forming, nonmotile, rod-shaped bacterium. It is resistant to the Gram stain due to the presence of large amount of mycolic acid on the cell surface. The Ziehl-Neelsen stain, or acid-fast stain as it is commonly known, is often used instead. *M. tuberculosis* is thus known as an AFB, and among mycobacterial species, it is known as a slow-growing organism, with a generation time between 15 and 20 h. It takes about 4–8 weeks to grow in conventional AFB cultures on solid media versus 12 plus or minus 4 days using liquid media on automated systems [3].

Pulmonary TB is by far the most common form of the disease. Peritoneal TB represents only 1–2% of all cases of TB [4], but it is the most common form of abdominal involvement.

Risk factors for developing peritoneal TB include history of cirrhosis, diabetes mellitus, AIDS, chronic use of systemic corticosteroids, treatment with antitumor necrosis factor agents, underlying malignancy, and continuous ambulatory peritoneal dialysis. Up to 20% of patients have no identifiable risk factors.

Peritoneal TB is commonly associated with a primary focus elsewhere. It is usually due to hematogenous spread from the lung, although surprisingly only in 33% of the cases there is evidence of pulmonary TB on a chest x-ray. It can also result from the reactivation of a latent tuberculous focus in the peritoneum, transmural invasion from infected bowel, lymphatic spread from affected lymph nodes, or contiguous spread of tuberculous salpingitis.

Clinical manifestations of peritoneal TB are nonspecific and usually develop over a period of several months. These include fever, malaise, anorexia, abdominal distension, and pain. The physical examination may show abdominal tenderness and indicate the presence of ascites.

The diagnosis is made by recovery of exudative ascitic fluid with a white blood cell count up to 4000/μL with a lymphocytic predominance. AFB stain and culture are positive in less than 3% and 20% of cases, respectively. Other tests include the measurement of adenosine deaminase level that may have a sensitivity of 100% and specificity of 97% (with a cutoff level of 33 U/L), nucleic acid probes and polymerase chain reaction (PCR) [5, 6], and measurement of CA-125 levels. The diagnosis is mainly achieved by direct visualization of the abdominal cavity with presence of thickened peritoneum studded with multiple whitish nodules or tubercles and adhesions [7]. This alone can be diagnostic in up to 95% of cases. The final diagnosis is made by targeted biopsies that reveal caseating or noncaseating granulomas in up to 95.5% of patients [8].

In some female patients, as in this case, the initial presentation, including history, physical examination, laboratory data with elevated CA-125, and radiological findings suggest a diagnosis of ovarian carcinoma [9]. Therefore, peritoneal tuberculosis should be considered in the differential diagnosis of ovarian carcinoma, especially in women immigrants from countries with a high prevalence of tuberculosis. CA-125 levels are elevated in cases of gynecologic cancers and in certain nonmalignant conditions [10] such as peritoneal TB. In most reported cases, the levels are <500 U/mL. Normalization of the CA-125 level correlates closely with response to antituberculous therapy and can be used a follow-up marker [11].

Mortality from tuberculous peritonitis remains high, up to 50% [12]. Standard anti-tubercular treatment is highly effective in curing this condition. Early diagnosis, although difficult, is the key to improving the outcome of this serious infection.

Key Points/Pearls

- Peritoneal TB, although it represents 1–2% of all cases of TB, is the most common presentation of extrapulmonary TB of the abdominal cavity.
- The diagnosis of peritoneal TB requires a high index of suspicion and should be considered in the differential diagnosis of women with suspected ovarian cancer who present with adnexal mass, peritoneal thickening, ascites, and elevated CA-125 levels, especially if they ever lived in an area of high prevalence of TB.
- Up to 95% of peritoneal TB cases can be diagnosed with direct visualization of the abdominal cavity by laparoscopy.
- Targeted peritoneal biopsy is diagnostic in almost 100% of the cases; AFB smear and culture are low yield.

- Standard antituberculous therapy can achieve cure in the majority of cases, and when elevated, the CA-125 level can be used as a marker for response to therapy.

References

1. Global Tuberculosis Report 2016. World Health Organization. http://www.who.int/tb/publications/global_report/en/. Accessed 22 June 2017.
2. Centers for Disease Control and Prevention. Reported tuberculosis in the United States, 2014. Atlanta: U.S. Department of Health and Human Services, CDC, October 2015. http://www.cdc.gov/tb/statistics/reports/2014. Accessed 22 June 2017.
3. Ghodbane R, Raoult D, Drancourt M. Dramatic reduction of culture time of *Mycobacterium tuberculosis*. Sci Rep. 2014;4:4236.
4. Mimidis K, Ritis K, Kartalis G. Peritoneal tuberculosis. Ann Gastroenterol. 2005;18(3):325–9.
5. Wang YC, Lu JJ, Chen CH, Peng YJ, Yu MH. Peritoneal tuberculosis mimicking ovarian cancer can be diagnosed by polymerase chain reaction: a case report. Gynecol Oncol. 2005;97:961–3.
6. Uzunkoy A, Harma M, Harma M. Diagnosis of abdominal tuberculosis: experience from 11 cases and review of literature. World J Gastroenterol. 2004;10(24):3647–9.
7. Apaydin B, Paksoy M, Bilir M, Zengin K, Saribeyoglu K, Taskin M. Value of diagnostic laparoscopy in tuberculous peritonitis. Eur J Surg. 1999;165:158–63.
8. Cavalli Z, Ader F, Valour F, et al. Clinical presentation, diagnosis, and bacterial epidemiology of peritoneal tuberculosis in two university hospitals in France. Infect Dis Ther. 2016;5(2):193–9.
9. Lataifeh I, Matalka I, Hayajneh W, Obeidat B, Al Zou'bi H, Abdeen G. Disseminated peritoneal tuberculosis mimicking advanced ovarian cancer. J Obstetr Gynaecol. 2014;34(3):268–71.
10. Eltabbakh GH, Belinson JL, Kennedy AW, Gupta M, Webster K, Blumenson LE. Serum CA-125 measurements > 65 U/mL. Clinical value. J Reprod Med. 1997;42(10):617–24.
11. Mas MR, Cömert B, Sağlamkaya U, et al. CA-125; a new marker for diagnosis and follow-up of patients with tuberculous peritonitis. Dig Liver Dis. 2000;32(7):595–7.
12. Chow KM, Chow VC, Hung LC, Wong SM, Szeto CC. Tuberculous peritonitis-associated mortality is high among patients waiting for results of mycobacterial cultures of ascitic fluid samples. Clin Infect Dis. 2002;35:409–13.

Pulmonary Infection in a Patient After Stem Cell Transplantation

Dima Dandachi and Vagish Hemmige

A 69-year-old male with a past medical history of hypertension, diabetes mellitus, and acute myelogenous leukemia (AML) who underwent allogeneic hematopoietic stem cell transplantation (HSCT) presented with recurrent fever and cough.

The patient had undergone allogeneic HSCT from a matched unrelated donor 17 months previously, conditioned by fludarabine, melphalan, and alemtuzumab. His posttransplant course was complicated by graft versus host disease and multiple central venous catheter infections with coagulase-negative *Staphylococcus* spp., vancomycin-resistant *Enterococcus*, *Lactobacillus*, and alpha-hemolytic *Streptococcus*. During his initial course, he also developed a nodular pneumonia, and the subsequent workup included a bronchoscopy that was nondiagnostic. The pneumonia resolved with empiric posaconazole treatment. Sixteen months after the transplant, the patient developed fatigue, low-grade fevers, and cough. Chest x-ray (CXR) showed a new, left lower lobe infiltrate. A sputum culture then grew fluoroquinolone-susceptible *Pseudomonas*, and the Oncology Service subsequently discharged the patient home on moxifloxacin alone. Three weeks later, he presented again with recurrent cough and fever and was readmitted. A CXR showed a new, right lower lobe infiltrate.

The patient had a remote history of symptomatic bradycardia for which he had undergone pacemaker placement. He was a former cigarette smoker (40 pack-years), but he denied any intravenous drug use. He was a retired automobile mechanic and lived at home with his wife and a dog. He had traveled recently to Las Vegas for a short trip to visit casinos.

His medications on admission included acyclovir, fluconazole, and dapsone prophylaxis. He previously had an adverse reaction to imipenem, which caused a rash, and to voriconazole, which caused visual hallucinations.

On physical examination, he was alert and oriented. His temperature was 100.5 °F, heart rate 86 beats per minute, blood pressure 134/94 mmHg, respiratory rate 20 breaths per minute, and oxygen saturation 90% on ambient air. He had mild bilateral crackles at the lung bases and a well-healed, non-tender, non-erythematous surgical scar at the site of the pacemaker pocket on the anterior chest wall. The remainder of his physical examination was unremarkable.

Laboratory values were significant for pancytopenia, with WBC count of 3500/μl, (76% neutrophils, 8% lymphocytes, and 12% monocytes), hemoglobin 11.6 g/dL (normal range, 13.5–17.5 g/dL), and platelet count of 122,000/μL (normal range, 150,000–450,000/μL). Other laboratory

D. Dandachi, M.D. • V. Hemmige, M.D. (✉)
Baylor College of Medicine, Houston, TX, USA
e-mail: Vagish.Hemmige@bcm.edu

© Springer International Publishing AG 2018
M. David, J.-L. Benoit (eds.), *The Infectious Disease Diagnosis*,
https://doi.org/10.1007/978-3-319-64906-1_26

studies, including the basic metabolic panel, liver function tests, lactate dehydrogenase (LDH), total protein, and albumin were normal. Two sets of blood cultures, peripheral blood for Epstein-Barr virus (EBV) and cytomegalovirus (CMV) polymerase chain reaction (PCR), serum *Aspergillus* antigen, *Legionella* urinary antigen test (UAT), pneumococcal-UAT, and *Histoplasma*-UAT were all negative. A nasal swab tested positive for parainfluenza on direct fluorescent antibody (DFA). A sputum culture grew normal flora. A high-resolution computed tomography (CT) scan of the lungs showed bilateral interstitial and nodular infiltrates (Fig. 26.1). Because the patient had fever on presentation, did not have signs of congestive heart failure, was not exposed to radiation, did not receive drugs known to cause lung injury, and did not receive any blood transfusion, we suspected that his symptoms were most likely due to an infection. When the parainfluenza virus (PIV) DFA test came back positive, it was therefore decided to treat him with empiric antibiotics to cover the common bacterial pathogens that cause pneumonia, such as *Staphylococcus aureus* and *Pseudomonas aeruginosa*. The differential diagnosis for diffuse interstitial infiltrates in immunocompromised patients is presented in Table 26.1.

The patient was treated with intravenous (IV) vancomycin, IV aztreonam, and inhaled ribavirin for 5 days; however, he became progressively more hypoxic over the next 10 days. Serial CXR demonstrated the development of an interstitial

Table 26.1 Differential diagnosis of diffuse pulmonary infiltrates in the immunocompromised patient [5]

Infectious causes
Bacteria
– *Mycoplasma pneumoniae*
– *Legionella* spp.
– *Nocardia* spp.
– *Staphylococcus aureus*
– *Pseudomonas aeruginosa*
Viruses
– Cytomegalovirus (CMV)
– Influenza
– Respiratory viruses, especially respiratory syncytial virus (RSV), parainfluenza viruses, adenovirus, and human metapneumovirus
Fungi
– *Pneumocystis jirovecii*
– *Aspergillus* spp.
– Mucormycosis agents
– Histoplasmosis (*Histoplasma capsulatum*)
– Blastomycosis (*Blastomyces dermatitidis*)
Mycobacteria
– *Mycobacterium tuberculosis*
– Nontuberculous mycobacteria, including *M. avium* Complex, *M. kansasii*, and *M. abscessus*
Noninfectious causes
Congestive heart failure
Acute respiratory distress syndrome
Malignancy (leukemic infiltrates, lymphoma, metastatic disease)
Pulmonary hemorrhage
Drug-induced lung injury
Engraftment syndrome
Transfusion-related lung injury
Radiation toxicity

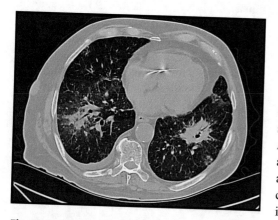

Fig. 26.1 CT scan of the lungs showing diffuse bilateral micronodular and interstitial infiltrates

pattern with diffuse infiltrates. An aminoglycoside was added to cover the possibility of antibiotic-resistant *Pseudomonas* pneumonia because he showed no significant improvement. Subsequently, he had a bronchoscopy without transbronchial biopsy to rule out other etiologies. A bronchoalveolar lavage (BAL) specimen was sent for Gram stain and bacterial culture, acid-fast bacillus (AFB) smear and culture, fungal and viral cultures, and *Pneumocystis jirovecii* DFA testing, which were all negative. We nevertheless began empiric therapy for *P. jirovecii* pneumonia (PJP) with clindamycin and primaquine and also restarted inhaled ribavirin. Over the next several days, the patient's dyspnea progressed, ultimately necessitating intubation. After extensive discussion, he underwent video-assisted thoracoscopy with lung biopsy. Histopathology findings were consistent with viral infection, and DFA testing was positive for *P. jirovecii*. Because the patient had deteriorated while on clindamycin and primaquine, this therapy was changed to trimethoprim/sulfamethoxazole (TMP-SMX).

Subsequently, he was successfully extubated, weaned to room air, and transferred to a rehabilitation facility. At a 6-month follow-up visit, he was doing well, confirming the efficacy of his PJP therapy and resolution of PIV pneumonia. One month later, unfortunately, he was readmitted to our hospital with sepsis. An extensive workup failed to reveal an etiology. He developed multisystem organ failure and he expired. An autopsy was not performed.

26.1 Parainfluenza Pneumonia in Immunocompromised Hosts

Parainfluenza viruses (PIV) are enveloped RNA viruses of the family Paramyxoviridae [1]. PIV are common respiratory pathogens known primarily to cause infection in children. However, immunity is incomplete and reinfection can occur [2]. PIV infection in immunocompromised patients, particularly in the setting of hematologic malignancy, solid organ transplantation, or HSCT [3], is increasingly recognized and can be associated with a wide spectrum of disease, ranging from mild upper respiratory symptoms to pneumonitis and severe respiratory failure. The mortality rate of PIV lower respiratory disease has varied among studies, reaching more than 50% in some reports [2, 3].

When PIV infection is suspected, the diagnosis is made primarily by detection of PIV antigen by direct or indirect fluorescence antibody testing from a nasopharyngeal wash, swab, or BAL, a test with limited sensitivity but high specificity. Viral culture is also used, but it may take several days to return positive. PIV PCR is highly sensitive and specific, but it may not be readily available or may take more time than antibody assays [4]. Recently multiplex

PCR testing has become available for multiple respiratory pathogens including parainfluenza viruses. The University of Chicago lab currently performs the PCR amplification method with analysis by automated nested multiplex PCR by a commercially available assay. The test is performed in house everyday with a 6- to 8-h turnover, and it detects the important respiratory viruses (influenza A; influenza A subtypes H1, H3, and H1-2009; influenza B; respiratory syncytial virus; parainfluenza viruses types 1–4; adenovirus; human metapneumovirus; coronavirus HKU1, NL63, and 229E; and enterovirus/rhinovirus) and three bacterial pathogens (*Mycoplasma pneumoniae*, *Chlamydophila pneumoniae*, and *Bordetella pertussis*).

CT scan of the lungs is usually the preferred imaging modality for identifying pulmonary abnormalities [5, 6]. Radiographic findings in PIV infection are variable; they can be focal or diffuse, interstitial, and alveolar-interstitial infiltrates [2, 7]. Some studies suggest that having multiple small, non-cavitating pulmonary nodules might be indicative of a viral etiology of pneumonia, such as PIV [6].

Currently, no antiviral is approved for treatment of PIV. Small studies and cases reports have shown mixed results regarding the clinical benefit of aerosolized or systemic ribavirin, with or without IV gamma globulin. The majority of studies to date have failed to demonstrate improved outcomes in treated patients in terms of progression to pneumonia, need for mechanical ventilation, duration of illness, or mortality [3, 8]. Many of the patients in these studies had other respiratory co-pathogens, which was associated with higher mortality. Organisms identified included mixed viral infection (e.g., CMV, adenovirus, or respiratory syncytial virus), superimposed bacterial or fungal infection (particularly aspergillosis), and mycobacterial infection [3, 8]. Dual infection with *P. jirovecii* and a respiratory virus has also been reported [9]. Recently, DAS181, a sialidase fusion protein that cleaves Neu5Ac alpha (2,3) and (2,6)-Gal linkages of sialic acid from respiratory endothelial cell surfaces, has been used in 16 HSCT recipients with PIV infection (14 with pneumonia), with complete clinical response in

9 patients and partial in 4. There was no control group in the study. The drug is administered either by oral inhalation using a dry powder inhaler or by nebulizer for intubated patients. It targets a host protein to which PIV binds rather than a viral structure [10].

26.2 Pneumocystis jirovecii Pneumonia (PJP) in Non-HIV-Infected Patients

PJP is caused by the fungus *P. jirovecii*, previously known as *P. carinii*. However, *P. carinii* is now understood to be a separate species that infects rodents, whereas *P. jirovecii* infects humans, hence the name change. Most *P. jirovecii* infections are diagnosed in persons infected with the human immunodeficiency virus (HIV) who have an absolute CD4+ T lymphocyte count below 200 cells/mm^3.

Non-HIV-infected immunocompromised patients are at increased risk for invasive fungal infection including *P. jirovecii* [11]. Consequently, prophylaxis has been recommended with TMP-SMX. However, TMP-SMX use has been limited by adverse reactions such as skin rash, nausea, vomiting, nephrotoxicity, and bone marrow suppression. Dapsone is considered an acceptable alternative despite a higher rate of breakthrough infection [12].

Non-HIV-infected patients who have PJP demonstrate a more acute clinical course, often with delays in treatment initiation and higher mortality compared to patients with HIV infection [13]. TMP-SMX remains the treatment of choice, based primarily on studies in HIV-infected patients [14].

P. jirovecii cannot be cultured, and the diagnosis requires identification of the organism by staining of fluid from an induced sputum, BAL, or lung biopsy specimen by microscopy. DFA staining has become the most commonly used method. In some studies among immunocompromised patients without HIV there was a lower organism burden and a poorer diagnostic yield of conventional staining of a specimen from induced sputum or BAL [15]. Although the *P. jirovecii*

real-time PCR has a higher sensitivity and specificity than DFA and can be particularly useful in this population [16], the test may not be able to differentiate colonization from true infection. Therefore, tissue sampling for diagnosis may be necessary to confirm PJP in non-HIV-infected patients [17].

Key Points/Pearls

- The differential diagnosis of pulmonary infiltrates in the immunocompromised host is broad, and a detailed history and workup are essential to establish a specific etiology.
- Tissue sampling is frequently needed to establish a definitive diagnosis of PJP in non-HIV-infected immunocompromised patients.
- Multiple simultaneous infectious and noninfectious pathologic processes are common in immunocompromised patients.
- PJP should be considered in the differential diagnosis of patients with HIV, as well as immunocompromised patients without HIV who are presenting with pneumonia.
- The mainstay of therapy for PIV infection remains supportive, given the lack of evidence supporting the use of ribavirin or IV gamma globulin, although DAS181, a sialidase fusion protein that cleaves Neu5Ac alpha (2,3) and (2,6)-Gal linkages of sialic acid from respiratory endothelial cell surfaces, has been used in 16 HSCT recipients with PIV infection, with good response in 13 patients.
- Multiplex PCR testing has become available for multiple respiratory pathogens including influenza A; influenza A subtypes H1, H3, and H1-2009; influenza B; respiratory syncytial virus; parainfluenza viruses types 1–4; adenovirus; human metapneumovirus; coronavirus HKU1, NL63, and 229E; enterovirus/rhinovirus; *Mycoplasma pneumoniae*; *Chlamydophila pneumoniae*; and *Bordetella pertussis*.
- In AIDS patients with PJP, the addition of steroids is recommended if the A-a gradient is >35 or PaO$_2$ < 70; the use of steroids in other immunocompromised patients with PJP who meet these criteria is also recommended.
- The most effective drug to treat PJP is high-dose trimethoprim/sulfamethoxazole;

alternatives are clindamycin plus primaquine (test for G6PD deficiency) or pentamidine (much more toxic).

- The prognosis of PJP in non-HIV-infected immunocompromised patients is worse, most likely due to a delay in diagnosis and a more acute presentation.

References

1. Henrickson KJ. Parainfluenza viruses. Clin Microbiol Rev. 2003;16(2):242–64.
2. Lewis VA, Champlin R, Englund J, et al. Respiratory disease due to parainfluenza virus in adult bone marrow transplant recipients. Clin Infect Dis. 1996;23(5):1033–7.
3. Chemaly RF, Hanmod SS, Rathod DB, et al. The characteristics and outcomes of parainfluenza virus infections in 200 patients with leukemia or recipients of hematopoietic stem cell transplantation. Blood. 2012;119(12):2738–45. Quiz 2969.
4. Kuypers J, Campbell AP, Cent A, Corey L, Boeckh M. Comparison of conventional and molecular detection of respiratory viruses in hematopoietic cell transplant recipients. Transpl Infect Dis. 2009;11(4):298–303.
5. Wingard JR, Hiemenz JW, Jantz MA. How I manage pulmonary nodular lesions and nodular infiltrates in patients with hematologic malignancies or undergoing hematopoietic cell transplantation. Blood. 2012;120(9):1791–800.
6. Ferguson PE, Sorrell TC, Bradstock K, Carr P, Gilroy NM. Parainfluenza virus type 3 pneumonia in bone marrow transplant recipients: multiple small nodules in high- resolution lung computed tomography scans provide a radiological clue to diagnosis. Clin Infect Dis. 2009;48(7):905–9.
7. Marcolini JA, Malik S, Suki D, Whimbey E, Bodey GP. Respiratory disease due to parainfluenza virus in adult leukemia patients. Eur J Clin Microbiol Infect Dis. 2003;22(2):79–84.
8. Falsey AR. Current management of parainfluenza pneumonitis in immunocompromised patients: a review. Infect Drug Resist. 2012;5:121–7.
9. Lehner PJ, Rawal B, Hoyle C, Cohen J. Dual infection with Pneumocystis carinii and respiratory viruses complicating bone marrow transplantation. Bone Marrow Transplant. 1992;9(3):213–5.
10. Salvatore M, Satlin MJ, Jacobs SE, et al. DAS181 for treatment of parainfluenza virus infections in hematopoietic stem cell transplant recipients at a single center. Biol Blood Marrow Transplant. 2016;22(5):965–70.
11. Harrison N, Mitterbauer M, Tobudic S, et al. Incidence and characteristics of invasive fungal diseases in allogeneic hematopoietic stem cell transplant recipients: a retrospective cohort study. BMC Infect Dis. 2015;15:584.
12. Stern A, Green H, Paul M, Vidal L, Leibovici L. Prophylaxis for Pneumocystis pneumonia (PCP) in non-HIV immunocompromised patients. Cochrane Database Syst Rev. 2014(10):CD005590.
13. Roux A, Canet E, Valade S, et al. Pneumocystis jirovecii pneumonia in patients with or without AIDS. France Emerg Infect Dis. 2014;20(9):1490–7.
14. Nickel P, Schürmann M, Albrecht H, et al. Clindamycin-primaquine for pneumocystis jiroveci pneumonia in renal transplant patients. Infection. 2014;42(6):981–9.
15. Thomas CF, Limper AH. Pneumocystis pneumonia: clinical presentation and diagnosis in patients with and without acquired immune deficiency syndrome. Semin Respir Infect. 1998;13(4):289–95.
16. Church DL, Ambasta A, Wilmer A, et al. Development and validation of a Pneumocystis jirovecii real-time polymerase chain reaction assay for diagnosis of Pneumocystis pneumonia. Can J Infect Dis Med Microbiol. 2015;26(5):263–7.
17. White DA, Wong PW, Downey R. The utility of open lung biopsy in patients with hematologic malignancies. Am J Respir Crit Care Med. 2000;161(3 Pt 1):723–9.

Moira McNulty

A 38-year-old African American man with a past medical history of human immunodeficiency virus (HIV) infection presented with 1 month of nausea, vomiting, and hiccups that had worsened over the past day. For the previous day he had emesis within 5 min of food intake and associated hiccups. He had one episode of fever prior to admission and noted a dry cough. He reported 20 lb of weight loss over the past month. He did not have dysphagia, odynophagia, hematemesis, or abdominal pain. He denied having chest pain, shortness of breath, palpitations, chills, night sweats, constipation, diarrhea, and urinary symptoms. He had no recent sick contacts and no travel out of the country. He reported that he was admitted 10 days before to a different hospital with the same complaints and was diagnosed with right lower lobe pneumonia and was treated with levofloxacin. He was discharged and was tolerating the medication until the day prior to admission.

His past medical history included HIV infection, which was diagnosed 5 years prior, but he did not seek treatment at the time. He also had hypertension. He had no past surgical history. His family history was significant for diabetes mellitus and

hypertension in his mother. He lived at home with his mother and her partner at the time of presentation, and he was sexually active with men. He worked as a bouncer, drank two shots of alcohol per week, and was in jail for 1 week several years before.

On physical examination he was found to have a temperature of 38.8 °C. His heart rate was 114 beats per minute, respiratory rate 18 breaths per minute, blood pressure 131/82 mmHg, and oxygen saturation 100% on room air. He was in no distress and appeared comfortable. His mouth had no thrush, and he had no cervical lymphadenopathy. No icterus was noted. He was tachycardic with a regular rhythm without murmurs. Crackles were noted in the upper lung fields bilaterally without wheezing. The abdomen was soft and non-tender. No rashes were noted. His joints had no swelling and a normal range of motion. He was alert and oriented with intact cranial nerves.

His labs showed a white blood cell (WBC) count of 4000/μL (normal range, 3500–11,000/μL) (77% neutrophils, 7% bands, 10% lymphocytes), hemoglobin 12.4 g/dL (13.5–17.5 g/dL), and platelets 473,000/μL (150,000–450,000/μL). The complete metabolic panel was remarkable for sodium of 126 mmol/L (normal range, 134–149 mmol/L), potassium 5.6 mmol/L (3.5–5.0 mmol/L), chloride 88 mmol/L (95–108 mmol/L), carbon dioxide 16 mmol/L (23–30 mmol/L), blood urea nitrogen (BUN)

M. McNulty, M.D.
Section of Infectious Diseases and Global Health,
Department of Medicine, University of Chicago,
Chicago, IL, USA
e-mail: moira.mcnulty@uchospitals.edu

© Springer International Publishing AG 2018
M. David, J.-L. Benoit (eds.), *The Infectious Disease Diagnosis*,
https://doi.org/10.1007/978-3-319-64906-1_27

30 mg/dL (7–20 mg/dL), and creatinine 2.3 mg/dL (0.5–1.4 mg/dL). His liver function tests (LFTs) demonstrated a normal bilirubin with elevated aspartate aminotransferase (AST) of 84 U/L (normal range, 8–37 U/L) and alanine aminotransferase (ALT) of 41 U/L (8–35 U/L). His CD4+ T-cell count was 15/μL (normal range, 515–1642/μL), and the blood HIV viral load was 79,593 copies/mL.

A chest x-ray showed upper-lobe predominant interstitial opacities and a nodule at the left costophrenic angle (Fig. 27.1). He then underwent computed tomography (CT) without contrast of the chest, which showed bilateral upper-lobe predominant ground glass opacities and cystic changes, with tree-in-bud nodules in the left lower lobe (Fig. 27.2).

He was started on intravenous (IV) cefepime, vancomycin, and azithromycin as well as high-dose trimethoprim-sulfamethoxazole (TMP-SMX). Bronchoscopy was performed, and the cell count showed 94 total cells with 28 red blood cells and 66 WBC (3% neutrophils, 97% macrophages). The bacterial culture grew normal respiratory flora, and the fungal and acid-fast bacilli (AFB) cultures had no growth. The *Pneumocystis* direct fluorescent antigen (DFA) assay was negative, but *Pneumocystis jirovecii* continued to be on the differential so a Fungitell assay was sent, which tests for β-D glucan found in fungal cell walls. Upon review by the pathologist, there were organisms morphologically consistent with *Pneumocystis* on microscopic examination, and therefore, the DFA assay was repeated and was positive. The Fungitell test came back positive as well.

The patient then developed rash, fevers, and leukopenia. He was found to have rapidly rising LFTs with AST of 1506 U/L and ALT of 734 U/L. He developed altered mental status and became tachypneic with episodes of hypoxia, and prednisone was started. TMP-SMX was discontinued due to rash and fevers. His glucose-6-phosphate dehydrogenase (G-6-PD) level was normal, and he was started on clindamycin with primaquine. The Hepatology Service was consulted and a liver biopsy was performed. He had persistent fevers and elevation of LFTs, and

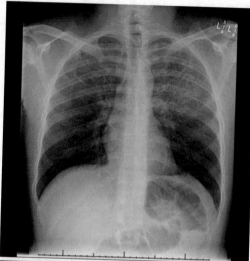
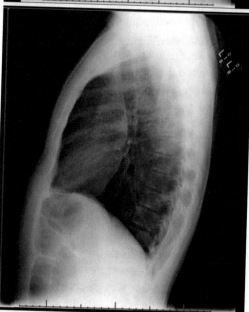

Fig. 27.1 Chest radiograph showing upper-lobe predominant interstitial opacities

therefore, IV acyclovir was initiated due to concern for herpes simplex virus (HSV) hepatitis.

With the initial signs of fever, rash, and rise in LFTs, there was concern that the patient had toxicity to TMP-SMX, which can cause liver injury [1, 2]. When the LFTs continued to rise despite discontinuation of TMP-SMX, it was felt that viral hepatitis could be the etiology. Since he had a rapid rise in AST and ALT with a normal serum bilirubin level, HSV hepatitis

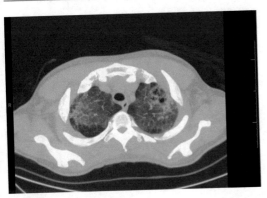

Fig. 27.2 Computed tomography (CT) of the chest with upper-lobe predominant ground glass opacities and cystic changes

was high on the differential. Additional viral studies were sent while awaiting the results of the liver biopsy. These included negative hepatitis A, B, and C antibodies, serum cytomegalovirus (CMV) polymerase chain reaction (PCR), and serum adenovirus PCR. In addition to a potential drug reaction and viral hepatitis, *P. jirovecii* infection of the liver was also a possibility, with concern that inflammation after starting treatment could be the source of the liver injury. Additional causes of acute hepatitis are listed in Table 27.1.

The liver biopsy showed patchy hepatocellular necrosis with small clusters of necrotic hepatocytes, with Gomori methenamine silver (GMS) stains positive for yeast forms consistent with *Pneumocystis*, and an immunohistochemical stain for HSV-1/2 that was positive in the patchy areas of necrosis. A diagnosis of *Pneumocystis* and HSV hepatitis was made. The patient's LFTs began to improve within 3 days of starting IV acyclovir. He continued IV acyclovir with resolution of rash, fevers, and encephalopathy. He was started on highly active antiretroviral therapy for HIV with tenofovir, emtricitabine, and raltegravir. He was discharged to complete a 14-day course of oral valacyclovir for HSV and a 21-day course of clindamycin, primaquine, and prednisone for *P. jirovecii* pneumonia (PJP). His LFTs had normalized at the time of follow-up in Infectious Diseases Clinic 3 weeks later. He continued to follow up in this Clinic and recovered with therapy.

Table 27.1 Differential diagnosis of acute hepatitis [1–3]

Noninfectious
Drug-induced[a]
Acetaminophen
Alcohol
Antibiotics
Isoniazid
Rifampin
Azole antifungals
Nitrofurantoin
Amoxicillin-clavulanate
Minocycline
Trimethoprim-sulfamethoxazole
Phenytoin
Herbal remedies
Ischemic hepatitis
Autoimmune hepatitis
Budd-Chiari syndrome
Wilson's disease
Acute fatty liver of pregnancy
Infectious
Hepatitis A, B, C, D, or E viruses
Cytomegalovirus (CMV)
Varicella zoster virus (VZV)
Epstein-Barr virus (EBV)
Herpes simplex virus (HSV) 1, 2
Adenovirus
Human immunodeficiency virus (HIV)
Yellow fever virus
Dengue
Typhoid fever (*Salmonella typhi*)
Q fever (*Coxiella burnetii*)
Brucellosis
Leptospirosis
Human herpesvirus 6 (HHV-6)
Parvovirus B19
Lyme disease (*Borrelia burgdorferi*)
Syphilis (*Treponema pallidum*)
Bartonellosis

[a]Partial list

27.1   *Pneumocystis jirovecii* in HIV

P. jirovecii is a fungal pathogen that most commonly affects immunocompromised individuals and is considered an opportunistic infection in individuals infected with HIV [3]. The likeli-

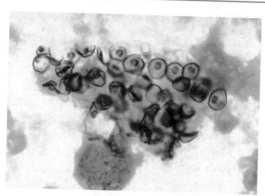

Fig. 27.3 Methenamine silver stain showing cysts of *Pneumocystis jirovecii* in a smear from bronchoalveolar lavage. Source: http://phil.cdc.gov/phil/details_linked.asp?pid=554 (Accessed June 22, 2017)

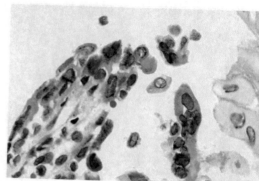

Fig. 27.4 Histopathology of an esophageal ulcer in a patient with AIDS showing intranuclear inclusions and multinucleation due to herpes simplex virus infection. Source: http://phil.cdc.gov/phil/details_linked.asp?pid=957 (Accessed June 22, 2017)

hood of *P. jirovecii* infection increases with lower CD4+ T-cell counts (usually with counts <200/μL) [3]. It most frequently manifests as pneumonia, but less commonly may have extrapulmonary manifestations in those with advanced HIV, affecting the lymph nodes, spleen, liver, eyes (chorioretinitis), and bone marrow [4]. Diagnosis of extrapulmonary infection is made by biopsy with pathology examination by GMS stain or fluorescent monoclonal antibody stain (Fig. 27.3) [3].

27.2 Herpes Simplex Virus (HSV) Hepatitis

Hepatitis is a rare complication of HSV infection, with HSV representing less than 1% of all cases of acute liver failure [5]. It is characterized by fever and abrupt elevation in transaminases with mild bilirubin elevation (usually anicteric), often without mucocutaneous lesions [3, 5]. It can lead to fulminant hepatic necrosis and may progress to liver failure requiring transplant or causing death if not recognized and treated promptly [6]. HSV hepatitis most commonly affects immunosuppressed and pregnant patients, but has been reported in healthy individuals [3]. Compromised cellular immunity is a major risk factor for severe and disseminated disease [7]. The diagnosis is

made by pathological examination of a liver biopsy specimen. Because HSV hepatitis is not frequently suspected, the diagnosis is often made after death [5]. If suspected, experts recommend immediate treatment with IV acyclovir [3].

Persistent and recurrent HSV infections are a common clinical presentation in patients infected by HIV, usually manifesting as mucocutaneous lesions [3]. Reactivation of HSV is more common in HIV-infected individuals and is associated with low CD4+ T-cell counts and high HIV viral load [3]. HSV can also cause esophagitis (Fig. 27.4), keratitis with large ulcers, and acute retinal necrosis in persons with HIV infection. Disseminated disease and hepatitis due to HSV are rare, however, even in advanced disease [8].

Key Points/Pearls
- Individuals with advanced HIV infection may experience more than one infection at any given time.
- HSV is an uncommon but severe cause of acute viral hepatitis, more often seen in immunocompromised hosts and pregnant women.
- If hepatitis due to HSV is suspected, prompt initiation of intravenous acyclovir is recommended.
- The diagnosis of HSV hepatitis is made by liver biopsy, and the case fatality rate is high.

References

1. Polson JE. Hepatotoxicity due to antibiotics. Clin Liver Dis. 2007;11:549–61.
2. Bernal W, Auzinger G, Dhawan A, Wendon J. Acute liver failure. Lancet. 2010;376:190–201.
3. Curry MP, Chopra S. Acute viral hepatitis. In: Mandell GL, Dolin R, Bennett JE, editors. Mandell, Douglas, and Bennett's principles and practice of infectious diseases. Philadelphia, PA: Churchill Livingstone; 2010. p. 1577–92.
4. U.S. Centers for Disease Control and Prevention. DPDx—Laboratory identification of parasitic diseases of public health concern: *Pneumocystis*. Page last updated 29 Nov 2013. http://www.cdc.gov/dpdx/pneumocystis/. Accessed 22 June 2017.
5. Norvell JP, Blei AT, Jovanovic BD, Levitsky J. Herpes simplex virus hepatitis: an analysis of the published literature and institutional cases. Liver Transpl. 2007;13(10):1428–34.
6. Gelven PL, Gruber KK, Swiger FK, Cina SJ, Harley RA. Fatal disseminated herpes simplex in pregnancy with maternal and neonatal death. South Med J. 1996;89(7):732–4.
7. Kaufman B, Gandhi SA, Louie E, Rizzi R, Illei P. Herpes simplex virus hepatitis: case report and review. Clin Infect Dis. 1997;24(3):334–8.
8. Panel on Opportunistic Infections in HIV-Infected Adults and Adolescents. Guidelines for the prevention and treatment of opportunistic infections in HIV-infected adults and adolescents: recommendations from the Centers for Disease Control and Prevention, the National Institutes of Health, and the HIV Medicine Association of the Infectious Diseases Society of America. http://aidsinfo.nih.gov/contentfiles/lvguidelines/adult_oi.pdf. Accessed 22 June 2017 [O1-O7].

28

A Real Nail-Biter

Jessica Ridgway

A 67-year-old man with multiple myeloma presented with neutropenic fever for 2 days and pain and swelling of his left third finger for 7 days. He had no history of trauma to the finger but admitted that he occasionally bit his fingernails. His oncologist had prescribed clindamycin 4 days before for treatment of finger cellulitis, but he had no improvement in his symptoms.

Two weeks before, he had received chemotherapy with cisplatin, cytoxan, doxorubicin, and etoposide. He had been neutropenic for 8 days. In addition to fever and finger swelling, he also reported mild oral mucositis. He denied headache, cough, rhinorrhea, diarrhea, or other localizing symptoms. He had no pets or exposure to animals. He was originally from the United Arab Emirates, but denied any recent travel. He reported no sick contacts.

His medications included prophylactic antibiotics that were prescribed per protocol for chemotherapy-induced neutropenia, including moxifloxacin, fluconazole, and acyclovir.

On physical examination, temperature was 38.3 °C, blood pressure 144/75 mmHg, heart rate 99 beats per minute, respiratory rate 18 breaths per minute, and oxygen saturation 99% on room air. He was in no acute distress. Oral exam revealed mild mucositis, a known side effect of his chemotherapy. He had no sinus tenderness or cervical lymphadenopathy. Cardiac, pulmonary, and abdominal examinations were normal. His left third finger showed evidence of paronychia with surrounding erythema, warmth, and tenderness. There was no fluctuance or drainage. He had a tunneled central line in the right side of his chest without surrounding erythema, warmth, tenderness, or drainage.

Complete blood count was remarkable for a white blood cell (WBC) count of 100/μL (4500–11,000/μL) with 20% neutrophils (50–60%), hemoglobin of 7.1 g/dL (13.5–17.5 g/dL), and platelets of 16,000/μL (150,000–450,000/μL). He was thus profoundly neutropenic with an absolute neutrophil count (ANC) below 100/μL. His electrolytes, creatinine, and blood urea nitrogen were within normal limits. The C-reactive protein was 164 mg/dL (<5 mg/dL). A chest x-ray was normal, and a left third finger x-ray showed soft tissue swelling but no bony abnormalities.

The patient was presumed to have a bacterial cellulitis as the cause of his neutropenic fever. The differential diagnosis for bacterial pathogens causing neutropenic fever is shown in Table 28.1 [1]. The patient was initially treated with intravenous (IV) vancomycin and IV imipenem for empiric coverage of neutropenic fever and cellulitis, and blood cultures were collected. The

J. Ridgway, M.D., M.S.
Section of Infectious Diseases and Global Health,
Department of Medicine, University of Chicago,
Chicago, IL, USA
e-mail: Jessica.Ridgway@uchospitals.edu

© Springer International Publishing AG 2018
M. David, J.-L. Benoit (eds.), *The Infectious Disease Diagnosis*,
https://doi.org/10.1007/978-3-319-64906-1_28

Table 28.1 Bacterial pathogens causing neutropenic fever

Gram-positive bacteria	Staphylococcus aureus
	Coagulase-negative Staphylococcus spp.
	Streptococcus spp.
	Enterococcus spp.
	Corynebacterium jeikeium
	Bacillus spp.
	Listeria monocytogenes
Gram-negative bacteria	Escherichia coli
	Pseudomonas aeruginosa
	Klebsiella spp.
	Enterobacter spp.
	Citrobacter spp.
	Acinetobacter spp.
	Stenotrophomonas maltophilia
	Proteus spp.
	Serratia spp.
	Capnocytophaga spp.
	Legionella spp.
	Moraxella spp.
	Neisseria meningitidis
Other	Clostridium difficile
	Other anaerobes
	Mycobacteria

patient defervesced on hospital day 3. He was treated with filgrastim (granulocyte colony-stimulating factor [G-CSF]), and his neutropenia resolved on day 4. A blood culture drawn on admission became positive on hospital day 5 for Gram-negative rods in the anaerobic bottle. It later speciated as *Capnocytophaga* species.

While *Capnocytophaga canimorsus* and *C. cynodegmi* are usually associated with dog or cat bites, other *Capnocytophaga* species are found in the oral flora of humans, such as *C. gingivalis*, *C. sputigena*, and *C. ochracea*. In immunocompetent hosts, *Capnocytophaga* can cause gingivitis and periodontal disease. In neutropenic patients, it is a rare cause of bacteremia. Severe mucositis is a risk factor for bacteremia in immunocompromised hosts. For the patient presented in this vignette, he likely acquired the infection by biting his fingernails, which led to paronychia, finger cellulitis, and secondary bacteremia. The patient was discharged home to complete a 14-day course of therapy with IV imipenem and recovered well.

28.1 *Capnocytophaga* Species

Capnocytophaga (*capno*, smoke, i.e., carbon dioxide requirement; *cytophaga*, cell eater, i.e., cell wall eater) is a facultative anaerobic, fastidious, slow-growing, fusiform, Gram-negative rod that grows better on blood agar and in the presence of 5–10% CO_2 and exhibits gliding motility. *Capnocytophaga* is found in the oral cavities of dogs, cats, and humans.

Two *Capnocytophaga* species are found in the oral cavity of dogs and cats. *C. canimorsus* (from the Latin words for dog bite), which is typically transmitted to humans via dog bites, can lead to septic shock, disseminated intravascular coagulation, purpura fulminans, and skin necrosis. *C. canimorsus* sepsis can affect immunocompetent individuals, but higher incidence is associated with asplenia, chronic liver disease, alcoholism, and immunocompromise. Mortality for *C. canimorsus* sepsis is approximately 25% [2]. *C. cynodegmi* (from the Greek words for dog bite) also is present in the oral cavity of dogs and cats, and can be transmitted by dog bites, but mostly causes skin and soft tissue infections, with rare case reports of bacteremia [3].

Other *Capnocytophaga* species are found in humans, including *C. gingivalis*, *C. granulosa*, *C. haemolytica*, *C. ochracea*, and *C. sputigena*. These species most commonly cause gingivitis, subgingival plaque, and periodontal disease, but they can also lead to bacteremia in neutropenic patients; endocarditis, subdural empyema, or brain abscess in immunocompetent patients after dental work; ocular infections in the elderly or immunosuppressed; or chorioamnionitis in pregnant women [4]. There are also case reports of *Capnocytophaga* spp. causing peritonitis, septic arthritis, soft tissue infections, osteomyelitis, pulmonary empyema, and liver abscess. *Capnocytophaga* spp. are susceptible to clindamycin, tetracycline, imipenem, and β-lactam/β-lactamase inhibitor combination drugs. These species have had an increasing incidence of β-lactamase production (up to 70% in one series). Fluoroquinolones, metronidazole, aminoglycosides, and macrolides have variable susceptibility [5].

Key Points/Pearls

- *Capnocytophaga* spp. are Gram-negative bacilli found in the oral cavities of dogs, cats, and humans.
- *C. canimorsus* from dog bites can cause septic shock with disseminated intravascular coagulation and purpura, and it is associated with a high mortality.
- *C. cynodegmi* usually causes local infection after dog bites.
- Other *Capnocytophaga* spp. are part of the normal human oral flora and typically cause gingivitis in immunocompetent hosts.
- *Capnocytophaga* spp. are a rare cause of bacteremia in neutropenic patients and are associated with severe mucositis.
- It is difficult to identify *Capnocytophaga* to the species level by conventional biochemical methods; 48–72-h incubation is required to identify the colonies.
- Matrix-assisted laser desorption/ionization time-of-flight mass spectrometry (MALDI-TOF MS) has been helpful in speeding up identification of the genus and species.
- Purpura fulminans (i.e., intravascular thrombosis with skin necrosis, disseminated intravascular coagulation, and hypotension) is a feature of septicemia due to *Neisseria meningitidis*, *Vibrio vulnificus*, *Capnocytophaga canimorsus*, and other Gram-negative bacilli; of rickettsioses like Rocky Mountain spotted fever (RMSF); occasionally of Gram-positive sepsis by *Staphylococcus aureus* and β-hemolytic streptococci; of disseminated viral infection in immunocompromised hosts including varicella-zoster virus and measles; and rarely of falciparum malaria.
- Dog and cat bites can lead to multiple infectious complications, including rabies (rare in the USA), as well as skin and soft tissue infections due to *Staphylococcus aureus*, β-hemolytic streptococci, *Fusobacterium*, and other anaerobes and important Gram-negative bacilli including *Pasteurella multocida* and *P. canis* (which cause rapidly progressive skin and soft tissue infection), *Capnocytophaga canimorsus*, and *C. cynodegmi*.
- Dogs carry ticks that can transmit RMSF.
- A tetanus booster is recommended for a dog bite [6].

References

1. Freifeld AG, Bow EJ, Sepkowitz KA, et al. Clinical practice guideline for the use of antimicrobial agents in neutropenic patients with cancer: 2010 update by the Infectious Diseases Society of America. Clin Infect Dis. 2011;52(4):e56–93.
2. Lion C, Escande F, Burdin JC. *Capnocytophaga canimorsus* infections in human: review of the literature and cases report. Eur J Epidemiol. 1996;12(5):521–33.
3. Khawari AA, Myers JW, Ferguson DA, et al. Sepsis and meningitis due to *Capnocytophaga cynodegmi* after splenectomy. Clin Inf Dis. 2005;40(11):1709–10.
4. Martino R, Ramila E, Capdevila JA, et al. Bacteremia caused by *Capnocytophaga* species in patients with neutropenia and cancer: results of a multicenter study. Clin Infect Dis. 2001;33(4):E20–2.
5. Jolivet-Gougeon A, Sixou JL, Tamanai-Shacoori Z, Bonnaure-Mallet M. Antimicrobial treatment of *Capnocytophaga* infections. Int J Antimicrob Agents. 2007;29(4):367–73.
6. Abrahamian FM, Goldstein EJC. Microbiology of bite infections. Clin Microbiol Rev. 2011;24(2):231–46.

29

Nodular Skin Lesions in a Patient with Leukemia

Daniela Pellegrini

A 45-year-old female with a history of breast cancer underwent curative chemotherapy and lumpectomy complicated by therapy-related acute lymphoblastic leukemia (ALL). At the time of presentation, she was suffering from a second relapse of ALL after multiple chemotherapy regimens over 3 years and a hematopoietic stem cell transplant (HSCT) approximately 6 months before. She had received intrathecal chemotherapy 3 days prior to her admission. She presented with 2 days of syncope, headaches, and generalized weakness.

Three years prior to the current presentation, she developed pancytopenia and was diagnosed with ALL by bone marrow biopsy. She promptly began chemotherapy at that time. Her subsequent course was complicated by neutropenic fevers and oral mucositis despite being on acyclovir and levofloxacin prophylaxis. She underwent a HSCT approximately 18 months after her ALL diagnosis, but the ALL relapsed. She restarted chemotherapy, and although her course was again complicated by neutropenic fevers, she was eventually discharged home. At the time of presentation, she was prescribed posaconazole prophylaxis.

On the morning of admission, the patient was walking down a flight of stairs at home when she lost consciousness for approximately 30 s. She had felt weak for 2 days prior. She was caught by her husband and did not fall or suffer any head trauma. There was no seizure-like activity, nor any bowel or urinary incontinence. The patient denied any fevers, chills, night sweats, or weight change. She had no vision or hearing changes, chest pain, shortness of breath, cough, abdominal pain, nausea, vomiting, diarrhea, constipation, dysuria, hematuria, myalgias, arthralgias, focal weakness, skin rash, changes in speech, memory problems, easy bruising, or bleeding.

Her medications included levofloxacin, posaconazole, acyclovir, hydroxyurea, allopurinol, and ergocalciferol. Her chemotherapy was on hold. Her past surgical history included a mastectomy, and her family history was not contributory. She was born in the United States and had no recent travel outside of the Midwest.

On physical examination, the tympanic temperature was 36.4 °C (97.5 °F). Her blood pressure was 103/71 mmHg and pulse 91 beats per minute. Her respiratory rate was 14 breaths per minute and oxygen saturation 98% on room air. She appeared uncomfortable lying in bed but was alert and cooperative. She had no conjunctival pallor or injection and there was no icterus. She had no nasal discharge, and her oropharynx was pink with moist mucous membranes. Her neck was supple with full range of motion. The cardiac,

D. Pellegrini, M.D.
Section of Infectious Diseases and Global Health,
Department of Medicine, University of Chicago,
Chicago, IL, USA
e-mail: Daniela.Pellegrini@uchospitals.edu

© Springer International Publishing AG 2018
M. David, J.-L. Benoit (eds.), *The Infectious Disease Diagnosis*,
https://doi.org/10.1007/978-3-319-64906-1_29

pulmonary, musculoskeletal, and neurologic examination was normal. No lower extremity edema was appreciated, and there were no rashes or bruises seen. She had no costophrenic angle or suprapubic tenderness. She had no appreciable lymphadenopathy, and her extremities were warm and well perfused.

The serum glucose was 117 mg/dL, alkaline phosphatase was 118 U/L, aspartate aminotransferase (AST) was 31 U/L (normal range, 8–37 U/L), and alanine aminotransferase (ALT) was 54 U/L (8–35 U/L), while the rest of the metabolic panel was within normal limits. The white blood cell (WBC) count was 6400/μL, hemoglobin was 18.4 g/dL (normal range, 13.5–17.5 g/dL), and platelets were 63,000/μL (150,000–450,000/μL). The prothrombin time (PT) was 13.6 s and the international normalized ratio (INR) was 1.0.

Computerized tomography (CT) of the head at the time of admission showed no acute intracranial hemorrhage and only mild thickening of the maxillary sinus mucosa with a mucous retention cyst, along with thickening of the ethmoid sinus. A chest x-ray and transthoracic echocardiogram were normal. A CT of the chest performed 1 week prior showed prominent mediastinal lymph nodes and splenomegaly with clear lungs.

On day 4 of admission, the Dermatology Service was consulted for a new rash of the right upper arm and anterior neck that was first noted 2 days prior (Fig. 29.1). One lesion on the right dorsal foot was violaceous. The lesions were firm, red, and tender to palpation but there was no pruritus. In addition her anterior legs were noted to have numerous scattered petechiae and ecchymoses in areas of trauma and bandaging.

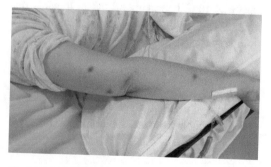

Fig. 29.1 Right upper extremity lesions

The patient was afebrile on admission but developed neutropenic fevers during the hospitalization. She had negative blood cultures and a normal lumbar puncture. There was concern for varicella zoster virus exposure in the Emergency Department, and the patient was therefore treated prophylactically with valacyclovir. Her WBC count steadily increased with an increasing number of blasts. Antimicrobial medications started empirically at that time were cefepime and micafungin in addition to valacyclovir.

A skin punch biopsy was obtained. The differential diagnosis is shown in Table 29.1. The Ear, Nose, Throat (ENT) Service was consulted given her mucosal thickening, and biopsies were taken. Upon further investigation, it was found that although posaconazole was prescribed prior to admission, it had not been taken as directed.

The patient was eventually found to have fungemia, with *Fusarium* growing from several blood cultures. She was also diagnosed with invasive fungal sinusitis by pathological examination of the ENT biopsies. The skin biopsy specimens also demonstrated the presence of fungi with hyphae. Given the concern for disseminated fungal infection, liposomal amphotericin B was added to micafungin several days prior to the diagnosis of fusariosis. The

Table 29.1 Differential diagnosis of skin lesions in neutropenic fever

Bacterial infections:
Ecthyma gangrenosum
Gram negatives, especially *Pseudomonas aeruginosa*
Septic emboli complicating bacteremia
Fungal infections
Yeast:
Candida spp.
Cryptococcus (uncommon)
Molds
Aspergillus spp.
Fusarium spp.
Zygomycetes (*Mucor, Rhizopus, Rhizomucor*, etc.)
Dimorphic (endemic) fungi (uncommon)
Viruses
Herpes simplex virus, type 1 (HSV-1)
Varicella zoster virus (VZV)
Noninfectious
Leukemia cutis
Sweet syndrome

patient had a central venous catheter in place that could not be removed given the lack of alternative vascular access. Her blood cultures cleared, but she developed respiratory failure, possibly due to volume overload. She was intubated and mechanically ventilated, and she unfortunately expired shortly thereafter.

29.1 *Fusarium* Species

Fusarium spp. are ubiquitous and found in soil and plant debris. They are also present worldwide in water. *Fusarium* can grow on a wide variety of surfaces and materials including soil [1]. The principle portable of entry for *Fusarium* species is the airways, followed by the skin at a site of tissue breakdown and possibly mucosal membranes. Airborne fusariosis is thought to be acquired by the inhalation of airborne fusarial conidia, leading to sinusitis and pneumonia in the absence of dissemination. Infections after skin trauma or other damage support this as a portal of entry as well [2]. Water-related activities such as showering appear to be an effective dispersion mechanism of airborne fusarial conidia [1].

29.2 Fusariosis: Clinical Presentation and Pathogenesis

Fusarium spp. infections in humans may present in a variety of ways. The dissemination of a *Fusarium* spp. infection within a host depends on the immune status and the portal of entry. *Fusarium* infections have been classified as locally invasive, superficial, and disseminated. Disseminated infections most often occur in immunocompromised patients [1, 2]. Prolonged neutropenia is a strong risk factor as it is for invasive aspergillosis and other invasive mold infections. Patients with fusariosis who have neutropenia have higher fungal burdens than immunocompetent hosts. Acute leukemia and HSCT are both risk factors for *Fusarium* infections. Locally invasive *Fusarium ssp.* infections may also develop after solid organ transplantation, usually after recovery from surgery; however, the literature suggests that the risk of fusariosis is higher among HSCT patients [1].

Disseminated fusariosis most commonly presents as a combination of characteristic skin lesions and blood cultures that are positive for *Fusarium* spp., with or without lung or sinus involvement. The prognosis is poor and determined by the degree of immunosuppression and the extent of infection. Mortality is nearly 100% in those who are persistently neutropenic with disseminated disease [1].

Fusarium spp. possess virulence factors including mycotoxins that suppress both humoral and cellular immunity. They may contribute to tissue breakdown during infection. These pathogens also produce proteases and collagenases. *Fusarium* spp. can adhere to prosthetic material, complicating therapy. Among immunocompetent hosts, keratitis (including as a complication of contact lens use) and onychomycosis are the most common infections. Less frequently, an infection may occur secondary to skin breakdown, as seen in burns or wounds. *Fusarium* spp. may also cause sinusitis, septic arthritis, osteomyelitis, peritonitis in the setting of peritoneal dialysis, pneumonia, endophthalmitis, thrombophlebitis, and fungemia with or without invasive disease of internal organs [1, 2].

Clinical manifestations of *Fusarium* in immunocompromised patients include endophthalmitis; sinusitis, which can be clinically indistinguishable from infections caused by *Aspergillus* species; pneumonia; and skin lesions that may appear erythematous and papular or nodular, may be painful, and frequently have central necrosis [1]. Target lesions may also be present; bullae are rarer. *Fusarium* spp. skin lesions evolve rapidly, usually over a few days. There is generally a predominance of lesions in the extremities, but they can involve any skin site. Lesions at different stages may be present in 30% of patients with concomitant myalgias (suggesting muscle involvement) in 15%. Skin lesions, in one study, were the source of diagnosis in the majority of patients who presented with the above described lesions [1, 2].

Positive blood cultures among patients with fusariosis are characteristic, in contrast to those with aspergillosis, who rarely have positive blood cultures. Occasionally, in fact, fungemia is the only manifestation of fusariosis in patients who have a central venous catheter in place.

29.3 Diagnosis and Treatment of Fusariosis

Diagnosis of fusariosis depends on the clinical form of the disease. As stated above, skin involvement and positive blood cultures suggest disseminated disease. Confirmation of the diagnosis may require histopathologic examination of tissue from a biopsy. The findings of hyphae and yeast-like structures together are highly suggestive of *Fusarium* species, distinguishing them from dimorphic (endemic) and other pathogenic fungi. The 1,3-β-D-glucan test is usually positive in invasive *Fusarium* spp. infections but cannot distinguish *Fusarium* from other fungal infections [1]. Skin lesions can be appreciated early in the disease and are often observed in disseminated cases [2].

Those with localized fusariosis are likely to benefit from surgical debridement. The optimal treatment strategy with severe infection remains unclear, given the lack of clinical trials and the critical role of immune reconstitution in fusariosis outcomes. For those with disseminated infections, it is recommended that initially amphotericin B and/or an effective azole antifungal drug (voriconazole, posaconazole, or isavuconazole) be started. This initial therapy can then be adjusted if necessary with the availability of susceptibility testing results. Surgical debridement of infected tissue and removal of infected foreign bodies are recommended when possible. The duration of therapy varies and depends on the site and extent of the disease, the immune status, and the response to therapy. Granulocyte colony-stimulating factor (G-CSF) is frequently used in immunocompromised patients, especially in the setting of persistent neutropenia. However, the role of G-CSF has not been established in randomized trials [1].

Key Points/Pearls

- Infections caused by *Fusarium* spp. are often disseminated or invasive in immunocompromised people, particularly those with prolonged or profound neutropenia.
- Clinical data to support the diagnosis of fusariosis often include skin lesions and positive blood cultures.
- Prognosis is poor in immunocompromised hosts with *Fusarium* spp. infections.
- Recommendations for treatment include antifungals, surgical debridement of infected tissue, removal of infected prosthetic materials when possible, and consideration of adjuvant therapy with G-CSF.
- Always request a skin biopsy in patients with neutropenic fever and skin nodules; also perform PCR for HSV and VZV when the rash is consistent.
- Molds rarely grow in blood cultures, but patients with fusariosis frequently have positive blood cultures.
- *Fusarium* is suspected when both hyphae and yeast-like structures are identified on skin biopsy or blood cultures.

References

1. Nucci M, Anaissie E. *Fusarium* infections in immunocompromised patients. Clin Microbiol Rev. 2007;20(4):695–704.
2. Gupta AK, Baran R, Summerball RC. *Fusarium* infections of the skin. Curr Opin Infect Dis. 2000;13(2):121–8.

Elderly Man with Fever and Cough: TB or Not TB?

30

Moira McNulty

An 81-year-old man presented with productive cough, subjective fevers, chills, and malaise for 5 days prior to admission to the hospital. He had paroxysms of productive cough accompanied by light-headedness and dizziness. He also had nasal congestion. He tried over-the-counter cough syrup without relief. He did not have shortness of breath or hemoptysis. He was treated for a similar episode approximately 10 months prior, at which time he was diagnosed with pneumonia due to a consolidation seen on chest x-ray. He was prescribed azithromycin. His symptoms improved, but his wife noticed that he was wheezing over the previous several months, although he was not known to have chronic lung disease. Of note, the patient remembered being diagnosed with tuberculosis in his teens and he was treated with home remedies. He recovered and did not have further pulmonary symptoms until soon before his presentation. On review of systems, he reported that he had no weight loss or night sweats. He had no sore throat, abdominal pain, nausea, vomiting, or diarrhea. He had chronic, mild, bilateral lower extremity edema.

The patient had a history of hypertension, type 2 diabetes mellitus, hyperlipidemia, psoriasis, osteoarthritis, and carpal tunnel syndrome.

Prior to admission he was taking a daily baby aspirin, metformin, rosuvastatin, and topical triamcinolone cream. He had no known medication allergies. His family history was significant for diabetes mellitus in his mother and sister. He was married with four grown children and two grandchildren. He was a retired physical education teacher and was very active, exercising daily. He did not use tobacco, alcohol, or illicit drugs. His hobbies included gardening, carpentry, and music, and he traveled extensively in the United States (US) and abroad, with his last international travel to Vietnam occurring 5 years prior.

On physical examination, his temperature was 38.5 °C, heart rate 102 beats per minute, blood pressure 115/90 mmHg, respiratory rate 22 breaths per minute, and oxygen saturation 93% on room air. He appeared well but fatigued. His oropharynx did not have exudate, and he had no cervical lymphadenopathy. His heart exam revealed tachycardia with a regular rhythm, and there were no murmurs noted. He had no increased work of breathing, but he did have decreased breath sounds at the bases of the lungs bilaterally, early expiratory wheezes in all lung fields, and crackles in the left lung. He had trace bilateral lower extremity pitting edema. His cranial nerves were intact and he had no sensory or strength deficits. He had no skin rash and his joints were normal without swelling or pain. He had a normal mood and affect.

M. McNulty, M.D.
Section of Infectious Diseases and Global Health, Department of Medicine, University of Chicago, Chicago, IL, USA
e-mail: moira.mcnulty@uchospitals.edu

© Springer International Publishing AG 2018
M. David, J.-L. Benoit (eds.), *The Infectious Disease Diagnosis*,
https://doi.org/10.1007/978-3-319-64906-1_30

His lab results showed a white blood cell (WBC) count of 5700/μL (normal range, 3500–11,000/μL) (67% neutrophils, 10% monocytes, and 22% lymphocytes), hemoglobin of 13.2 g/dL (13.5–17.5 g/dL), and platelets of 165,000/μL (150,000–450,000/μL). The complete metabolic panel showed normal electrolytes, the blood urea nitrogen (BUN) was 17 mg/dL (normal range, 7–20 mg/dL), and the creatinine was 1.5 mg/dL (0.5–1.4 mg/dL). His liver function tests demonstrated a normal bilirubin with a slightly elevated aspartate aminotransferase (AST) of 42 U/L (normal range, 8–37 U/L) and normal alanine aminotransferase (ALT). He had a lactase dehydrogenase level of 319 U/L (normal range, 116–245 U/L). Urine *Legionella* and *Streptococcus pneumoniae* antigens were negative. Blood cultures were negative. He had a positive interferon gamma release assay (used to diagnose active or latent *Mycobacterium tuberculosis* infection), non-reactive human immunodeficiency virus (HIV) antibody test, and a positive polymerase chain reaction (PCR) test for influenza A virus.

His chest radiograph (Fig. 30.1) showed a left upper lobe airspace opacity consistent with pneumonia, but an underlying mass or malignancy could not be ruled out. Computed tomography (CT) of the chest (Fig. 30.2) was performed and showed a consolidation of the left upper lobe and a large mass that narrowed the left upper lobe

bronchi, along with two areas of ill-defined opacity in the right lower lobe. The CT also showed mediastinal lymphadenopathy and bilateral non-specific adrenal gland nodularity.

His acute presentation was believed to be due to influenza A pneumonia with possible superimposed bacterial pneumonia, so he was started on ceftriaxone, vancomycin, azithromycin, and oseltamivir. The differential diagnosis (Table 30.1) for the lung mass included infectious causes such as *M. tuberculosis*, atypical mycobacterial infection, endemic fungal infections (e.g., blastomycosis, coccidioidomycosis, or histoplasmosis), lung abscess, and septic emboli. Possible non-infectious causes included primary lung cancer, metastatic cancer, lymphoma, and sarcoidosis.

The patient was placed on airborne precautions due to the possibility of active pulmonary tuberculosis, and three daily sputum samples were collected for acid-fast bacilli (AFB) smear and culture. He was tested for *Blastomyces* antibody and urinary *Histoplasma* antigen, which were negative. He underwent bronchoscopy with transbronchial biopsies performed in the left upper lobe as well as bronchoalveolar lavage (BAL) for cytology and bacterial, fungal, and AFB cultures. He underwent a positron emission tomography (PET) scan (Fig. 30.3), which showed increased activity in a cavitary lesion in the superior segment of the right lower lobe, the

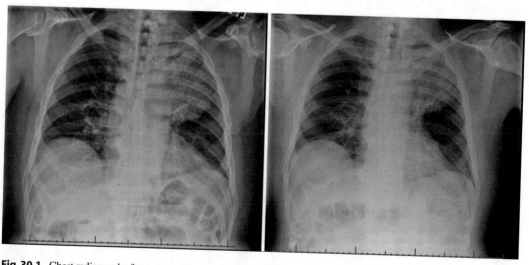

Fig. 30.1 Chest radiographs from current hospital admission (*left*) and from 10 months prior (*right*), showing persistent left upper lobe airspace opacity

left upper lobe, mediastinal and supraclavicular lymph nodes, the spleen, and both adrenal glands, findings which were suspicious for neoplasm.

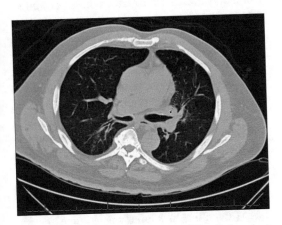

Fig. 30.2 Computed tomography (CT) of the chest showing narrowing of the left upper bronchus due to mass effect

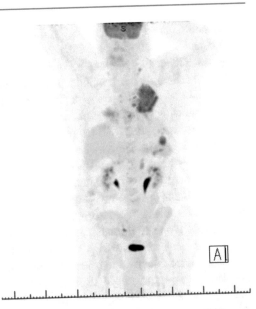

Fig. 30.3 Positron emission tomography (PET) scan with increased activity in a lesion in the superior segment of the right lung lower lobe, the left lung upper lobe, mediastinal and supraclavicular lymph nodes, spleen, and adrenal glands

Table 30.1 Differential diagnosis of persistent lung consolidation [1]

Noninfectious
Primary lung cancer
Metastatic cancer
Lymphoma
Sarcoidosis
Churg-Strauss syndrome
Granulomatosis with polyangiitis
Cryptogenic organizing pneumonia (COP)
Pulmonary hemorrhage
Pneumonitis associated with systemic lupus erythematosus, anti-synthetase syndrome, and other autoimmune conditions
Drug-induced infiltrates (e.g., amiodarone)
Interstitial lung diseases
Infectious
Mycobacterium tuberculosis
Non-tuberculous mycobacterial infection
Histoplasmosis (*Histoplasma capsulatum*)
Blastomycosis (*Blastomyces dermatitidis*)
Coccidioidomycosis (*Coccidioides immitis*)
Cryptococcosis (*Cryptococcus spp.*)
Aspergillosis (*Aspergillus spp.*)
Lung abscess
Septic emboli
Nocardia spp.
Pulmonary actinomycosis

Sputum and BAL samples revealed 1+ AFB on smear. Due to concern for advanced disseminated tuberculosis infection, he was started empirically on rifampin, isoniazid, pyrazinamide, and ethambutol (RIPE) therapy along with pyridoxine. Bacterial BAL cultures grew normal flora, and fungal cultures were negative. He completed a course of ceftriaxone for bacterial pneumonia and oseltamivir for influenza. Hematopathology results from the transbronchial biopsy showed a B cell lymphoma consistent with marginal zone lymphoma.

He was continued on RIPE therapy and his symptoms improved with no further cough and improved energy. Several weeks later, *Mycobacterium kansasii* grew in culture from the BAL. Pyrazinamide was discontinued, and he continued on rifampin, isoniazid, and ethambutol, which he tolerated well. He was not immediately started on therapy for lymphoma because his symptoms improved on treatment for *M. kansasii*. A CT of the chest and abdomen was repeated 3 months after initiation of *M. kansasii* treatment and showed a stable left upper lobe pulmonary consolidation, right lower lobe cavitary lesions, unchanged enlarged lymph nodes, and enlarged splenic and adrenal masses with new enlarged peritoneal adenopathy. Treatment for *M. kansasii* was continued, and after 6 months of therapy his sputum cultures were negative. A PET scan was repeated showing progression of his lesions, and he developed weight loss and fatigue despite therapy for *M. kansasii*. Biopsy of a left neck mass showed transformation to diffuse large B cell lymphoma (DLBCL), so his hematologist initiated chemotherapy with low-dose cyclophosphamide, doxorubicin, vincristine, prednisone (mini-CHOP), and rituximab. He completed six cycles and achieved remission of the DLBCL with significant improvement in his symptoms. He also underwent a total of 18 months of treatment for *M. kansasii*, completing 12 months of therapy after his sputum cultures cleared.

30.1 *Mycobacterium kansasii* Pulmonary Infection

M. kansasii is a slow-growing non-tuberculous mycobacterium (NTM) that is endemic in parts of the USA, recovered from tap water consistently and also rarely from other environmental sources [2, 3]. In the USA *M. kansasii* is the second most common NTM to cause human infections after *M. avium* complex and seems to predominate in the southern and central parts of the country [3]. It can affect individuals of any age, sex, or race but has been most frequently reported in middle-aged white men [3]. *M. kansasii* most commonly occurs as pulmonary disease. Its presentation is variable, but symptoms are similar to pulmonary tuberculosis including cough with or without sputum production, fatigue, malaise, fever, hemoptysis, chest pain, and weight loss [2, 3]. Risk factors for pulmonary infection include structural lung disease, such as bronchiectasis, pneumoconiosis, and chronic obstructive lung disease, and previous mycobacterial disease including prior tuberculosis infection, malignancy, gastroesophageal reflux disease, alcoholism, steroid use, and other immunocompromising conditions [2–5]. *M. kansasii* can also occur as a disseminated infection, primarily in patients with acquired immunodeficiency syndrome (AIDS) or other immunocompromising conditions such as hematologic malignancy and stem cell transplantation. It less commonly presents as isolated skin or bone infection [2, 3].

Guidelines for diagnosis of *M. kansasii* and other NTM pulmonary infections include both clinical and microbiologic findings. Clinical findings consist of pulmonary symptoms, chest radiograph with nodular or cavitary opacities or CT that shows multifocal bronchiectasis with small nodules, and exclusion of other diagnoses. Microbiologic criteria include positive culture results from at least two sputum samples or positive culture results from at least one BAL or lung biopsy with mycobacterial histopathologic features (granulomatous inflammation or AFB) and positive culture [3]. Patients who are suspected of having NTM pulmonary infection but do not meet diagnostic criteria should be followed closely until the diagnosis can be made or excluded [3]. *M. kansasii*, along with *M. marinum* and *M. szulgai*, can produce a positive interferon gamma release assay, a test used to diagnose active or latent tuberculosis [6].

First-line antibiotics for treatment of pulmonary infection with *M. kansasii* include rifampin, ethambutol, and isoniazid, although clarithromycin may be substituted for rifampin in the event of resistance or intolerance [2, 3, 7]. Treatment failure is associated with rifampin resistance, so initial susceptibility testing is recommended for rifampin and clarithromycin. If rifampin resistance is present, then further susceptibility testing should be performed and treatment chosen based on those results [2, 3, 7]. Treatment is continued until respiratory cultures are negative on therapy for 12 months [3].

Key Points/Pearls

- *M. kansasii* is a slow-growing non-tuberculous mycobacterium (NTM) that can be found in environmental sources such as tap water.
- *M. kansasii* most frequently causes pulmonary disease although it can also cause disseminated disease in immunocompromised individuals and less frequently skin or bone infections.

- Diagnosis of *M. kansasii* pulmonary infection is based on a combination of clinical and microbiologic criteria.
- *M. kansasii*, *M. marinum*, and *M. szulgai* may produce a positive interferon γ release assay (IGRA), an in vitro test that measures the release of interferon γ by lymphocytes in response to specific *M. tuberculosis* antigens (ESAT-6 and CFP-10).
- IGRA is used to help diagnose active or latent tuberculosis infection.
- *M. kansasii* is effectively treated by the combination of rifampin, isoniazid, and ethambutol, which are included in the empiric RIPE treatment for tuberculosis.
- When a diagnostic culture identifies *M. kansasii*, empiric pyrazinamide should be stopped, because this drug is inactive in NTM infection.

References

1. Pappas PG. Chronic pneumonia. In: Mandell GL, Dolin R, Bennett JE, editors. Mandell, Douglas, and Bennett's principles and practice of infectious diseases. Philadelphia, PA: Churchill Livingstone; 2010. p. 931–45.
2. Brown-Elliott BA, Wallace RJ. Infections due to nontuberculous mycobacteria other than *Mycobacterium avium-intracellulare*. In: Mandell GL, Dolin R, Bennett JE, editors. Mandell, Douglas, and Bennett's principles and practice of infectious diseases. Philadelphia, PA: Churchill Livingstone; 2010. p. 3191–8.
3. Griffith DE, Aksamit T, Brown-Elliott BA, et al. An official ATS/IDSA statement: diagnosis, treatment, and prevention of nontuberculous mycobacterial diseases. Am J Respir Crit Care Med. 2007;175(4):367–416.
4. Maliwan N, Zvetina JR. Clinical features and follow up of 302 patients with *Mycobacterium kansasii* pulmonary infection: a 50 year experience. Postgrad Med J. 2005;81:530–3.
5. Prevots DR, Marras TK. Epidemiology of human pulmonary infection with nontuberculous mycobacteria: a review. Clin Chest Med. 2015;36(1):13–34.
6. Andersen P, Munk ME, Pollock JM, Doherty TM. Specific immune-based diagnosis of tuberculosis. Lancet. 2000;356(9235):1099–104.
7. CLSI. Susceptibility testing of mycobacteria, nocardiae, and other aerobic actinomycetes; approved standard—second edition. CLSI document M24-A2. Wayne, PA: Clinical and Laboratory Standards Institute; 2011.

Malaise, Fever, and Nausea in a Man with Marfan Syndrome

Dima Dandachi and Vagish Hemmige

A 37-year-old male with Marfan syndrome was admitted to the hospital with several weeks of low-grade fevers. At age 21 years, he had a type A thoracic aortic dissection for which he underwent an aortic valve replacement with a St. Jude mechanical valve and aortic root repair, and then at the age of 36 years, he was diagnosed with an abdominal aortic aneurysm (AAA) dissection requiring a bypass graft repair. Extensive evaluation including transesophageal echocardiogram (TEE) was unrevealing; however, his fevers resolved with empiric antibiotics, and he was diagnosed with presumed culture-negative prosthetic valve endocarditis. He was discharged on intravenous (IV) ceftriaxone and vancomycin administered through a peripherally inserted central catheter (PICC) with oral rifampin. Rifampin was subsequently discontinued when he developed symptomatic hemolytic anemia with associated fever.

Four weeks later, he presented with a 1-week history of fatigue, malaise, and intermittent fever. He also complained of chills, night sweats, mild headache, and nausea. On admission, he was afebrile, with a temperature of 98.6 °F, heart rate 95 beats per minute, blood pressure 120/68 mmHg,

respiratory rate 18 breaths per minute, and oxygen saturation 99% on room air. Cardiovascular exam revealed a III/VI systolic heart murmur at the right upper sternal border, mechanical sound of S2, and no jugular venous distention. His lungs were clear to auscultation bilaterally. The abdominal exam showed a well-healed, midline scar, and the abdomen was soft, non-tender, and not distended, with normal bowel sounds and no evidence of hepatosplenomegaly. The lower extremities were warm and well perfused without edema. The PICC insertion site was clean, non-tender, and non-erythematous.

The white blood cell (WBC) count was 7000 cells/μL, hemoglobin 11.4 g/dL, and platelet count 295,000/μL. Other laboratory studies, including the basic metabolic panel, were normal. C-reactive protein was elevated at 44 mg/L (normal range, <3 mg/L). Two sets of blood cultures obtained on admission grew a yeast, and therefore the patient was started empirically on liposomal amphotericin B (AmB) and flucytosine. The PICC line was removed. The yeast was identified as *Candida lusitaniae*, and the antifungal coverage was changed to IV micafungin. Repeat TEE did not demonstrate any vegetation on the valves or any mass lesions. A high-resolution computed tomography (CT) of the chest, abdomen, and pelvis with contrast showed stable aortic aneurysm after thoracic repair and abdominal aortic bypass graft. The patient

D. Dandachi, M.D. • V. Hemmige, M.D. (✉)
Baylor College of Medicine, Houston, TX, USA
e-mail: Vagish.Hemmige@bcm.edu

cleared his candidemia after 5 days of treatment. He was discharged on IV micafungin in stable condition.

However, 2 weeks after discharge, the patient presented again with similar symptoms of fever, chills, nausea, and fatigue. This time, blood cultures were positive for *Pseudomonas fluorescens/putida* and coagulase negative *Staphylococcus* spp. He was treated with IV vancomycin and piperacillin-tazobactam and was continued on IV micafungin. Surveillance blood cultures were obtained to evaluate for resolution of the bacteremia. Surprisingly, blood cultures again grew *C. lusitaniae* and remained positive for more than 2 weeks. A repeat TEE was again negative. CT of the chest, abdomen, and pelvis showed emboli in the liver and spleen. Because of concern for seeding of the aortic mechanical valve or the aortic graft, an indium-tagged leucocyte scan was performed but was negative. The Cardiothoracic Surgery Service was consulted, but considering the patient's multiple previous aortic operations, they felt that the patient's operative risk was prohibitive. In light of persistent candidemia, oral flucytosine 25 mg/kg/dose four times daily and oral fluconazole 800 mg daily were added to IV micafungin, with subsequent clearing of blood cultures. The patient received a total of 6 weeks of flucytosine, micafungin, and high-dose fluconazole and 6 further weeks of micafungin and fluconazole dual therapy. He was then changed to a suppressive dose of oral fluconazole. The patient had multiple readmissions in subsequent years for other medical conditions including bowel obstruction, incarcerated hernia, and subarachnoid hemorrhage with no evidence of recurrence of the *Candida* infection.

31.1 *Candida lusitaniae*

While more than 20 *Candida* spp. cause human disease, 90% of all invasive disease is caused by just five *Candida* spp. listed in Table 31.1. Despite an increase in non-albicans *Candida* spp. invasive infections, *C. lusitaniae* remains uncommon [1, 2]. For most cases of invasive *C. lusitaniae* infection reported in the literature, the organism was

Table 31.1 Most common *Candida* species

Species	Characteristics
C. albicans	The most common species causing invasive *Candida* infection in the USA
	Incidence of resistance remains low
C. krusei	Strongly associated with prior fluconazole prophylaxis and neutropenia
	Intrinsically resistant to fluconazole
	Usually susceptible to posaconazole and echinocandins
	Decreased susceptibility to amphotericin B
	Usually resistant to flucytosine
C. glabrata	Associated with prior fluconazole use
	Many isolates are resistant to fluconazole and are generally resistant to voriconazole
C. parapsilosis	Emerged as nosocomial pathogen, frequently associated with central venous catheters and blood stream infection
	Susceptible to most antifungal agents
C. tropicalis	Associated with poor outcomes in neutropenic patients
	Usually susceptible to the azoles, amphotericin B, and the echinocandins

isolated from blood cultures. Major risk factors for candidemia were the presence of an indwelling intravenous catheter, recent abdominal surgery, and use of broad-spectrum antibiotics [3]. *Candida* spp. in the blood should not be considered a contaminant and should prompt initiation of therapy and a search for a focus of infection.

Different classes of systemic antifungal therapy used for *Candida* infection are listed in Table 31.2. In vitro antifungal susceptibility testing is becoming increasingly important to guide therapy because of increasing resistance. However, in vitro susceptibility does not always correlate with favorable clinical response [4]. In addition, a standard method for testing susceptibility has been developed by the Clinical and Laboratory Standards Institute (CLSI) and the European Committee on Antimicrobial Susceptibility Testing (EUCAST), but clinical breakpoints for susceptibilities have not been established for all *Candida* spp. and all drugs [2].

Table 31.2 Classes of systemic antifungal agents used in the treatment of candidiasis [11]

Antifungal class			
Triazoles	Echinocandins	Polyenes	Flucytosine
• Fluconazole • Itraconazole • Voriconazole • Posaconazole • Isavuconazole	• Caspofungin • Anidulafungin • Micafungin	• AmB deoxycholate • Lipid formulations of AmB (liposomal AmB, AmB lipid complex)	• Flucytosine
Mechanism of action			
Inhibits the cytochrome P450-dependent enzyme lanosterol 14-α-demethylase converting lanosterol to ergosterol (component of the fungal cellular membrane)	Inhibits of the synthesis of 1,3-β-D-glucan (component of the fungal cell wall)	Binds to ergosterol and forms pores leading to leakage of cellular components	Interferes with both DNA and RNA synthesis of fungal cells after uptake and conversion into 5-fluorouracil
Common adverse events			
As a class GI SE, hepatitis, prolongation of QT interval on electrocardiogram	Well tolerated, rare histamine-mediated facial flushing or swelling	Nephrotoxicity, acute infusion- related reaction (fever, chills, rigors), hypokalemia, hypomagnesemia; fewer SE with lipid formulations	Bone marrow suppression, GI SE, hepatitis
Spectrum of activity			
Active against many *Candida* spp. Fluconazole is less active against *C. glabrata* and inactive against *C. krusei*	Active against most *Candida* spp. including azole-resistant strains Resistance appears to be on the rise, most notably among *C. glabrata* isolates *C. parapsilosis* may be less responsive to the echinocandins	Broadest antifungal activity, active against most *Candida* spp.; however *C. lusitaniae* can be resistant	Broad antifungal activity against most *Candida* spp., except for *C. krusei* Resistance can develop rapidly if used as monotherapy

AmB amphotericin B, *GI* gastrointestinal, *SE* side effects

C. lusitaniae has a unique antifungal susceptibility pattern that is different from other Candida spp. The pattern varies among studies depending on the methodology used and the population studied, posing a therapeutic challenge. Most studies have shown either a high rate of AmB resistance or acquired resistance on therapy following exposure to AmB [5, 6]. Isolates with acquired resistance to AmB can also develop cross resistance to fluconazole and itraconazole [7]. However, despite some reported resistance, the majority of isolates are still susceptible to triazoles, including posaconazole and voriconazole [8]. Echinocandin resistance in *C. lusitaniae*, particularly to caspofungin, is rare but has been described [8]. Decreased susceptibility of *C. lusitaniae* to flucytosine has been demonstrated

in some studies, and induced fluconazole resistance has also been reported [8, 9]

31.2 Treatment of Candidemia

Candidemia can be a complication of an infected vascular catheter or a manifestation of deep-seated infection. Recent guidelines recommend echinocandins as first-line therapy for candidemia in non-neutropenic patients based on studies showing an improved survival when compared to AmB or triazole therapy and fewer drug-related adverse events [10]. As an alternative, fluconazole can be used as initial therapy when the patient is not critically ill and unlikely to have resistant *Candida* spp. infection. AmB use should be considered in cases of intolerance or resistance to other antifungals [11]. A step-down approach to fluconazole after initial therapy is recommended if patient is clinically stable, has negative blood cultures, and has a susceptible *Candida* isolate [11].

Duration of therapy for candidemia without a metastatic focus has not been studied well; however, guidelines published in 2016 by the Infectious Diseases Society of America (IDSA) recommend 2 weeks of therapy after blood cultures have become negative. When blood cultures remain positive, it is recommended to seek out a focus of infection in order to attain source control [11].

Whether combination antifungal therapy is more effective than monotherapy for invasive candidiasis, including candidemia, remains controversial; moreover, there are theoretical concerns that AmB and azoles may interact antagonistically [12]. However, antagonism was not noted in a large study comparing AmB combined with fluconazole to fluconazole monotherapy in the treatment of candidemia. In Kaplan-Meier analysis, 30-day success was not significantly different between the two arms ($p = 0.08$); however, failure to clear candidemia was more prevalent in the monotherapy group (17%) than the combination group (6%) [13]. Flucytosine is usually used in combination with AmB in the treatment of refractory cases, *Candida* endocarditis and central nervous system candidiasis [11] because of in vitro synergism and because resistance develops rapidly when flucytosine is used as monotherapy [14]. Successful outcomes have been reported with other antifungal combinations such as azoles with echinocandins and polyenes with echinocandins, but data are limited [15].

Suppressive therapy with lifelong fluconazole after treatment has been described in patients with *Candida* endocarditis for whom cardiac surgery was contraindicated, as well as patients with infected artificial implants that cannot be removed, as for the patient in the present case [11, 16].

Key Points/Pearls

- In recent years, there has been an increase in incidence of *Candida* spp. infections caused by more resistant non-albicans species.
- Echinocandins are the first-line empirical therapy for candidemia, but antifungal susceptibility testing is increasingly used to guide therapy.
- Antifungal susceptibility for *C. lusitaniae* is unique: the yeast is often resistant to or quickly acquires resistance on therapy with amphotericin B.
- *Candida* spp. produce biofilm that allow them to stick to foreign bodies, such as prosthetic heart valves, vascular grafts, intravascular catheters, and cardiac devices; removal of the foreign body is required to cure infection, but when this is not possible, suppression with oral azole therapy is an option.
- In cases of candidemia, it is recommended to obtain an ophthalmology evaluation to rule out endophthalmitis, which may cause blindness and requires a combination of surgery and prolonged therapy with antifungal agents that reach adequate concentrations within the eyes.

References

1. Pfaller MA, Andes DR, Diekema DJ, Horn DL, Reboli AC, Rotstein C, et al. Epidemiology and outcomes of invasive candidiasis due to non-albicans species of *Candida* in 2,496 patients: data from the Prospective Antifungal Therapy (PATH) registry 2004–2008. PLoS One. 2014;9(7):e101510.
2. Pfaller MA, Messer SA, Woosley LN, Jones RN, Castanheira M. Echinocandin and triazole antifungal susceptibility profiles for clinical opportunistic yeast and mold isolates collected from 2010 to 2011: application of new CLSI clinical breakpoints and epidemiological cutoff values for characterization of geographic and temporal trends of antifungal resistance. J Clin Microbiol. 2013;51(8):2571–81.
3. Kullberg BJ, Arendrup MC. Invasive candidiasis. N Engl J Med. 2015;373(15):1445–56.
4. Fernández-Ruiz M, Aguado JM, Almirante B, Lora-Pablos D, Padilla B, Puig-Asensio M, et al. Initial use of echinocandins does not negatively influence outcome in *Candida parapsilosis* bloodstream infection: a propensity score analysis. Clin Infect Dis. 2014;58(10):1413–21.
5. Miller NS, Dick JD, Merz WG. Phenotypic switching in *Candida lusitaniae* on copper sulfate indicator agar: association with amphotericin B resistance and filamentation. J Clin Microbiol. 2006;44(4):1536–9.
6. Atkinson BJ, Lewis RE, Kontoyiannis DP. *Candida lusitaniae* fungemia in cancer patients: risk factors for amphotericin B failure and outcome. Med Mycol. 2008;46(6):541–6.
7. Favel A, Michel-Nguyen A, Peyron F, Martin C, Thomachot L, Datry A, et al. Colony morphology

switching of *Candida lusitaniae* and acquisition of multidrug resistance during treatment of a renal infection in a newborn: case report and review of the literature. Diagn Microbiol Infect Dis. 2003;47(1):331–9.

8. De Carolis E, Sanguinetti M, Florio AR, La Sorda M, D'Inzeo T, Morandotti GA, et al. In vitro susceptibility to seven antifungal agents of *Candida lusitaniae* isolates from an Italian University Hospital. J Chemother. 2010;22(1):68–70.

9. Chapeland-Leclerc F, Bouchoux J, Goumar A, Chastin C, Villard J, Noël T. Inactivation of the FCY2 gene encoding purine-cytosine permease promotes cross-resistance to flucytosine and fluconazole in *Candida lusitaniae*. Antimicrob Agents Chemother. 2005;49(8):3101–8.

10. Andes DR, Safdar N, Baddley JW, Playford G, Reboli AC, Rex JH, et al. Impact of treatment strategy on outcomes in patients with candidemia and other forms of invasive candidiasis: a patient-level quantitative review of randomized trials. Clin Infect Dis. 2012;54(8):1110–22.

11. Pappas PG, Kauffman CA, Andes DR, Clancy CJ, Marr KA, Ostrosky-Zeichner L, et al. Clinical practice guideline for the management of candidiasis: 2016 update by the Infectious Diseases Society of America. Clin Infect Dis. 2016;62(4):e1–50.

12. Sugar AM. Use of amphotericin B with azole antifungal drugs: what are we doing? Antimicrob Agents Chemother. 1995;39(9):1907–12.

13. Rex JH, Pappas PG, Karchmer AW, Sobel J, Edwards JE, Hadley S, et al. A randomized and blinded multicenter trial of high-dose fluconazole plus placebo versus fluconazole plus amphotericin B as therapy for candidemia and its consequences in nonneutropenic subjects. Clin Infect Dis. 2003;36(10):1221–8.

14. Barchiesi F, Arzeni D, Caselli F, Scalise G. Primary resistance to flucytosine among clinical isolates of *Candida* spp. J Antimicrob Chemother. 2000;45(3):408–9.

15. Johnson MD, MacDougall C, Ostrosky-Zeichner L, Perfect JR, Rex JH. Combination antifungal therapy. Antimicrob Agents Chemother. 2004;48(3):693–715.

16. Lye DC, Hughes A, O'Brien D, Athan E. *Candida glabrata* prosthetic valve endocarditis treated successfully with fluconazole plus caspofungin without surgery: a case report and literature review. Eur J Clin Microbiol Infect Dis. 2005;24(11):753–5.

Diarrhea Leads to Pneumonia and Hematuria in the Intensive Care Unit

32

Lindsay A. Petty

A 26-year-old male with a past medical history of Crohn's disease, in remission for more than 10 years, presented to the Medical Intensive Care Unit (MICU) with diarrhea, hematuria, left-sided pulmonary infiltrates, transaminitis, and rapid-onset respiratory failure with acute kidney injury (AKI). The patient was well until 7 days prior to ICU admission, when he developed severe non-bloody diarrhea, approximately 20 times daily. Three days prior, he presented to an emergency department (ED) and was sent home after rehydration with normal saline with a reportedly normal chest x-ray (CXR). Two days prior, he presented to his primary care provider with continued diarrhea and fever to 39.4 °C, and he was sent home with anti-diarrheal medications. One day prior, he returned to the ED with chest tightness, shortness of breath, and cough productive of dark sputum, and he was found to have a new left-sided infiltrate on CXR, consistent with a pneumonia. He also reported dark urine and anorexia. He denied nausea, vomiting, abdominal pain, rash, or dysuria. In the ED, he was noted to be febrile with a temperature of 40.6 °C, tachycardic with a heart rate of 140 beats per minute, tachypneic with a respiratory rate of 29 breaths per minute and blood pressure of 115/65 mmHg, and hypoxic with an oxygen saturation of 93% on 4 L per minute of oxygen supplementation. He was transitioned to bilevel positive airway pressure (BIPAP) due to his increased work of breathing and hypoxia and received empiric antibiotic therapy and steroids, including intravenous (IV) ceftriaxone, azithromycin, and linezolid. He was then transferred to the University of Chicago Medicine MICU. His respiratory status worsened, and after about 5 h he was intubated. The patient had eaten no recent restaurant foods and had no known sick contacts. He worked as a pipe fitter. He denied having pets, unusual hobbies, or travel within the previous 6 months.

On physical examination, his heart rate was 150 beats per minute, blood pressure 100/50 mmHg, temperature 39.1 °C, and respiratory rate 28 breaths per minute. He was intubated and sedated. He did not have any cervical adenopathy, and his conjunctivae were injected. His pulmonary exam demonstrated crackles bilaterally, and cardiovascular exam revealed a normal S1 and S2 with no murmurs. Pulses were equal, but capillary refill was slow, approximately 3 s. Abdominal exam showed normal liver and spleen to palpation and was nontender. He did not have any rashes.

Initial serum laboratory results on transfer to the MICU included white blood cell (WBC) count of 11,900/μL (92% neutrophils, 3% lymphocytes), hemoglobin of 14.1 g/dL, and platelet count of 195,000/μL. The basic metabolic panel was within

L.A. Petty, M.D.
University of Michigan, Ann Arbor, MI, USA
e-mail: lindsay.a.petty@gmail.com

normal limits, with blood urea nitrogen of 16 mg/dL and creatinine of 1.0 mg/dL. Liver function tests showed elevated transaminases, with an alanine aminotransferase (ALT) of 1353 U/L (normal range, 8–35 U/L) and an aspartate aminotransferase (AST) of 356 U/L (8–37 U/L).

Seven hours later, his creatinine had risen to 1.9 mg/dL (normal range, 0.5–1.4 mg/dL) and the transaminases to ALT of 1877 U/L and AST of 501 U/L. He also had a markedly elevated creatine kinase (CK) of 180,620 U/L (9–185 U/L) and elevated lactate of 4.5 mmol/L (0.6–2.2 mmol/L). Urinalysis revealed 3+ blood, 3+ protein, 3–5 red blood cells (RBC), and 0 WBC, raising the question of rhabdomyolysis given the elevation in CK and the 3+ blood on urinalysis with only 3–5 RBCs. Further infectious labs known at this point are in Table 32.1; they were significant for only a positive polymerase chain reaction (PCR) for adenovirus from a nasopharyngeal swab. By this time, his chest imaging had worsened with bilateral airspace opacities and consolidations, as well as a left-sided effusion (Fig. 32.1).

Given the combination of pneumonia, diarrhea, transaminitis, and acute kidney injury (AKI), the diagnostic picture appeared to be a disseminated infection. It was clarified that the patient was not at that point, nor had he ever been treated with immunosuppressive medications for Crohn's disease. The differential diagnosis for his constellation of symptoms is shown in Table 32.2. When a disseminated infection is found in an immunocompetent host, one should question if there is an unknown underlying immunodeficiency, and undiagnosed human immunodeficiency virus (HIV) should be considered. His HIV antibody test from blood was negative, but the question of acute HIV remained, so a serum viral load was also checked that was also negative. Given his residence in the Midwest, histoplasmosis and blastomycosis were the

Table 32.1 Laboratory results

Laboratory test	Result	Normal values
Blood urea nitrogen	24 mg/dL	7–20 mg/dL
Creatinine	1.9 mg/dL	0.5–1.4 mg/dL
Total bilirubin	0.4 mg/dL	
Alanine aminotransferase	1877 U/L	8–35 U/L
Aspartate aminotransferase	501 U/L	8–37 U/L
Alkaline phosphatase	75 mg/dL	30–120 U/L
White blood cell count	8200/μL	3500–11,000/μL
Creatine kinase	180,620 U/L	9–185 U/L
Lactate, blood	4.5 mmol/L	0.6–2.2 mmol/L
Urinalysis	3 + blood/3 + protein/3–5 red blood cells/0 white blood cells	
2 blood cultures	No growth	
2 respiratory cultures	Normal flora	
Urine culture	No growth	
Stool culture	No growth	
Rotavirus antigen, stool	Negative	
C. difficile stool polymerase chain reaction (PCR)	Negative	
Human immunodeficiency virus (HIV) serology	Nonreactive	
Respiratory viral panel, PCR[a]	Adenovirus positive	
Cytomegalovirus PCR, blood	Negative	
Epstein-Barr virus (EBV) PCR, blood	Negative	
Legionella antigen, urine	Negative	

[a]Polymerase chain reaction test for the following pathogens: adenovirus, coronavirus 229E, coronavirus HKU1, coronavirus OC43, coronavirus NL63, human metapneumovirus, human rhinovirus/enterovirus, influenza A, influenza A/H1, influenza A/H1-2009, influenza A/H3, influenza B, parainfluenza 1, parainfluenza 2, parainfluenza 3, parainfluenza 4, respiratory syncytial virus (RSV), Bordetella pertussis, Chamydophila pneumoniae, and Mycoplasma pneumoniae

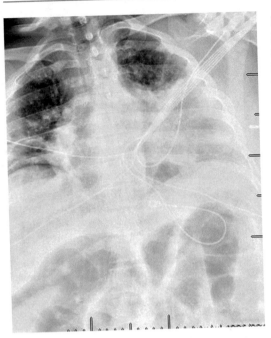

Fig. 32.1 Chest radiograph at time of intubation, showing airspace opacities and consolidations, as well as a left-sided pleural effusion

Table 32.2 Differential diagnosis for diarrhea, pneumonia, transaminitis, and hematuria

Hemophagocytic lymphohistiocytosis or immune reaction to adenovirus
Histoplasmosis (*Histoplasma capsulatum*)
Blastomycosis (*Blastomyces dermatitidis*)
Cytomegalovirus (CMV)
Epstein-Barr virus (EBV)
Disseminated adenovirus infection
Hepatitis B virus
Hepatitis C virus
Herpes simplex virus (HSV)
Acute human immunodeficiency virus (HIV) infection
Legionella pneumonia with rhabdomyolysis

endemic infections considered. Most of the diseases listed in Table 32.2 are more likely to cause disseminated disease in an immunocompromised host, but they occasionally cause disseminated disease in the absence of an immunocompromising condition.

Given the positive result of the nasopharyngeal qualitative PCR sample for adenovirus, a serum quantitative adenovirus PCR was emergently run in the microbiology laboratory. It was also positive, with 1,967,036 viral copies per mL. The patient was treated with cidofovir, and hemodialysis was initiated for what was determined to be rhabdomyolysis. Over the next week, his viral load decreased and he was extubated. He was discharged from the hospital still on hemodialysis, but with hope for recovery of renal function.

32.1   Adenovirus

Adenovirus was first isolated from human adenoid tissue in 1950 [1]. The virus was initially detected in military recruits in the setting of acute respiratory illnesses but was later found to have a broad spectrum of disease manifestations, including gastroenteritis, hepatitis, keratoconjunctivitis, meningoencephalitis, cystitis, upper and lower respiratory tract infections, and myocarditis [2].

Adenoviruses are non-enveloped, lytic, double-stranded DNA viruses responsible for typically self-limited illness. Children, military recruits, and college students are the most commonly affected groups [3]. Adenovirus infections occur worldwide, year-round, and infect most individuals by age 10 years. The virus is spread via aerosol droplets, by fecal-oral spread, by contact with contaminated fomites, through cervical/perinatal transmission, and by solid organ transplantation (kidney and liver). Adenoviruses are non-enveloped, so they can survive on surfaces for a prolonged period, and they are resistant to lipid disinfectants.

There are at least 54 known serotypes of human adenovirus, and the subgroups share similar disease presentations. For example, subgroup F, serotypes 41 and 42, is associated with infantile gastroenteritis [2, 3], while others typically cause respiratory disease.

Disseminated adenovirus infections occur more commonly in immunocompromised patients, in particular stem cell transplant (SCT) patients, but they have significant mortality rates in both immunocompromised and immunocompetent populations. The mortality rate for disseminated adenovirus infections in SCT patients is up to 70% [3], while in immunocompetent children it is up to 60% [4]. Importantly, immunocompromised hosts can shed adenovirus in stool for an extended period of time, after symptoms of clinical disease have resolved.

Diagnosis is most commonly made using qualitative and quantitative PCR [3]. The quantitative number can be used to assess response to treatment, but one must also consider asymptomatic viral shedding and take into account the entire clinical picture. Disseminated disease is definitively diagnosed by histopathology.

Some viral infections have been associated with myositis and rhabdomyolysis, including influenza, coxsackievirus, herpes simplex virus, and Epstein-Barr virus [5]. Case reports have described rhabdomyolysis with adenovirus infection [5, 6]. In the patient described in the present case, the elevated CK and the AKI were most likely attributable to rhabdomyolysis.

Typically, treatment for adenovirus consists of supportive care. In the setting of severe adenovirus pneumonia or disseminated disease, there is some literature supporting the use of cidofovir [2, 3, 7], as was used in the patient described.

Key Points/Pearls

- Elevated CK, AKI, and gross hematuria with a urinalysis demonstrating only 0–5 RBC should prompt consideration of rhabdomyolysis.
- Adenovirus has a broad range of clinical presentations, including acute upper respiratory illness, pneumonia, diarrhea, hepatitis, keratoconjunctivitis, and disseminated disease.
- Adenovirus can also cause hemorrhagic cystitis in immunocompetent and transplant patients (in the latter BK virus and CMV are in the differential diagnosis).
- Certain serotypes of adenovirus are associated with different clinical presentations.
- In the setting of severe disease, cidofovir should be considered for treatment.

References

1. Rowe WP, Huebner RJ, Gilmore LK, Parrott RH, Ward TG. Isolation of a cytopathogenic agent from human adenoids undergoing spontaneous degeneration in tissue culture. Proc Soc Exp Biol Med. 1953;84(3):570–3.
2. Lion T. Adenovirus infections in immunocompetent and immunocompromised patients. Clin Microbiol Rev. 2014;27(3):441–62.
3. Sandkovsky U, Vargas L, Florescu DF. Adenovirus: current epidemiology and emerging approaches to prevention and treatment. Curr Infect Dis Rep. 2014;16(8):416.
4. Munoz FM, Piedra PA, Demmler GJ. Disseminated adenovirus disease in immunocompromised and immunocompetent children. Clin Infect Dis. 1998;27(5):1194–200.
5. Meshkinpour H, Vaziri ND. Acute rhabdomyolysis associated with adenovirus infection. J Infect Dis. 1981;143(1):133.
6. Wright J, Couchonnal G, Hodges GR. Adenovirus type 21 infection. Occurrence with pneumonia, rhabdomyolysis, and myoglobinuria in an adult. JAMA. 1979;241(22):2420–1.
7. Kim SJ, Kim K, Park SB, Hong DJ, Jhun BW. Outcomes of early administration of cidofovir in non-immunocompromised patients with severe adenovirus pneumonia. PLoS One. 2015;10(4):e0122642.

Pain and Rash in a Stem Cell Transplant Recipient

Eric Bhaimia and Nirav Shah

A 40-year-old male with a past medical history of chronic myelogenous leukemia (CML) who had undergone a hematopoietic stem cell transplant (HSCT) presented with left leg pain. The pain began as left thigh cramping approximately 3 weeks prior to presentation, followed by the development of a petechial rash on the medial and posterior aspects of the left thigh. The pain then extended into the left calf and progressively increased in severity. On the day of presentation, the pain was so severe that he was not able to move his leg. He denied paresthesias of the affected extremity, fever, chills, nausea, vomiting, and abdominal pain. He also denied recent trauma to the left lower extremity. Review of systems was significant for a chronic cough, with acute onset shortness of breath starting the day prior to presentation. He had undergone thoracentesis the week prior. The pleural fluid was bloody with negative cytological studies and cultures.

The patient was diagnosed with CML 12 years prior to presentation, and he underwent multiple chemotherapy regimens followed by an allogeneic HSCT approximately 10 years after the initial diagnosis. His disease course was complicated by relapse identified by bone marrow biopsy 1 year after the HSCT. He received a donor lymphocyte infusion 1 month later, and his course was complicated by graft versus host disease affecting the liver. He had a history of *Streptococcus pneumoniae* meningitis, localized herpes zoster, and a subdural hematoma. His past surgical and family history were unremarkable. The social history was significant for birth in the Philippines and migration to the United States (US) at the age of 20 years. Medications included budesonide, fluconazole, trimethoprim-sulfamethoxazole, valacyclovir, and tacrolimus. He was intolerant of voriconazole, which caused visual hallucinations. He denied recent travel or having pets in the household. He had been unemployed since receiving the diagnosis of CML.

On physical examination, the temperature was 98.2 °F, heart rate was 140 beats per minute, blood pressure was 87/43 mmHg, respiratory rate was 29 breaths per minute, and oxygen saturation was 96% breathing room air. He appeared in mild respiratory distress with supraclavicular retractions and intermittent dry cough. The mucous membranes were moist and the neck supple. Auscultation of the heart revealed tachycardia, without murmur, rub, or gallop. Lungs were clear to auscultation. The abdomen was soft, non-tender, and not distended, with normal bowel sounds and no evidence of hepatosplenomegaly. The left knee was flexed at the knee and could not be extended

E. Bhaimia, D.O. • N. Shah, M.D., M.P.H. (✉)
Department of Medicine, NorthShore University
HealthSystem, Evanston, IL, USA

University of Chicago Medicine, Chicago, IL, USA
e-mail: nss197@gmail.com

© Springer International Publishing AG 2018
M. David, J.-L. Benoit (eds.), *The Infectious Disease Diagnosis*,
https://doi.org/10.1007/978-3-319-64906-1_33

due to pain. No significant erythema of the joint was noted, and the skin was appropriately warm to touch. Dermatologic exam was notable for a dry, petechial rash over the medial left thigh and bullous lesions over the medial left calf, with palpable purpura interspersed among the bullous lesions (Fig. 33.1). The left calf was exquisitely tender to palpation. Dorsalis pedis pulses were 2+ in both feet, and sensation to light palpation was intact. Strength testing was limited by pain.

Complete blood count revealed a white blood cell (WBC) count of 2900 cells/μL (normal range, 4500–11,000 cells/μL), with a differential of 91% neutrophils and 3% lymphocytes, hemoglobin 8.7 g/dL (13.5–17.5 g/dL), and platelet count of 22,000/μL (150,000–450,000/μL). The basic metabolic panel was within normal limits. Liver function tests revealed a direct hyperbilirubinemia (total bilirubin 3.9 mg/dL and direct bilirubin 3.0 mg/dL; normal ranges, 0.3–1.9 mg/dL and 0.0–0.3 mg/dL, respectively), alkaline phosphatase of 215 U/L (44–147 U/L), alanine aminotransferase of 60 U/L (7–55 U/L), and aspartate aminotransferase of 38 U/L (8–48 U/L). Lactate dehydrogenase was elevated at 498 U/L (105–333 U/L), creatine kinase was normal at 26 U/L, and C-reactive protein was elevated at 325 mg/dL (0–10 mg/dL). Urinalysis revealed 3+ blood, 2+ protein, >20 red blood cells (RBC), and 10–20 WBC. Computed tomography (CT) of the chest revealed sub-centimeter nodules of the lower lobe of the right lung.

The differential diagnosis for palpable purpura is presented in Table 33.1. Palpable purpura is caused by inflammation of the small blood vessels. This inflammation can occur as the result of infectious or inflammatory etiologies which include Rocky Mountain spotted fever, meningococcemia, disseminated gonorrhea, ecthyma gangrenosum, and small-vessel vasculitis due to Henoch-Schönlein purpura, polyarteritis nodosa, leukocytoclastic vasculitis, microscopic polyangiitis, or mixed essential cryoglobulinemia. Further laboratory testing included an autoimmune workup, viral studies, imaging of the involved extremity, and a skin biopsy. Results from further work-up are shown in Table 33.2. CT of the left lower extremity showed edema and thickening of the dermis but no evidence of abscess or subcutaneous gas. Findings of pathological examination of the skin biopsy specimen were consistent with occlusive vasculopathy. Hepatitis B surface antigen (HBsAg) was reactive, hepatitis B viral load in the blood was >150,000,000 U/mL by polymerase chain reaction (PCR), and the serum cryoglobulin level was elevated, together confirming the diagnosis of cryoglobulinemia secondary to hepatitis B infection.

The patient's hepatitis serologies prior to HSCT were notable for a negative HBsAg, positive hepatitis B surface antibody (HBsAb), and positive hepatitis B core IgG (HBcAb), indicating

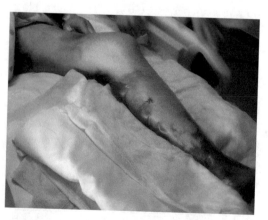

Fig. 33.1 Left medial leg displaying purpura, petechiae, and bullae

Table 33.1 Differential diagnosis for palpable purpura

Rocky Mountain spotted fever
Acute or chronic meningococcemia
Disseminated gonococcal infection
Ecthyma gangrenosum
Vasculitis syndromes
• Henoch-Schönlein purpura
• Polyarteritis nodosa
• Leukocytoclastic vasculitis
• Microscopic polyangiitis
• Mixed essential cryoglobulinemia
– Human immunodeficiency virus (HIV)
– Hepatitis C virus
– Hepatitis B virus
– Multiple myeloma
– Waldenström's macroglobulinemia

Table 33.2 Laboratory results, blood, or serum (normal values in parentheses)

Lactate dehydrogenase	498 U/L (105–333 U/L)
C-reactive protein	325 mg/L (0–10 mg/dL)
Lactate	4.6 mg/dL (<2 mmol/L)
Creatine kinase	26 U/L (52–336 U/L)
Complement component 3	53 mg/dL (88–252 mg/dL)
Complement component 4	14 mg/dL (12–72 mg/dL)
Cytomegalovirus (CMV) PCR	Negative
Epstein-Barr virus (EBV) PCR	Negative
Adenovirus PCR	Negative
Hepatitis C antibody	Negative
Hepatitis B surface antigen (HBsAg)	Reactive
Hepatitis B surface antibody (HBsAb)	Nonreactive
Hepatitis B viral load (PCR)	150,000,000 U/mL (<20 U/mL)
Serum cryoglobulin	1.0% volume (undetectable)
Rheumatoid factor	<8 IU/mL (<15 IU/mL)
Sjogren's Ss-A	16 AU/mL (<100 AU/mL)
Sjogren's Ss-B	2 AU/mL (<100 AU/mL)
Serum viscosity	1.3 cP (1.4–1.8 cP)

PCR polymerase chain reaction

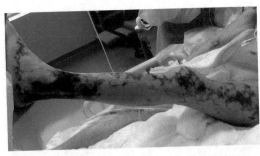

Fig. 33.2 Left lateral leg displaying purpura and petechiae later in hospital course

ening neuropathic chest pain and hemolytic anemia. He developed septic shock due to pansusceptible *Escherichia coli* bacteremia, suspected invasive pulmonary aspergillosis treated with micafungin, and progressive renal and hepatic failure that ultimately resulted in death 28 days after admission.

33.1 Hepatitis B Virus

Hepatitis B virus is a member of the *Hepadnaviridae* family (see Fig. 33.3). It can be transmitted via exposure to infected blood or body fluids. In highly endemic regions, perinatal transmission is the most common route of spread. In the United States (USA), intravenous drug use and sexual intercourse are frequent routes of infection. There were an estimated 19,200 cases of acute hepatitis B in 2014 with an incidence rate of 0.9 cases per 100,000 population in the USA [2]. There were 850,000–2.2 million cases of chronic hepatitis B in the USA in 2014 [3]. Chronic hepatitis B prevalence is high in sub-Saharan Africa and East Asia (5–10% of the adult population), in the Amazon and the southern parts of eastern and central Europe, and in the Middle East and the Indian subcontinent (2–5% of the population). Hepatitis B can cause both acute and chronic disease. The spectrum of acute disease ranges from patients with subclinical disease to mild hepatitis to fulminant hepatitis resulting in liver failure. The chronic disease spectrum includes asymptomatic carriers, chronic hepatitis, cirrhosis, and hepatocellular carcinoma. Extrahepatic manifestations can occur in both acute and chronic infections [4]. Dermatologic manifestations include

resolved infection with immunity. With the HSCT and donor infused lymphocytes, our patient lost his immunity to hepatitis B and then seroconverted from reactivation of latent HBV within the liver secondary to immune suppression. Of note, he carried the hepatitis Be antigen (HBeAg) but tested negative for the hepatitis Be antibody, indicating that he was in the early phase of hepatitis B infection with active replication and high infectivity.

Because the patient had an elevated hepatitis B viral load and was HBeAg positive, he was started on dual therapy for hepatitis B with entecavir and tenofovir [1]. He developed acute renal insufficiency, with a rising creatinine, and tenofovir was therefore eventually discontinued. Rituxan and plasmapheresis were initiated for cryoglobulinemia. The course was complicated by progression of the rash with involvement of the lateral aspect of the left leg (Fig. 33.2), wors-

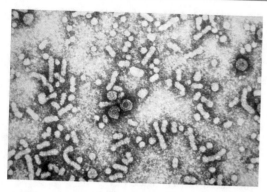

Fig. 33.3 Scanning electron micrograph of hepatitis B virus (Source: CDC Public Health Image Library. Accessed at https://phil.cdc.gov/phil/details.asp. Accessed on June 22, 2017)

polyarteritis nodosa, bullous pemphigoid, lichen planus, Gianotti-Crosti syndrome and cryoglobulinemia. Diagnosis is determined by serologic assays and PCR for hepatitis B virus viral load.

Acute hepatitis is generally managed with supportive care, but there may be subgroups of patients who benefit from antiviral therapy [5]. Patients with HBsAg or HBcAb positivity are at risk of reactivation with immunosuppressants and should be considered for antiviral therapy to reduce the risk of reactivation [6]. Chronic hepatitis B infections can be treated with interferon, entecavir, tenofovir, lamivudine, adefovir, and telbivudine. While these agents are currently first-line therapy, new clinical trials may result in a shift in practice in the near future. The decision to treat is made to reduce the risk of progressive liver disease, transmission, and other long-term complications. Vaccination against hepatitis B is the best way to prevent infection. Universal vaccination of newborns is recommended in the United States.

33.2 Cryoglobulinemia

Cryoglobulin consists of immunoglobulins and complement components that precipitate upon refrigeration of plasma and serum and that dissolve upon re-warming. Cryoglobulinemia is the term often applied to the systemic inflammatory syndrome in which a predominantly small to medium vessel vasculitis occurs in the setting of cryoglobulin-containing immune complex deposition. Cryoglobulins containing more than one immunoglobulin component are referred to as mixed cryoglobulins [7]. The Brouet classification scheme is used to sub-type cryoglobulinemia (Table 33.3) [8]. Clinical manifestations of the mixed cryoglobulinemia syndrome (associated with cryoglobulinemia types II and III) include palpable purpura, renal disease, arthralgias, and other nonspecific symptoms including weakness, cough, and peripheral neuropathy. The classical Meltzer triad, consisting of palpable purpura, weakness, and arthralgia, is present in up to 25–30% of patients with cryoglobulinemia. The majority of renal disease can be characterized by microscopic hematuria and sub-nephrotic proteinuria or nephrotic syndrome with or without chronic renal insufficiency. Pulmonary symptoms are reported in 40–50% of patients and may range from dyspnea and cough to pleurisy. Peripheral neuropathy occurs in approximately two-thirds of

Table 33.3 The Brouet classification scheme of cryoglobulinemia [11]

Cryoglobulinemia type	Criteria	Associated conditions
1	Monoclonal Ig	Multiple myeloma Waldenström's macroglobulinemia
2	Polyclonal Ig + monoclonal Ig, with RF	Viral infections (HCV, HIV)
3	Polyclonal Ig without monoclonal Ig component	Autoimmune disorders Lymphoproliferative disorders HBV, HCV Proposed viral infections: CMV, EBV, Parvovirus B19

CMV cytomegalovirus, *EBV* Epstein-Barr virus, *HCV* hepatitis C virus, *HIV* human immunodeficiency virus, *Ig* immunoglobulin, *RF* rheumatoid factor

patients with mixed cryoglobulinemia. This most commonly affects sensation in the distal extremities and is mediated by immune complex deposition of the vasa nervorum.

The diagnosis of mixed cryoglobulinemia syndrome is made on the basis of history, typical clinical manifestations as described above, and the presence of serum cryoglobulins. Biopsy of purpuric skin lesions may reveal the presence of a leukocytoclastic vasculitis. Testing for HIV, HBV, and HCV should be performed in all patients in whom the diagnosis is suspected. Treatment focuses on initial immunosuppressive therapy as well as therapy for the underlying disease process. Immunosuppression is used as initial therapy in patients with a rapidly progressive, organ- or life-threatening clinical course, regardless of the underlying etiology. This therapy usually involves a short course of glucocorticoids combined with either rituximab or cyclophosphamide [9]. In some patients, plasmapheresis may also be attempted [10]. Prognosis is dependent on the underlying disease state and the development of complications.

Key Points/Pearls

- Hepatitis B can cause numerous extrahepatic manifestations including polyarteritis nodosa and dermatologic conditions such as cryoglobulinemia.
- Hepatitis B reactivation may occur in immunocompromised patients who are HBsAg negative and HBcAb is positive, whether they are HBsAb positive or negative. This occurs, for example, in immunosuppression due to organ transplant, chemotherapy, CD20-directed cytolytic antibodies (ofatumumab and rituximab), or high-dose steroids.
- Persons with hepatitis C virus (HCV) who are co-infected with hepatitis B virus (HBV) may be at risk for reactivation of HBV infection during or following HCV treatment with directly acting antivirals; this includes those who are hepatitis B surface antigen (HBsAg) and hepatitis B surface antibody (HBsAb or anti-HBs) negative, but hepatitis B core antibody (HBcAb or anti-HBc) positive.

- The Meltzer triad—palpable purpura, weakness, and arthralgia—is present in up to 25–30% of patients with mixed cryoglobulinemia.
- Cryoglobulinemia therapy requires treatment of the underlying cause and in severe cases may require immunosuppressive therapy or plasmapheresis.

References

1. Lok AS, Trinh H, Carosi G, Akarca US, Gadano A, Habersetzer F, et al. Efficacy of entecavir with or without tenofovir disoproxil fumarate for nucleos(t)ide-naïve patients with chronic hepatitis B. Gastroenterology. 2012;143(3):619–28.e1.
2. Commentary | U.S. 2014 surveillance data for viral hepatitis | statistics & surveillance | Division of Viral Hepatitis | CDC [Internet]. https://www.cdc.gov/hepatitis/statistics/2014surveillance/commentary.htm#bkgrndB. Accessed 22 June 2017.
3. Roberts H, Kruszon-Moran D, Ly KN, Hughes E, Iqbal K, Jiles RB, et al. Prevalence of chronic hepatitis B virus (HBV) infection in U.S. households: National Health and Nutrition Examination Survey (NHANES), 1988-2002. Hepatology. 2016;63(2):388–97.
4. Kappus MR, Sterling RK. Extrahepatic manifestations of acute hepatitis B virus infection. Gastroenterol Hepatol (NY). 2013;9(2):123–6.
5. Lok ASF, McMahon BJ. Chronic hepatitis B: update 2009. Hepatology. 2009;50(3):661–2.
6. Loomba R, Rowley A, Wesley R, Liang TJ, Hoofnagle JH, Pucino F, et al. Systematic review: the effect of preventive lamivudine on hepatitis B reactivation during chemotherapy. Ann Intern Med. 2008;148(7):519–28.
7. Gorevic PD, Kassab HJ, Levo Y, Kohn R, Meltzer M, Prose P, et al. Mixed cryoglobulinemia: clinical aspects and long-term follow-up of 40 patients. Am J Med. 1980;69(2):287–308.
8. Brouet JC. [Cryoglobulinemias]. Presse Med 1983;12(47):2991–6.
9. Terrier B, Krastinova E, Marie I, Launay D, Lacraz A, Belenotti P, et al. Management of noninfectious mixed cryoglobulinemia vasculitis: data from 242 cases included in the CryoVas survey. Blood. 2012;119(25):5996–6004.
10. Ramos-Casals M, Robles A, Brito-Zerón P, Nardi N, Nicolás JM, Forns X, et al. Life-threatening cryoglobulinemia: clinical and immunological characterization of 29 cases. Semin Arthritis Rheum. 2006;36(3):189–96.
11. Dispenzieri A, Gorevic PD. Cryoglobulinemia. Hematol Oncol Clin North Am. 1999;13(6):1315–49.

A 2-Year-Old Girl with a Limp

Daniel Glikman

A 2-year-old girl was transferred from another hospital to our tertiary care medical center for evaluation of a limp. She had been healthy until a month prior, when she was noted to be limping on her right leg. The difficulty in walking progressed and she refused to walk 3 weeks later. Her mother recalled that the child fell while walking about a week before the symptoms started. The child had a mild fever for 2 days during the illness. There was no history of upper airway illness, cough, diarrhea, skin rash, sick contacts, travel, or animal exposure. Her past medical history was unremarkable. She was healthy, up-to-date with immunizations, lived with both parents and two siblings in Chicago, and did not attend day care.

At the first hospital, she was noted to be afebrile and in good general condition but with a right swollen knee. The knee was warm without erythema, and movements of the joint were restricted. Plain radiographs of her chest and leg were reported as normal. The knee was aspirated, yielding a small amount of clear fluid. Intravenous (IV) clindamycin was administered, but because the culture of the aspirated fluid had no growth, and no improvement was noted, she was transferred to our center.

On physical examination, she appeared comfortable with no signs of distress. The temperature was 37.2 °C, the heart rate 112 beats per minute, the respiratory rate 24 breaths per minute, and the blood pressure 95/55 mmHg. Her examination was normal except for the mildly swollen right knee with limited range of motion and some local tenderness without erythema. The rest of the skeletal examination was normal.

Laboratory evaluation revealed a C-reactive protein of 3 mg/L (normal range < 5 mg/L), erythrocyte sedimentation rate of 38 mm/h, and white blood cell count of 3900/mm^3 with 32% neutrophils, 9% bands, and 48% lymphocytes. The hemoglobin was 10.2 g/dL (normal range, 11.5–14 g/dL) and the platelets 223,000/mm^3. The aspartate aminotransferase was 89 U/L (normal range, 8–37 U/L) and the alanine aminotransferase 54 U/L (8–35 U/L); the rest of the blood chemistries were normal. Computerized tomography (CT) scan of the right knee and a magnetic resonance imaging (MRI) scan revealed a 2.4-cm ovoid lesion in the medial femoral epiphysis with a small knee effusion (Fig. 34.1). Osteomyelitis was suspected, although the differential diagnosis was broad, as listed in Table 34.1.

A diagnostic test was performed.

D. Glikman, M.D.
Pediatric Infectious Diseases Unit, Galilee Medical Center, Nahariya, and The Faculty of Medicine in the Galilee, Bar-Ilan University, Safed, Israel
e-mail: DannyG@gmc.gov.il

Fig. 34.1 Computerized tomography of the right knee demonstrating a 2.4 cm ovoid lesion in the medial femoral epiphysis (*arrow*)

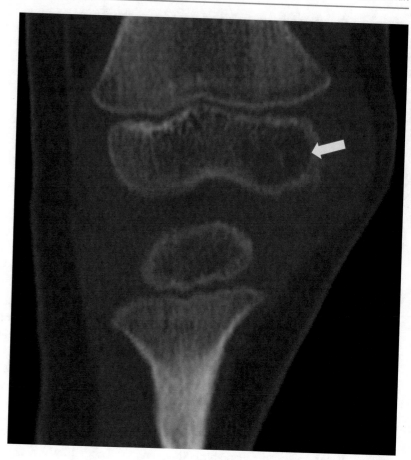

Table 34.1 Differential diagnosis in a child with a limp and a fever

Osteomyelitis with or without secondary involvement of a joint
Trauma
Pyomyositis
Malignancy, such as leukemia, neuroblastoma, or a bone tumor
Bone infarction in sickle cell disease
Arthritis
Septic arthritis
Reactive arthritis
Arthritis associated with autoinflammatory or immunologic disorders such as:
Crohn's disease
Juvenile idiopathic arthritis
Kawasaki disease

34.1 Osteomyelitis in Children

Osteomyelitis in children is primarily of hematogenous origin. Infecting organisms enter the bone through the nutrient artery and are deposited in the metaphysis where the blood flow is slow. Age-related differences in the anatomy of the bone and its blood supply influence the clinical manifestations of osteomyelitis. Transphyseal vessels are present in most children younger than 18 months of age, providing a vascular connection between the metaphysis and the epiphysis. As a result, in infants, infection originating in the metaphysis can spread to the epiphysis and the joint space. After the age of 2 years, the cartilaginous growth plate usually prevents extension of infection into the joint space [1].

Radiologic diagnosis of osteomyelitis can be achieved by using radionuclide imaging (such as a technetium-99 bone scan) or MRI, although the changes detected are not specific for osteomyelitis and can be seen with malignancy, fracture, or infarction. Bone changes in osteomyelitis are detected late in the course of infection on plain films, usually after 7–14 days. Therefore, the microbiologic diagnosis of osteomyelitis has importance in confirming the diagnosis and providing adequate targeted antimicrobial therapy. Most cases of osteomyelitis are of bacterial origin. The pathogen can be identified in ~80% of cases when multiple samples are taken for culture from blood and the affected bone or joint [1].

Staphylococcus aureus is the most common cause of acute hematogenous osteomyelitis (Table 34.2). *Kingella kingae, Streptococcus pneumoniae,* and *Streptococcus pyogenes* are isolated in most other cases. *Kingella kingae* and *Streptococcus pneumoniae* are most common in young children (up to the age of 5 and 2 years, respectively). *Haemophilus influenzae* (type b) (Hib) was a relatively common cause of osteomyelitis before the widespread use of the Hib conjugate vaccine. *Bartonella henselae* causes granulomatous infection of the bone and should be suspected in chil-

dren who play with cats and dogs and when cultures of blood and bone do not yield a pathogen. *Salmonella* spp. can infect infarcted bone in children with sickle cell disease. Skeletal lesions occur in approximately 1% of children with tuberculosis; infection can persist for years before clinical signs are apparent. Chest radiographs may be normal, but the tuberculin skin test is positive in about 90% of cases. Puncture wounds of the foot, especially through sports shoes, can cause bacterial osteochondritis. The offending pathogens are mainly *S. aureus* (early onset: 3–5 days after trauma) and *Pseudomonas aeruginosa* (late onset: after 5 days following trauma). Osteoarticular involvement is the predominant manifestation of brucellosis in children. It should be suspected in certain geographic areas and when history of contact with animals or ingestion of unpasteurized milk or milk products is elicited. Infection with *Serratia* spp. and *Aspergillus* spp. should be considered in children with chronic granulomatous disease.

34.2   Diagnosis: Brucellosis with Skeletal Involvement

A bone biopsy was performed in our patient from the lesion in the medial femoral epiphysis, demonstrating erosion of the bone cortex and inflammation within the bone (Fig. 34.2), compatible with osteomyelitis. The blood cultures taken at the first hospital and at our tertiary care medical center were positive after 4–6 days for small, Gram-negative coccobacilli, identified as *Brucella melitensis*.

Clues to the diagnosis were obtained with additional social history. The family was originally from Mexico. The 2-year-old daughter was born in Chicago and never traveled outside the region. Her father returned from a visit to his village in Mexico about a month before his daughter's illness started. He brought back with him a traditional Mexican cheese from a farm in the village, made of goat's milk. All family members ate the cheese. Only the daughter and her mother had symptoms. The mother had 10 days of fever and chills but refused to go to a physician.

Table 34.2 Pathogens of concern beyond the neonatal age group in pediatric osteomyelitis

Common pathogens
Staphylococcus aureus (including methicillin-susceptible and methicillin-resistant strains)
Streptococcus pyogenes
Kingella kingae
Other pathogens
Streptococcus pneumoniae
Haemophilus influenzae
Bartonella henselae
Mycobacterium tuberculosis
Salmonella spp.
Pseudomonas aeruginosa
Brucella spp.
Serratia spp.
Aspergillus spp.

Fig. 34.2 A bone biopsy was performed from the lesion in the medial femoral epiphysis, demonstrating erosion of the bone cortex (**a**) and inflammation within the bone (**b**), compatible with osteomyelitis

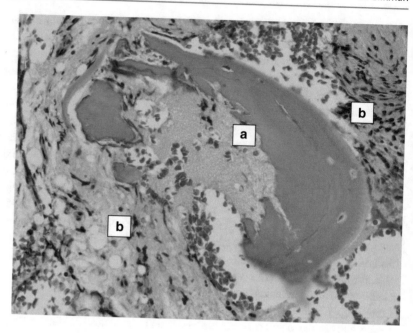

34.3   Brucellosis

Brucellosis is a zoonosis caused by small, Gram-negative coccobacilli of the genus *Brucella*, which consists of six species classified according to their preferred natural hosts. *Brucella melitensis* is the most common species in goats and sheep. *Brucella* spp. are facultative intracellular pathogens capable of replicating and surviving within host phagocytes, mainly in the reticuloendothelial system [2, 3].

Brucellosis exists worldwide but is highly prevalent in the Arabian Peninsula, Indian subcontinent, Mediterranean region, Eastern Europe, and parts of Mexico and Central and South America. Brucellosis is not common in the United States (US); the estimated incidence per 100,000 per year is 0.02–0.09, whereas in Mexico the incidence is 25 per 100,000, and in the Mediterranean region, the incidence ranges from 1.4 to 70 per 100,000 [4]. Of note, in the US, in states bordering Mexico, the incidence of brucellosis is eight times higher than elsewhere in the country [2].

Humans are accidental hosts, contracting the disease by direct contact with infected animals or ingestion of their milk or milk products. Many cases are linked to ingestion of fresh goat milk or goat dairy products, such as unpasteurized soft cheeses, imported from endemic countries. Hence, brucellosis can occur even with no history of direct animal contact, as we suspected in the present case.

In children and adults, brucellosis is a systemic illness. After an incubation period ranging from 3 to 4 weeks to several months, various nonspecific symptoms are described with a paucity of physical findings. The onset can be acute or gradual. Fever, malaise, lethargy, anorexia, and joint pains are the most common complaints in children. In young children with brucellosis, refusal to bear weight on an extremity is common. Fever can be prolonged, and brucellosis should be in the differential diagnosis of fever of unknown origin (FUO). On physical examination fever is evident in 80% and osteoarticular abnormalities in 50% (more common in children compared with adults). Hepatosplenomegaly is not as common in children (16%) as in adults (35%) [2, 5].

Nearly every organ system can be involved. Osteoarticular involvement predominates. In adults, sacroiliitis is more common and in children the large peripheral joints are the most often affected. Osteomyelitis may affect the vertebrae and long bones. Other organ systems involved may include the central nervous (meningitis, encephalitis, myelitis, or brain abscess), cardiovascular (endocarditis), genitourinary (orchitis or glomerulonephritis), and respiratory (pneumonia) systems. The liver is probably always involved. Acute hepatitis with or without focal necrosis, noncaseating granulomas, and abscesses are described. Hepatic enzymes commonly are only mildly elevated. Other routine laboratory tests are not helpful except for the white blood cell count, which tends to be normal or low. Death is caused mainly from complications of neurobrucellosis or endocarditis [2].

A definitive diagnosis of brucellosis requires recovering *Brucella* on culture from blood, bone marrow, or other tissues. Blood cultures are positive in 60–70% of patients, usually within 3–5 days of incubation [5]. Bone marrow cultures are probably more sensitive. Indirect diagnosis is by serology (serum agglutination test or enzyme immunoassay). No single antibody titer is diagnostic; however, most patients with brucellosis will have a titer of ≥1:160 [2].

Combination therapy with at least two antimicrobials is recommended, as monotherapy is associated with a high relapse rate. Treatment should be given for 6 weeks for uncomplicated brucellosis and 4–6 months for complicated disease. The combination of tetracyclines (especially doxycycline) given for 6 weeks with aminoglycosides (usually gentamicin) for 5–14 days is the regimen associated with the lowest relapse rate. An all-oral regimen of doxycycline and rifampin for 45 days is a more convenient treatment option but is associated with a higher relapse rate and is less effective for complications such as spondylitis. Children under the age of 8 years pose a special problem because an optimal regimen has not been studied. Combinations of trimethoprim-sulfamethoxazole (TMP-SMX) with gentamicin and/or rifampin are often used [2, 3].

Prevention of disease in animals is by immunization with a live-attenuated vaccine. Humans can be protected against food-borne infection by only ingesting pasteurized milk and dairy products and by cooking meat from susceptible animals until well done [2, 3].

The 2-year-old girl in the present case was treated with a combination of TMP-SMX and gentamicin with clinical and laboratory improvement. After a few days, she was able to walk without limping, the erythrocyte sedimentation rate decreased, and repeat blood cultures were sterile. She was treated for 2 weeks intravenously and discharged to complete an additional 4 weeks of oral TMP-SMX and rifampin.

Key Points

- Brucellosis is a zoonosis caused by *Brucella*, a small, Gram-negative coccobacillus.
- *Brucella melitensis* in goats and sheep is the most prevalent species causing human disease.
- Brucellosis is prevalent in the Arabian Peninsula, Indian subcontinent, Mediterranean region, Eastern Europe, and parts of Mexico and Central and South America.
- In the United States, in states bordering Mexico, the incidence of brucellosis is eight times greater than elsewhere in the country, where the disease is rare.
- Many brucellosis cases are linked to ingestion of unpasteurized milk or dairy products, imported from endemic countries; brucellosis can thus occur even with no history of direct animal contact.
- Fever, malaise, anorexia, and joint pains are the most common complaints; osteoarticular involvement is frequent.
- Combination therapy with at least two antimicrobials is recommended.
- Treatment should be given for 6 weeks for uncomplicated brucellosis and longer for complications.
- Tetracycline and aminoglycoside combination therapy has the lowest relapse rate.
- Food-borne infection can be prevented by pasteurization of milk and milk-containing dairy products and thorough cooking of meat from susceptible animals.
- Brucellosis may cause prolonged fever of unknown origin and culture-negative endocarditis, as well as neurobrucellosis with protean manifestations.
- Other pathogens to consider with a history of ingestion of unpasteurized milk or dairy product include *Mycobacterium bovis* (bovine tuberculosis), brucellosis, *Listeria*, *Campylobacter*, *Escherichia coli* O157:H7, *Salmonella*, and *Cryptosporidium*.

References

1. Gutierrez K. Osteomyelitis. In: Long SS, Pickering LK, Prober CG, editors. Principles and practice of pediatric infectious diseases. 4th ed. New York: Elsevier Saunders; 2012. p. 469–77.
2. Young EJ. *Brucella* species (Brucellosis). In: Long SS, Pickering LK, Prober CG, editors. Principles and practice of pediatric infectious diseases. 4th ed. New York: Elsevier Saunders; 2012. p. 861–5.
3. Pappas G, Akritidis N, Bosilkovski M, Tsianos E. Brucellosis. N Engl J Med. 2005;352:2325–36.
4. Dean AS, Crump L, Greter H, Schelling E, Zinsstag J. Global burden of human brucellosis: a systematic review of disease frequency. PLoS Negl Trop Dis. 2012;6:e1865.
5. Megged O, Chazan B, Ganem A, Ayoub A, Yanovskay A, Sakran W, et al. Brucellosis outbreak in children and adults in two areas in Israel. Am J Trop Med Hyg. 2016;95:31–4.

An Elderly Woman with a Fever After Traveling

35

Oana Denisa Majorant and Sara Hurtado Bares

A 74-year-old female presented to the Emergency Department because of a febrile illness of 1 week's duration. She reported daily fevers up to 104 °F (40 °C), rigors, and sweats. She also reported a dry cough without shortness of breath, sinus congestion, headache, abdominal pain, nausea, vomiting, diarrhea, dysuria, or urinary frequency. The patient's past medical history was remarkable for hypertension and left bundle branch block, invasive melanoma (with an excision approximately 4 years prior), and a remote history of Lyme disease many years before. She had never had a blood transfusion. She took verapamil daily and had no drug allergies. The patient resided in Illinois and had vacation homes in the Northwestern United States (U.S.) and coastal New England. She had traveled extensively during the last year, not only within the U.S. but also in Europe, Africa, and South America. Her most recent international trip was to South Africa, approximately 8 months earlier where she had visited Kruger National Park and participated in game drives and walking safaris. She had also visited Kenya 1 year before. She had not taken malaria prophylaxis for any of those trips. She denied any recent sick contacts or insect bites.

On physical examination, the patient appeared diaphoretic, but was not in any acute distress. The temperature was 104.7 °F (40.4 °C), blood pressure 122/69 mmHg, pulse 68 beats per minute, respirations 18 breaths per minute, and oxygen saturation by pulse oximetry 94% while breathing room air. There were fine crackles in the bases of both lungs, and the examination was otherwise normal.

Laboratory tests were notable for a hemoglobin of 12.0 g/dL, white blood count 4400/μL (61% neutrophils, 32% lymphocytes, and 6% monocytes), and platelet count 52,000/μL (normal range, 150,000–450,000/μL). The aspartate aminotransferase was 193 U/L (8–37 U/L) and alanine aminotransferase was 157 U/L (8–35 U/L). Results of a urinalysis and other routine laboratory tests were normal. The blood cultures and the urine cultures sent on admission remained negative. A chest radiograph revealed small bilateral pleural effusions (Fig. 35.1).

This case and images were contributed by Sara Hurtado Bares M.D., Jean-Luc Benoit M.D., and James Vardiman M.D., University of Chicago, Department of Medicine, Chicago, IL, and presented at Fellows' Day during IDWeek 2012, a joint effort of Infectious Diseases Society of America (IDSA), HIV Medicine Association, Pediatric Infectious Diseases Society (PIDS), and the Society for Healthcare Epidemiology of America (SHEA). Copyright Infectious Disease Society of America (IDSA), 2012, and previously published on the Partners Infectious Disease Images web as Case #12009: 2012 ID Week Case: An elderly woman with a fever. [Internet]. Partners Infectious Disease Images. Available from: http://www.idimages.org/idreview/case/caseid=474 (http://www.idimages.org/idreview/case/caseid=229). Used with permission, all rights reserved.

O.D. Majorant, M.D. • S.H. Bares, M.D. (✉)
University of Nebraska Medical Center,
Omaha, NE, USA
e-mail: sara.bares@unmc.edu

© Springer International Publishing AG 2018
M. David, J.-L. Benoit (eds.), *The Infectious Disease Diagnosis*,
https://doi.org/10.1007/978-3-319-64906-1_35

Fig. 35.1 Chest radiograph with increased hilar markings and without evidence of lobar consolidation

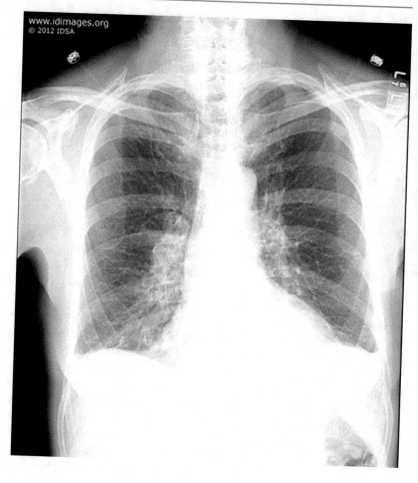

The differential diagnosis at this time was broad and included infections acquired both domestically and abroad (see Table 35.1). Given her extensive travel history, thick and thin peripheral blood smears were obtained. Both of these blood smears (shown in Figs. 35.2, 35.3, and 35.4) revealed intraerythrocytic protozoa, described as small ring forms including multiple forms in some red blood cells. The infected red blood cells were of normal size, and there were no parasites with brown pigment, no ameboid trophozoites, no schizonts, and no gametocytes. There were no cytoplasmic Schüffner's dots within the infected red blood cells. All these features ruled out malaria due to either *Plasmodium vivax* or *Plasmodium ovale*, which can cause malaria relapses from liver hypnozoites (dormant

Table 35.1 Differential diagnosis for a returning traveler with fever, anemia, thrombocytopenia, and abnormal liver function tests

Malaria (*Plasmodium* spp.)
Babesiosis (*Babesia* spp.)
Ehrlichiosis (*Ehrlichia chaffeensis* or *Ehrlichia ewingii*)
Lyme disease (*Borrelia burgdorferi*)
Spotted fever rickettsiae
Disseminated histoplasmosis (*Histoplasma capsulatum*)
Viral hepatitis
Acute human immunodeficiency virus (HIV) infection
Dengue fever
Chikungunya
Cytomegalovirus (CMV) infection
Epstein-Barr virus (EBV) infection

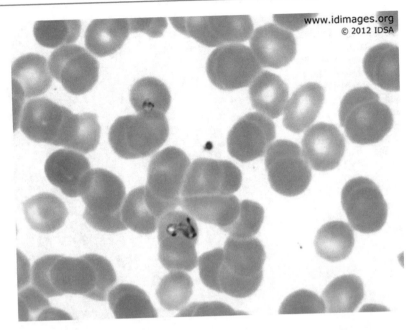

Fig. 35.2 Peripheral smear, Wright-Giemsa stain, ×1250 magnification; note the intraerythrocytic ring forms, including one multiple-infected red blood cell with a vacuole

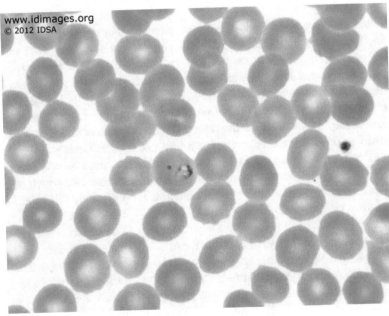

Fig. 35.3 Peripheral smear, Wright-Giemsa stain, ×1250 magnification; note the intraerythrocytic ring form with vacuoles

forms) up to a few years after infection. Malaria due to *Plasmodium malariae*, which can cause low-grade chronic infection, was also unlikely due to the relatively high parasitemia and the lack of band forms, schizonts, and pigment. The patient had not traveled to an area where zoonotic monkey malaria due to *Plasmodium knowlesi* has been described.

The pathologist identified the intraerythrocytic protozoa as *Plasmodium falciparum*. This protozoon is quite different from non-falciparum species, because older parasites induce the formation of knobs carrying the *Plasmodium falciparum* erythrocyte membrane protein 1 (Pfemp1) on the surface of red blood cells. This enables binding to receptors on the postcapillary venules

Fig. 35.4 Peripheral smear, Wright-Giemsa stain, ×1250 magnification; note the intraerythrocytic ring forms at the edges of the red blood cell, which is more typical of *P. falciparum* but can be seen with *B. microti* as well

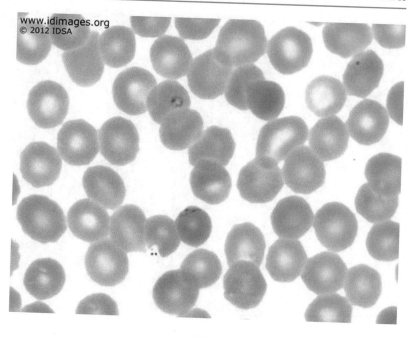

within various organs. Consequently, only small ring forms are typically identified on the peripheral blood smear; mature trophozoites and schizonts are not identified, and pigment is not seen. Occasionally, banana-shaped gametocytes, which are pathognomonic for *Plasmodium falciparum*, may be identified on the smear. The ring forms of *Plasmodium falciparum* are tiny and usually appear as two dots of chromatin and a thin ring of cytoplasm. Multiple infections of normal-sized red blood cells are often identified. Another characteristic finding is that the cytoplasm ring is frequently found at the periphery of the red blood cell (accolé or appliqué form).

This patient's smear was not typical of *Plasmodium falciparum* because many of the protozoa had a vacuole, and there was great variation in their shape (polymorphism). Ultimately, the differential diagnosis was between malaria due to *Plasmodium falciparum* and babesiosis due to *Babesia microti*. In babesiosis, the protozoa divide in a binary manner, which can led to protozoa pairs, triads, and tetrads. The latter are called Maltese crosses (after the cross portrayed on the Maltese flag).

As noted above, the pathologist initially identified the intraerythrocytic parasites as *Plasmodium falciparum* with 1.11% parasitemia.

Atovaquone 1000 mg and proguanil hydrochloride 400 mg were administered daily by mouth for 3 days. On the evening of the first day, fevers persisted, and the level of parasitemia decreased slightly, to 0.83%. On the second day, the maximum temperature was 104.2 °F (40.1 °C). The platelet count was 62,000/µL, and the level of parasitemia was 0.74%.

Because of the persistent fevers, the infectious diseases team reviewed the peripheral smears and ultimately felt babesiosis was more likely given the unusually long incubation period for falciparum malaria in conjunction with the patient's history and morphology, in spite of the lack of Maltese crosses. Given this diagnostic uncertainty, the patient was treated for both falciparum malaria and babesiosis while additional testing was performed. Malaria polymerase chain reaction (PCR) performed on the patient's serum was negative for *Plasmodium falciparum* and *Plasmodium vivax*. Serum *Babesia* PCR was positive for *Babesia microti*. *Babesia microti* IgG and IgM were elevated at >1:1024 (reference range < 1:64) and >1:320 (<1:20), respectively. The patient was thus diagnosed with babesiosis due to *Babesia microti*, which she most likely acquired from an *Ixodes scapularis* deer tick bite while visiting her vacation home in New England.

She ultimately completed a 7-day course of therapy for babesiosis with atovaquone 750 mg twice daily and azithromycin 500 mg on day 1 followed by 250 mg daily, with subsequent resolution of the patient's fever, parasitemia, thrombocytopenia, and elevated transaminases.

35.1   Babesiosis

Babesiosis is a tick-borne febrile illness caused by a protozoan parasite that can infect a wide range of mammals. It is an obligate intracellular organism that lives inside the red blood cells. It was named after Victor Babeş (1854–1926), a Romanian physician and bacteriologist who in 1888 was the first to describe a parasitic sporozoan of ticks that caused febrile hemoglobinuria in cattle [1]. For many years, babesiosis was considered an animal disease, until 1957, when a Yugoslav cattle farmer who had had a splenectomy contracted babesiosis.

Most cases of babesiosis in the USA are caused by *Babesia microti*, which is transmitted primarily by the nymphs of the *Ixodes scapularis* deer tick, the same tick that transmits the Lyme disease pathogen *Borrelia burgdorferi* and the etiology of human granulocytic anaplasmosis, *Anaplasma phagocytophilum*. Babesiosis can also be transmitted via organ transplantation and blood transfusion, which is of increasing concern given that the blood supply is not routinely screened for *Babesia* species [2].

The clinical manifestations of babesiosis derive from infection of erythrocytes, which leads to subsequent hemolysis and splenic sequestration. Symptoms can range from asymptomatic to severe illness and may include fever, chills, sweats, headache, myalgias, arthralgias, and anorexia as well as manifestations of hemolysis (jaundice and hemoglobinuria).

Multiorgan system failure (acute respiratory distress syndrome, disseminated intravascular coagulation, congestive heart failure, and renal failure) can occur, but is rarely seen in the absence of risk factors such as age > 50 years, asplenia, or underlying immunocompromising conditions. Laboratory testing usually reveals evidence of hemolytic anemia (e.g., low hemoglobin, high lactate dehydrogenase, high indirect bilirubin, and decreased haptoglobin). The thick and thin peripheral blood smears usually reveal the parasite in symptomatic patients, but may be negative. Serology or PCR testing can be performed to confirm the diagnosis.

35.2   Distinguishing Malaria and Babesiosis

As demonstrated in this case, differentiating between malaria caused by *Plasmodium* species and babesiosis can sometimes prove to be a difficult task [3]. *Babesia* and *Plasmodium* species are both transmitted by insect vectors (hard ticks and *Anopheles* mosquitoes, respectively), and both live inside the erythrocytes and may present with hemolysis, thrombocytopenia, and fever [1].

One key differentiating factor is the geographical areas of endemicity. Malaria is endemic outside the USA, with areas of transmission in Africa, Asia, and South America. Babesiosis, on the other hand, is often acquired in the USA, with the overwhelming majority of cases occurring in the Northeast and Upper Midwest. The diagnosis may prove to be challenging in patients such as the one presented above, who have traveled extensively and visited areas in which both organisms are endemic.

The incubation period for *Babesia* species usually ranges from 1 to 6 weeks after the infecting tick bite. In contrast, the incubation period for *Plasmodium* species usually ranges from 8 to 25 days, but may occasionally be much longer depending on multiple factors: the immune status of the infected person, the strain and the species of *Plasmodium*, the dose of sporozoites, and especially the effects of partially effective chemoprophylaxis. Thus, a careful interview in which time periods of travel and symptom onset are clarified may be helpful in distinguishing between the two pathogens.

The blood smear examination is an important step in diagnosis, but, as seen in this case, differentiating between the two protozoa based on morphology alone may be quite difficult (see

Table 35.2 Morphological comparison of *B. microti* and *P. falciparum*

	Babesia microti	*Plasmodium falciparum*
Number of parasitic forms per erythrocyte	Multiple parasites form pairs, triads, or tetrads (Maltese cross)	Multiple ring forms (no tetrads)
Shape, size, and location within the red cell	Polymorphism, including small rings and elongated forms; vacuoles	Small rings with two dots of chromatin; scant cytoplasm; location in the periphery (accolé or appliqué form)
Extraerythrocytic forms	Seen occasionally in heavily infected and asplenic patients	Not seen
Gametocytes	None	Banana-shaped (pathognomonic), but not seen early in travelers

Table 35.2). As noted above, intraerythrocytic ring forms can be seen in both *Plasmodium falciparum* and *Babesia* infections. Banana-shaped gametocytes and schizonts, which are occasionally seen on the peripheral blood smear in *P. falciparum* infection, are never seen in *Babesia* infection. A pathognomonic finding in *Babesia* infection is an intraerythrocytic tetrad of merozoites, appearing in a "Maltese cross" configuration, but this is only seen in a minority of cases, and it was not present in our patient's smear [4].

Serum indirect fluorescent antibody (IFA) and PCR testing are both available and may be used to establish the final diagnosis. Antibody and molecular testing are more sensitive than blood smear examination and can be particularly useful in the setting of low-level parasitemia or when the morphological characteristics observed on microscopy do not allow for a clear differentiation between *Babesia* and *Plasmodium*.

35.3 Babesiosis Treatment

Treatment of babesiosis varies depending on the severity of the disease. Those with asymptomatic disease do not require treatment. For patients with mild to moderate disease, the combination of atovaquone and azithromycin for 7–10 days is preferred [5]. The standard of care for those with severe disease remains clindamycin plus quinine. This combination is well studied and effective, but associated with more side effects (e.g., gastrointestinal upset, tinnitus, and vertigo) than atovaquone and azithromycin. In patients with parasitemia levels >10% or with clinical evidence

of end organ dysfunction, additional interventions such as blood transfusion, exchange transfusion, or hemodialysis may be needed.

Key Points/Pearls

- Babesiosis is a relatively common protozoan tick-borne illness in the USA, where most cases occur in the Northeast and Upper Midwest caused by *B. microti*; babesiosis due to different species is also present in other areas of the USA, Europe, and Asia.
- *Babesia* and *Plasmodium falciparum* are not always easily differentiated by morphological characteristics alone, and both infections must be considered in a patient with dual risk factors.
- The differing incubation periods for *Babesia* and *Plasmodium* species can help narrow the differential.
- It is reasonable to initiate treatment for the more severe of the two diseases (in this case, falciparum malaria) or for both diseases while awaiting confirmatory testing.
- Serologic and molecular testing may be necessary to definitively identify the causative organism and are especially useful in cases of low-level parasitemia and inconclusive morphological characteristics.
- Because babesiosis may be asymptomatic, transfusion-associated transmission occurs; in cases of exposure to infected blood, transfused recipients are screened with PCR and followed closely for the onset of symptoms.
- *Ixodes scapularis* deer ticks transmit *Borrelia burgdorferi* (Lyme disease), *Anaplasma phagocytophilum* (human granulocytic ana-

plasmosis), *Babesia microti* (babesiosis), *Borrelia miyamotoi* (an emerging pathogen that causes a febrile illness), and the Powassan flavivirus (a cause of encephalitis).

References

1. Gelfand JA, Vannier EG. *Babesia* species. In: Mandell GL, Bennett JE, Dolin R, editors. Mandell, Douglas, and Bennett's principles and practice of infectious diseases. 8th ed. Philadelphia, PA: Churchill Livingstone/Elsevier; 2015. p. 3165–72.

2. Levin AE, Krause PJ. Transfusion-transmitted babesiosis: is it time to screen the blood supply? Curr Opin Hematol. 2016;23(6):573–80.

3. Clark IA, Jacobson LS. Do babesiosis and malaria share a common disease process? Ann Trop Med Parasitol. 1998;92(4):483–8.

4. U.S. Centers for Disease Control and Prevention (CDC), DPDX Laboratory identification of parasites of public health concern. http://www.dpd.cdc.gov/dpdx/HTML/Babesiosis.htm. Accessed 30 Apr 2017.

5. Krause PJ, Lepore T, Sikand VK, Gadbaw J Jr, Burke G, Telford SR III, et al. Atovaquone and azithromycin for the treatment of babesiosis. N Engl J Med. 2000;343(20):1454–8.

Internationally Adopted HIV-Infected Toddler with Skin Rash

Linda J. Walsh

A 2-year-old female who was perinatally infected by the human immunodeficiency virus (HIV) and recently adopted from Ethiopia by a family in the United States (USA) presented to the International Adoption Clinic for a routine follow-up visit. Her parents reported a new complaint of irritation and drainage on the right lateral shoulder. They described a gradual increase in redness and swelling of the area, which felt firm and fluctuant. They denied any fever, change in behavior, vomiting, or other skin rash. The child was eating, sleeping, and voiding normally. The toddler had arrived in the USA 1 month earlier with her new adoptive family and already completed a baseline laboratory workup. She had also been treated for bilateral acute otitis media with a 10-day course of amoxicillin.

In Ethiopia, the child was initially found to be HIV positive when screened 5 months earlier. She had been started on trimethoprim/sulfamethoxazole for *Pneumocystis jiroveci* prophylaxis, but was naïve to highly active antiretroviral therapy (HAART) at the time of her adoption. At her screening in Ethiopia, she reportedly tested negative for syphilis, hepatitis B, and hepatitis C. Three months prior to presentation, she had a CD4+ T cell count of 1273 cells/mm^3 (30%). Before leaving Ethiopia, the child was seen at a US State Department clinic where she had documentation of a normal chest x-ray, a negative tuberculosis skin test (no reaction), and acid-fast bacillus (AFB) sputum smear results on 3 consecutive days that were all negative. There was documentation of two doses of diphtheria, tetanus, and pertussis (DTP), inactivated polio virus (IPV), *Haemophilus influenzae* type B (HIB), pneumococcal conjugate (PCV-7), and hepatitis B vaccines, as well as one dose of measles, mumps, and rubella (MMR) vaccine.

The patient was abandoned by her birth mother at about age 12 months and was purportedly cared for by a foster mother in a remote part of Ethiopia. The adoptive parents reported that a variety of "traditional or ritualistic treatments" were administered to the child by the foster mother and had resulted in scarring of the child's inner thighs and skin above her left eyebrow. The adoptive family consisted of the mother, father, and their two biological children, aged 6 and 8 years.

On physical examination, the patient was in no acute distress. The oxygen saturation was 100% on room air, temperature 36 °C, heart rate 140 beats per minute (crying), respiratory rate 32 breaths per minute, and blood pressure

L.J. Walsh, N.P.
Section of Pediatric Infectious Diseases, Department of Pediatrics, University of Chicago Medicine, Chicago, IL, USA
e-mail: lwalsh@peds.bsd.uchicago.edu

© Springer International Publishing AG 2018
M. David, J.-L. Benoit (eds.), *The Infectious Disease Diagnosis*,
https://doi.org/10.1007/978-3-319-64906-1_36

109/79 mmHg. Her weight was 12 kg (30th %), height 80.3 cm (5th %), and head circumference 48.3 cm (75th %), all according to World Health Organization growth curves. She had clear nasal discharge but her oropharynx was without evidence of lesions or thrush. There was no otorrhea or pre/postauricular tenderness noted. Her lungs were clear to auscultation, her heart had a regular rhythm without any murmur, and her abdomen was soft but distended. There were multiple healed scars on her skin including on the bilateral inner thighs and a keloid above the upper eyelid. Over her right deltoid area was a 3 × 3 cm annular area of erythema, edema, and fluctuance, from which about 5 mL of greenish, purulent material was expressed. There was no lymphadenopathy noted in the right axilla or elsewhere. The patient was started empirically on a course of oral clindamycin for presumed bacterial skin abscess and cellulitis.

The child's laboratory studies are summarized in Table 36.1. They were notable for an HIV serum viral load of 181,487 copies/mL and a nearly normal CD4+ T cell count of 1246 cells/mm^3 (26%). She also had a low prealbumin of 13 mg/dL (normal range, 20–40 mg/dL) and ferritin of 7 ng/mL (10–220 ng/mL), indicative of malnutrition and iron deficiency, respectively. Kidney, liver, and thyroid function were all within normal limits; her white blood cell (WBC) count was 8800/µL. Her serologies for hepatitis A, B, and C as well as tests for syphilis and malaria were negative. An HIV genotype revealed resistance to non-nucleoside reverse transcriptase inhibitors (NNRTI) but susceptibility to all tested protease inhibitors (PI) and nucleoside reverse transcriptase inhibitors (NRTI). She had a normal chest x-ray and a tuberculosis skin test that was positive for an immunocompromised child, with 5 mm of induration. She had two stool specimens evaluated; one was positive for nonpathogenic *Entamoeba coli* and a second for *Giardia lamblia*

cysts and trophozoites. Gram stain of the wound drainage from the right shoulder showed many WBCs with a few red blood cells (RBCs) but no bacteria. There was no growth on routine bacterial culture. Further drainage was therefore sent for AFB and fungal cultures. The fungal culture was negative. *Toxoplasma* serum IgG, *Histoplasma* urine antigen, and cryptococcal serum antigen were all negative.

Five weeks after the initial right deltoid wound drainage, positive AFB culture results were reported, and the patient was started on oral isoniazid and rifabutin for 3 months. The rifabutin dosing was decreased by 75% as the patient was also started on initial HAART regimen with two NRTIs, lamivudine and zidovudine, and a boosted PI, lopinavir/ritonavir. Gradually, the right deltoid skin lesion became smaller and began to heal (Figs. 36.1, 36.2, and 36.3). Final results of AFB wound culture revealed *Mycobacterium bovis* BCG that was susceptible to rifampin, ethambutol, and isoniazid, but resistant to pyrazinamide. Her HIV viral load decreased by 2.4 logs in less than 1 month and was undetectable 6 months after starting appropriate HAART.

The differential diagnosis of a draining skin wound in an HIV-infected child is presented in Table 36.2. Cryptococcosis and other invasive fungal infections, *Nocardia brasiliensis*, *Leishmania aethiopica*, *Mycobacterium avium-intracellulare* (MAI), cutaneous tuberculosis, and BCG infection were on the differential diagnosis in this child. The bacterial and fungal cultures sent from the skin drainage were both negative. There were no tissue or skin biopsies obtained to assess for *Nocardia or Leishmania* infection. Testing for both *Histoplasma* and *Cryptococcus* was negative. MAI is unlikely in the setting of this child's high CD4+ T cell count. Although there was no documentation of this patient receiving Bacille Calmette-Guerin (BCG) vaccine, the location of the single skin lesion

Table 36.1 Laboratory results presented in the case

Laboratory test (blood)	Results	Normal range and comments
White blood count	8800/μL	5000–15,800/μL
Hemoglobin	11.2 g/dL	11.3–13.2 g/dL
Hematocrit	35.1%	34–40%
Platelet count	435,000/μL	150,000–450,000/μL
Creatinine	0.6 mg/dL	0.5–1.4 mg/dL
Alanine aminotransferase	24 U/L	8–35 U/L
Aspartate aminotransferase	46 U/L	8–37 U/L
% CD4+ / CD3+	25.96%	28–47%
Absolute CD4	1245.54 UL	700–2200 UL
HIV-1 viral load	181,487 copies/mL	In untreated HIV: Linear range 20–10,000,000 copies/mL
HIV genotype	RT mutations: K103 N, Y181C, Y188C, G190A Protease mutations: M36I	The patient was perinatally infected with HIV resistant to NNRTIs
Hepatitis B surface antigen	Nonreactive	Nonreactive
Hepatitis B core antibody	Nonreactive	Nonreactive
Hepatitis B surface antibody	Nonreactive	Nonreactive
Hepatitis C antibody	Nonreactive	Nonreactive
Rapid plasma reagin (RPR)	Nonreactive	Nonreactive
Prealbumin	13 mg/dL	21–41 mg/dL
Ferritin	7 ng/mL	10–220 ng/mL
Iron	41 μg/dL	40–160 μg/dL
Total iron binding capacity	397 μg/dL	230–430 μg/dL
% iron saturation	10.3%	14–50%
Stool ova and parasites #1	*Entamoeba coli* cysts	*Entamoeba coli* is a nonpathogenic amoeba
Stool ova and parasites #2	*Giardia lamblia* cysts and trophozoites	*Giardia lamblia* is a pathogenic intestinal protozoon
Chest x-ray	Normal	
Malaria smear, peripheral blood	No parasites seen on thin or thick smears	
Wound drainage culture and stain	Many WBCs, few RBCs, no organisms seen on Gram's stain; no growth	
Fungal culture of wound drainage	No growth after 28 days of incubation	
Histoplasma antigen urine	Negative	Negative
Cryptococcal antigen, blood	Negative	Negative
Fluid, right shoulder	Acid-fast bacilli smear positive; acid-fast culture positive	
Mycobacterium bovis BCG antimicrobial susceptibilities (MIC, μg/mL)	Rifampin (1.0) S Ethambutol (5) S Ethambutol (8) S Isoniazid (0.1) S Isoniazid (0.4) S Pyrazinamide (300) R	*Mycobacterium bovis* BCG is expected to be resistant to pyrazinamide

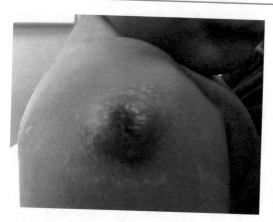

Fig. 36.1 Initial presentation of a fluctuant, erythematous lesion on the right shoulder

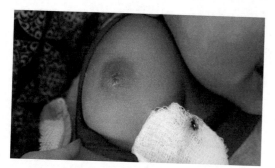

Fig. 36.2 Right shoulder lesion 10 days after drainage at initial presentation

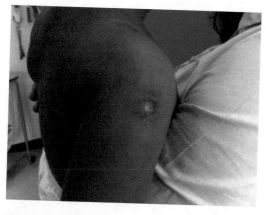

Fig. 36.3 Right shoulder lesion 8 weeks after initial presentation

Table 36.2 Differential diagnosis of a purulent skin infection in an HIV-infected Ethiopian child

Bacterial cellulitis, ecthyma, carbuncle, abscess, or pyomyositis
Infected insect bite
Phagedenic tropical ulcer (*Fusobacterium* spp., *Bacillus fusiformis*, and *Treponema vincenti*)
Cutaneous diphtheria (*Corynebacterium diphtheriae*)
Cutaneous anthrax (*Bacillus anthracis*)
Cutaneous tuberculosis (*Mycobacterium tuberculosis*)
Mycobacterium bovis BCG disease
Mycobacterium avium-intracellulare infection
Other nontuberculous mycobacterial infection including Buruli ulcer (*M. ulcerans*)
Cryptococcosis (*Cryptococcus* spp.)
Invasive skin fungus (e.g., blastomycosis [*Blastomyces dermatitidis*], histoplasmosis [*Histoplasma capsulatum*], or coccidioidomycosis [*Coccidioides immitis*])
Nocardia brasiliensis
Mycetoma (due to fungi or actinomycetes)
Cutaneous leishmaniasis (ulcerative lesion)
Myiasis (African tumbu fly *Cordylobia anthropophaga*)
Skin infections that do not usually look like an abscess, but may rarely be misdiagnosed as one • Crusted scabies • Bacillary angiomatosis (*Bartonella* spp.) • Leprosy (*Mycobacterium leprae*) • Creeping eruption • Herpes simplex virus infection • Varicella zoster virus (shingles)

36.1 BCG Disease in HIV-Infected Children

BCG vaccine, a live, attenuated strain of *M. bovis*, is considered safe and is routinely given to infants in much of the world to protect against tuberculosis-related illness [1, 2]. However, the risk of disseminated BCG disease after BCG vaccine has been shown in some studies to be hundredfold increased in HIV-infected infants [3–5]. In May 2007 the World Health Organization recommended that BCG not be given to HIV-infected asymptomatic infants regardless of tuberculosis prevalence or risk. This practice has been shown not to be feasible in countries such as South Africa, where the prevalence of both HIV and tuberculosis is very high and early HIV diagnosis in infants is not always possible [6].

made in the setting of HIV infection made cutaneous tuberculosis or BCG infection most likely. The definitive diagnosis was made by culture of the drainage, and so a biopsy was not necessary.

The prevalence of disseminated BCG disease in HIV-infected infants and children is unknown, and selective withholding of BCG vaccine may increase the risk of severe tuberculosis for both HIV-exposed and infected infants [7].

Up to 15% of HIV-infected infants who have received BCG vaccine develop BCG immune reconstitution inflammatory syndrome (BCG-IRIS) after the initiation of HAART [5, 6, 8]. These effects are often seen with a precipitous drop in HIV viral load and slow increase in CD4+ T cell count and can happen either early (within 3 months) or late (up to 2 years) after starting HAART. The Talbot classification system stratifies BCG disease into regional disease (ulcer, abscess, and/or lymphadenopathy at the inoculation site), extra-regional localized disease (infection at single site outside of the inoculation region), and disseminated disease (isolation of BCG on culture, positive culture, or evidence of infection at two or more sites beyond the area of inoculation and a systemic syndrome compatible with mycobacterial disease) [1].

36.2 Treatment of BCG Disease in HIV-Infected Children

There are no specific guidelines for the treatment of BCG disease in HIV-infected children, but there are preliminary recommendations based on the classification of BCG disease. Experts advocate for close monitoring of HIV-infected children who have received BCG vaccine, along with early initiation of HAART [1, 5, 6]. For local or regional disease, medical management is recommended with traditional tuberculosis medications (i.e., isoniazid, rifampicin, ethambutol, and ofloxacin) along with therapeutic aspiration or excisional biopsy if possible (ideally cultured for mycobacteria). It is important to pay close attention to dosing recommendations with concomitant HAART regimens and to monitor liver function regularly. For suspected or confirmed distant or disseminated disease, the same medication management is recommended along with expedited initiation of HAART [1]. It is important to note that *M. bovis BCG* is resistant to pyrazinamide [5].

Key Points/Pearls

- Bacille Calmette-Guerin (BCG) vaccine is safe and provides some protection against severe tuberculosis in immune competent children, but can pose significant risk for localized or disseminated disease in HIV-infected and other immunocompromised children.
- BCG disease is often associated with immune reconstitution inflammatory syndrome (BCG-IRIS) in HIV-infected children started on highly active antiretroviral therapy (HAART).
- BCG is resistant to pyrazinamide.
- When treating BCG disease with both antitubercular agents and antiretrovirals, care must be taken to adjust dosing appropriately based on drug-drug interactions.
- Early initiation of HAART has shown to decrease the severity of BCG-IRIS in HIV-infected children.
- The duration of treatment with antitubercular agents is not standardized, and consultation with a pediatric infectious diseases specialist is indicated.

References

1. Hesseling A, Rabie H, Marais B. Bacille Calmette-Guerin vaccine-induced disease in HIV-infected and HIV-uninfected children. Clin Infect Dis. 2006;42:548–58.
2. Mak TK, Hesseling A, Cotton MF, Hussey GD. Making BCG vaccination programmes safer in the HIV era. Lancet. 2008;372:786–7.
3. Hesseling A, Cotton M, Marais B. BCG and HIV reconsidered: moving the research agenda forward [Letter to the editor]. Vaccine. 2007;25(36):6565–8.
4. Hesseling A, Marais B, Gie RP. The risk of disseminated bacilli Calmette-Guerin (BCG) disease in HIV-infected children. Sci Dig. 2007;25:14–8.
5. Nuttall JJ, Davies MA, Hussey GD, Eley BS. Bacillus Calmette-Guerin (BCG) vaccine-induced complications in children treated with highly active antiretroviral therapy. Int J Infect Dis. 2008;12:e99–e105.
6. Rabie H, Violari A, Duong T. Early antiretroviral treatment reduces risk of bacilli Calmette-Guerin immune reconstitution adenitis. Int J Tub Lung Dis. 2011;15(9):1194–200.
7. de Souza Campos Fernandes RC, Medina-Acosta E. BCG-itis in two antiretroviral-treated HIV-infected infants. Int J STD AIDS. 2010;21(9):662–3.
8. Azzopardi R, Bennett C, Graham S, Duke T. Bacille Calmette-Guerin vaccine related disease in HIV-infected children: a systematic review. Int J Tub Lung Dis. 2009;13(11):1331–44.

37 A Pediatric Patient with a Progressive Chest Wall Mass

Colleen B. Nash

An 11-year-old autistic but otherwise healthy boy presented with a right chest wall mass of unknown duration. Intermittent tactile fever and cough were noted during the 4 days prior to presentation. Retrospectively, the parents noted decreased energy and an unwillingness of the boy to wear his school backpack, associated with complaints of right chest and rib pain over the past several months. He had no weight gain or loss and no other respiratory symptoms.

The boy had a history of periodontal disease, requiring general anesthesia for teeth extractions and the placement of fillings, crowns, and a spacer 9 months prior to presentation. His immunizations were current and he was not taking any medications. He lived in a suburban Midwest with his parents, both of whom were born in China. He was born in the United States and traveled only domestically to Washington, DC, and Orlando (Disney World) in the past year. The boy's parents had never been treated for active or latent tuberculosis. The boy had no other known tuberculosis exposures. There was no relevant family history, including malignancy. There were no household pets or other animal exposures.

Physical examination revealed an anxious but well-appearing patient. He was afebrile, hemodynamically stable, and saturating well on room air. An 8 × 10 cm firm, immobile mass was noted superior and medial to the right nipple, with overlying erythema and localized tenderness to touch, without evidence of ulceration, drainage, sinus tract formation, or crepitus. There was no tenderness beyond the margin of noted erythema. Breath sounds were diminished in the right middle and lower lung fields. Crowns were present over the most posterior mandibular molars bilaterally. The surrounding gingival mucosa was healthy and without evidence of inflammation. The remaining exam was unremarkable.

A complete blood count was significant for a white blood cell count of 16,000/μL (normal range, 3500–12,300/μL), hemoglobin 9.1 g/dL (11.3–15.2 g/dL), and platelets 512,000/μL (15,000–450,000/μL). Differential showed 79% neutrophils (35–80%). C-reactive protein was 5 mg/L (<5 mg/L) and erythrocyte sedimentation rate 46 mm/h (0–15 mm/h). Tuberculin skin test showed no induration. QuantiFERON-TB Gold test was negative, with a TB-antigen result of 0.03 IU/mL (<0.35 IU/mL). *Histoplasma* urine antigen by enzyme immunoassay (EIA), *Histoplasma* serum antibody by immunodiffusion, and *Blastomyces* serum antibody screen by EIA were negative.

A chest radiograph showed a poorly defined right upper and middle lobe opacity with a small right pleural effusion (Fig. 37.1). Computed tomography of the chest showed a right chest soft tissue mass-like opacity (6 × 7 × 8.5 cm) involving the right upper and middle lobes (Fig. 37.2a, b). There

C.B. Nash, M.D., M.P.H.
Rush University Medical Center, Rush University Children's Hospital, Chicago, IL, USA
e-mail: Colleen_Nash@rush.edu

© Springer International Publishing AG 2018
M. David, J.-L. Benoit (eds.), *The Infectious Disease Diagnosis*,
https://doi.org/10.1007/978-3-319-64906-1_37

Fig. 37.1 Chest radiograph, posterior-anterior view: Poorly defined right upper and middle lobe opacity with a small right pleural effusion

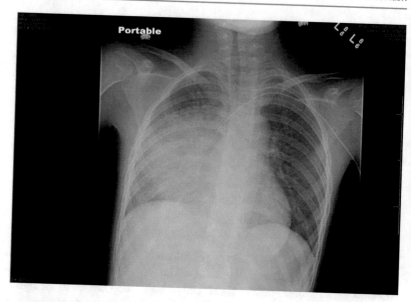

Fig. 37.2 Chest CT scan with contrast, lung window: (**a** and **b**) Right chest soft tissue mass-like opacity (measuring 6 × 7 × 8.5 cm) involving the right upper and middle lobes; mass seen with associated asymmetric thickening of the anterior chest wall subcutaneous tissues and periostitis of the interposed ribs; prominent pretracheal, subcarinal, and right peribronchial lymph nodes

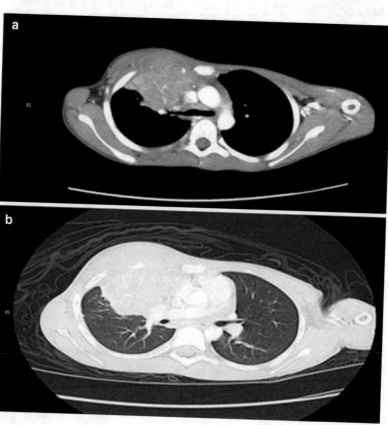

was asymmetric thickening of the anterior chest wall subcutaneous tissues and periostitis of the interposed ribs. The trachea, associated bronchi, and vasculature remained patent without evidence of compression. Transthoracic echocardiography was normal.

Open biopsy of the chest lesion was performed, and pathology showed skeletal muscle and fibro-

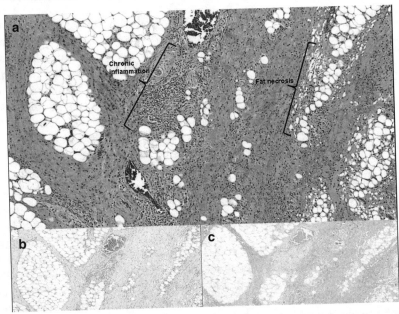

Fig. 37.3 Chest biopsy pathology: (**a**) Hematoxylin and eosin stain, ×10 magnification; portions of skeletal muscle and adipose tissue with severe chronic lymphocytic inflammation and secondary atrophic changes and focal fat necrosis; no bacterial colonies present. (**b**) Chest biopsy pathology slide: Fite stain, ×10 magnification; negative for acid-fast bacilli. (**c**) Chest biopsy pathology slide: Grocott's methenamine silver stain, ×10 magnification; negative for fungal organisms

adipose tissue with chronic inflammatory infiltrate of mostly small, mature lymphocytes and plasma cells. There was no evidence of malignant neoplasia. No granulomas or giant cells were seen. Hematoxylin and eosin, Fite, and Grocott's methenamine silver stains were negative for bacterial, mycobacterial, and fungal elements, respectively (Fig. 37.3). Samples were prepared for bacterial aerobic and anaerobic, fungal and mycobacterial culture. Six days after the biopsy, heavy growth of one organism was reported.

37.1   Differential Diagnosis

This child had a soft tissue mass of the chest wall with underlying pulmonary involvement, which was subacute and had likely evolved slowly over months as the patient had vague complaints of right rib pain and not wanting to wear his school backpack or have other things touch the area months prior to presentation. His parents also noted that he did not like to be helped with bathing or dressing, so they did not observe the patient's skin or chest wall routinely.

In addition to infectious etiologies in the differential diagnosis, it is important to consider and rule out an oncologic process (e.g., rhabdomyosarcoma, peripheral neuroectodermal tumor). Then there are several infectious organisms to consider that cause tissue invasion. This patient appeared to have a primary intrathoracic process leading to destruction of the anterior chest wall tissues. Our infectious differential included organisms that spread across tissue planes (Table 37.1).

Actinomycosis is a chronic granulomatous disease caused by an anaerobic, filamentous Gram-positive bacillus, most commonly *Actinomyces israelii*. *Actinomyces* may reside in the oropharynx, gastrointestinal, and genitourinary tract. Infection is often associated with contiguous spread, allowing abscess and sinus tract formation and soft tissue destruction [1, 2]. Sulfur granules, which are larger colonies of the organism, may be appreciated on histopathology. Clinical forms of disease include orocervicofacial, thoracic, and abdominopelvic disease [2]. Orocervicofacial disease is often a result of trauma to the face or mouth or from dental manipulation. Thoracic

Table 37.1 Pathogens that may cause chest wall mass

Mycobacterium tuberculosis
Nontuberculous mycobacteria
Actinomyces spp.
Aggregatibacter actinomycetemcomitans
Porphyromonas gingivalis
Fusobacterium spp.
Nocardia spp.
Pyogenic bacteria causing abscess (e.g., *Staphylococcus aureus*)
Blastomyces spp.
Histoplasma spp.
Aspergillus spp.

disease results from an extension of orocervicofacial or abdominal disease, aspiration, perforation, or hematogenous spread. Abdominopelvic disease often results from the presence of a foreign body (e.g., intrauterine device), perforation, or surgical manipulation. The boy's clinical presentation was most consistent with thoracic actinomycosis, possibly secondary to his periodontal disease. It is possible that the major dental procedure months prior was the cause of his infection. The empiric choice of penicillin was based on *Actinomyces'* known reliable susceptibility to penicillin [1, 3].

The boy's symptoms also prompted consideration of *Mycobacterium tuberculosis* infection. Pulmonary tuberculosis can mimic thoracic actinomycosis; both can appear as a cavitary mass with surrounding infiltrate [4]. Chest wall tuberculosis is much less common than pulmonary tuberculosis, but it is a well-described clinical entity often involving the sternum, ribs, and vertebrae [5]. While the boy's family members were born in an endemic region, there were no known exposures to persons with active tuberculosis. Additionally, his tuberculin skin test and interferon-gamma release assay were negative, and no acid-fast bacilli were detected on direct smear or grown in culture after 8 weeks.

Fungal organisms were also considered, namely, the thermally dimorphic fungi, *Blastomyces dermatitidis* and *Histoplasma capsulatum*, and the opportunistic fungus, *Aspergillus*. *Blastomyces* and *Histoplasma* are endemic to the Midwest, where the patient

resided. Both can produce large pulmonary mass-like and cavitary lesions, disseminate, and produce complicated infection. *Blastomyces* more typically disseminates to the skin, producing well-circumscribed skin lesions rather than invading into surrounding soft tissues [6, 7]. Complications of pulmonary histoplasmosis, including mediastinal fibrosis, mediastinal granuloma, and broncholithiasis, can cause local invasion, but this primarily involves airways and vasculature within the lungs [1]. This patient did not have skin findings suggestive of disseminated blastomycosis, nor did he have invasion into his airways or lung vasculature to suggest complicated histoplasmosis. *Histoplasma* urine antigen screen and serum antibody screens for *Histoplasma* and *Blastomyces* were all negative. Frequent cross-reactivity with other fungi and limited sensitivity is seen using these tests, making diagnosis less reliable without a positive culture. Our fungal culture remained negative. Invasive aspergillosis is characterized by angioinvasion, thrombosis, and infarction of the lung parenchyma with cavitation and necrosis [7]. While *Aspergillus* species may cause local invasion, they are more typically seen in patients with immunodeficiency, which was not evident in this child. Also, his chest imaging did not show evidence of vascular invasion, making the diagnosis of invasive aspergillosis unlikely.

37.2 Findings in This Case

Heavy growth of *Aggregatibacter actinomycetemcomitans* was found in three of three anaerobic cultures that were sent. Several attempts at susceptibility testing were unsuccessful. Although not included in the initial differential diagnosis, *Aggregatibacter* (*Actinobacillus*) *actinomycetemcomitans* infection has been reported as a clinical entity similar to actinomycosis. *Aggregatibacter* is a fastidious, anaerobic Gram-negative coccobacillus requiring incubation in a carbon dioxide-enhanced environment. It is one of the "HACEK" organisms, including *Haemophilus* species, *Aggregatibacter actinomycetemcomitans*, *Cardiobacterium hominis*, *Eikenella corrodens*, and *Kingella* species. It is an oral commensal and often the cause of periodontal pathology [8]. *Aggregatibacter* can be isolated in cases of actinomycosis (hence its name) or may occur on its own [8–10]. Its clinical presentation is similar to that of actinomycosis, but it is also an important pathogen in infective endocarditis. Thoracic infection has often been linked to dental manipulation and periodontal disease [5]. *Aggregatibacter* infection typically is not well resolved by normal host defenses as it resists phagocytosis and killing by neutrophils [11]. Variable antimicrobial susceptibility makes the choice of empiric therapy more challenging. *Actinomyces* and most HACEK organisms are largely susceptible to penicillin. *Aggregatibacter*, however, is most reliably susceptible to amoxicillin-clavulanate and tetracycline and variably resistant to penicillin, amoxicillin, clindamycin, and metronidazole [3].

The presence of sulfur granules on pathology (which were not found in the present case) and the spread of infection across anatomical barriers are highly consistent with actinomycosis. Prolonged antibiotic therapy is required for cure of actinomycosis [12].

Once it was clear his biopsy was not suggestive of malignancy, the boy was empirically started on intravenous (IV) penicillin for presumptive *Actinomyces* infection. The initial choice of penicillin was based on *Actinomyces'* known susceptibility to penicillin as the drug of choice [10]. After growth of *Aggregatibacter*, however, the antimicrobial agent was changed to IV ampicillin-sulbactam, which was continued for 8 weeks. The boy completed 16 additional weeks of oral amoxicillin-clavulanate and his recovery was complete.

Key Points/Pearls

- *Actinomyces* spp. are present in the oral flora with other potential pathogens, such as *Aggregatibacter actinomycetemcomitans*, *Eikenella corrodens*, *Capnocytophaga*, and *Fusobacterium*; therefore the isolation of *Actinomyces* spp. in a mixed infection of the mouth, neck, and lungs does not necessarily prove that the patient has actinomycosis.

- Actinomycosis may involve not only *Actinomyces* spp. but also "companion microbes," and the latter may be easier to isolate in culture because *Actinomyces* spp. may not grow on antibiotics and may require keeping the cultures longer.
- The presence of sulfur granules on pathology and the spread of infection across anatomical barriers are consistent with actinomycosis.
- *Aggregatibacter actinomycetemcomitans* is an oral commensal that can act alone or in concert with other oral commensals (namely, *Actinomyces*) to produce orofacial and thoracic pathology.
- Periodontal disease history is an important element in the evaluation of any patient with pulmonic disease involving invasion of chest wall.
- *Aggregatibacter actinomycetemcomitans* may have a variable antibiotic susceptibility profile compared with *Actinomyces*, making penicillin a less reliable empiric agent.

References

1. Wheat LJ, Conces D, Allen SD, et al. Pulmonary histoplasmosis syndromes: recognition, diagnosis, and management. Semin Respir Crit Care Med. 2004;25:129–44.
2. Wong VK, Turmezei TD, Weston VC. Actinomycosis. BMJ. 2011;343:d6099.
3. Kulik EM, Lenkeit K, Chenaux S, et al. Antimicrobial susceptibility of periodontopathogenic bacteria. J Antimicrob Chemother. 2008;61:1087–91.
4. Yeung VHW, Wong QHY, Chao NSY, et al. Thoracic actinomycosis in an adolescent mimicking chest wall tumor or pulmonary tuberculosis. Pediatr Surg Int. 2008;24:751–4.
5. Morris BS, Maheshwari M, Chalwa A. Chest wall tuberculosis: a review of CT appearances. Br J Radiol. 2004;77:449–57.
6. Fang W, Washington L, Kumar N. Imaging manifestations of blastomycosis: a pulmonary infection with potential dissemination. Radiographics. 2007;27:641–55.
7. Smith JA, Kauffman CA. Pulmonary fungal infections. Respirology. 2012;17:913–26.
8. Wang CY, Wang HC, Li JM, et al. Invasive infections of *Aggregatibacter* (*Actinobacillus*) *actinomycetemcomitans*. J Microbiol Immunol Infect. 2010;43(6):491–7.
9. Kaplan AH, Weber DJ, Oddone EZ, et al. Infection due to *Actinobacillus actinomycetemcomitans*: 15 cases and review. Rev Infect Dis. 1989;11:46–63.

10. Morris JF, Sewell DL. Necrotizing pneumonia caused by mixed infection with *Actinobacillus actinomycetemcomitans* and *Actinomyces israelii*: case report and review. Clin Infect Dis. 1994;18:450–2.

11. Permpanich P, Kowolich MJ, Galli DM. Resistance of fluorescent-labelled *Actinobacillus actinomycetem-comitans* strains to phagocytosis and killing by human neutrophils. Cell Microbiol. 2006;8(1):72–84.

12. Valour F, Sénéchal A, Dupieux C, et al. Actinomycosis: etiology, clinical features, diagnosis, treatment, and management. Infect Drug Resist. 2014;7:183–97.

Diffuse Lymphadenopathy in a Patient After Stem Cell Transplantation

Leona Ebara

A 59-year-old man with past medical history of chronic myelomonocytic leukemia (CMML) following a haplo-cord stem cell transplant (SCT) a year prior presented as a transfer from an outside hospital with new fever and cervical lymphadenopathy. He had been in his usual state of health until 2 days prior to the admission, when he noted feeling more tired than usual. On the day of admission to the outside hospital, his temperature at home was 101 °F, and he decided to go to the emergency department. On physical examination, he was febrile at 100.9 °F with a heart rate of 116 beats per minute, and his blood pressure was 106/62 mmHg. He was in no acute distress and breathing comfortably. He had no rash, no conjunctival pallor or injection, and no nasal discharge. His oropharynx was without lesions or abnormalities, but he had diffuse cervical lymphadenopathy. The heart, lung, abdominal, and neurological examination was normal. He had no edema in the lower extremities. His thought process was clear.

The white blood cell count was 2800/μL (normal range, 3500–11,000/μL), absolute neutrophil count 1050/μL (1120–6720/μL), hemoglobin 9.3 g/dL (13.5–17.5 g/dL), platelet count 67,000/μL (150,000–450,000/μL), sodium 128 mEq/L (134–149 mEq/L), potassium 3.8 mEq/L, chloride 94 mEq/L (95–108 mEq/L), carbon dioxide 19 mEq/L (23–30 mEq/L), blood urea nitrogen 17 mg/dL, creatinine 0.9 mg/dL, glucose 99 mg/dL, and calcium 10.7 mg/dL (8.4–10.2 mg/dL). The liver function tests were normal, and the stool *Clostridium difficile* toxin polymerase chain reaction (PCR) test was negative.

The patient was started on intravenous levofloxacin at the outside hospital. Blood and urine cultures had no growth prior to hospital transfer. Computed tomography (CT) of the chest without contrast demonstrated diffuse lymphadenopathy, a loculated anterior pericardial effusion, liver cysts, and concentric thickening of the antral wall of the stomach, suggestive of tumor infiltration. CT of the sinuses was unremarkable. He was transferred to our tertiary care hospital for continuity of care. CT of the neck and chest with contrast showed extensive cervical, supraclavicular, intrathoracic, and abdominopelvic lymphadenopathy (Fig. 38.1). A positron emission tomography (PET) scan showed widespread, markedly hypermetabolic tumor with extensive involvement of lymph nodes from the neck to the pelvis (Fig. 38.2). The differential diagnosis is presented in Table 38.1.

Further workup was performed including serum Epstein–Barr virus (EBV) PCR and cervical lymph node biopsy. The patient's blood EBV PCR was initially negative, but on repeated testing it became strongly positive, with 43,800 copies/mL during the first week of the admission. It increased to 252,000 copies/mL the following

L. Ebara, M.D.
Section of Infectious Diseases and Global Health,
Department of Medicine, University of Chicago,
Chicago, IL, USA
e-mail: Leona.Ebara@uchospitals.edu

© Springer International Publishing AG 2018
M. David, J.-L. Benoit (eds.), *The Infectious Disease Diagnosis*,
https://doi.org/10.1007/978-3-319-64906-1_38

Fig. 38.1 CT with contrast of the neck showing extensive cervical and supraclavicular lymphadenopathy; most lymph nodes appear homogeneous, but a few appear to be necrotic

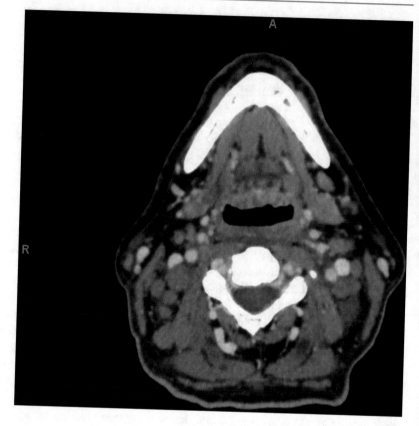

Fig. 38.2 Positron emission tomography (PET) scan showing widespread, markedly hypermetabolic tumor involving lymph nodes from the neck to pelvis as well as involvement of liver, spleen, and lungs with at least one osseous lesion

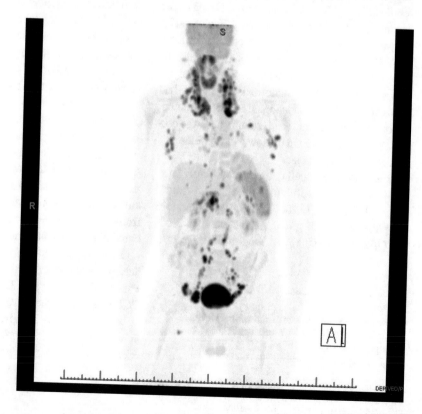

Table 38.1 Differential diagnosis for diffuse lymphadenopathy in the immunocompromised host such as after stem cell transplantation

Posttransplant lymphoproliferative disease (PTLD)
Lymphoma
Tuberculosis (*Mycobacterium tuberculosis*)
Atypical mycobacterial infection
Cytomegalovirus (CMV)
Epstein-Barr virus (EBV)
Toxoplasmosis (*Toxoplasma gondii*)
Bacillary angiomatosis due to *Bartonella henselae* (cat scratch disease pathogen) or *B. quintana* (trench fever pathogen)
Human immunodeficiency virus (HIV)
Kikuchi's disease
Head or neck malignancy
Brucellosis (*Brucella spp.*)
Coccidioidomycosis (*Coccidioides immitis*)
Histoplasmosis (*Histoplasma capsulatum*)
Blastomycosis (*Blastomyces dermatitidis*)

week. Pathological examination of the cervical lymph node biopsy specimen showed that its architecture was effaced by proliferation of medium to large atypical lymphoid cells with irregular nuclei, one to several prominent nucleoli and moderate amphophilic cytoplasm growing in sheets associated with clearly demonstrated mitotic activity. There were scattered tingible body macrophages and focal areas of necrosis with numerous apoptotic bodies. In some areas the large atypical lymphoid cells showed immunoblastic/plasmablastic features. This was consistent with a diagnosis of EBV-associated monomorphic B cell posttransplant lymphoproliferative disorder (PTLD) (diffuse large B cell lymphoma).

The patient was treated with intravenous rituximab and was discharged to home with a plan for weekly rituximab for a total of four doses with close follow-up in the Oncology Clinic.

38.1 Posttransplant Lymphoproliferative Disease (PTLD)

PTLD is a well-recognized complication of both solid organ transplantation (SOT) and allogeneic hematopoietic SCT as a result of immunosuppression. It is characterized by lymphoid and/or plasmacytic proliferation and is a serious and potentially fatal complication. The majority of these cases are related to EBV infection. There are three types of PTLD: (1) early lesion (infectious mononucleosis-type acute illness without evidence of malignant transformation), (2) polymorphic PTLD (with evidence of malignant transformation but poly- or oligoclonal and does not meet all of the criteria for B/T/NK cell lymphoma); and (3) monomorphic PTLD (which is monoclonal and meets criteria for B/T/NK cell lymphoma).

PTLD develops when B cell proliferation is induced by EBV infection in chronic immunosuppression and in the setting of decreased T cell surveillance. In the immunocompetent host, EBV viral antigen is expressed by B cells and elicits a T cell response that eliminates the majority of the infected B cells. In the immunocompromised host, in contrast, a small subset of the infected B cells downregulates viral antigen expression, escapes immune surveillance, and persists lifelong if T cell function wanes. Patients can then develop PTLD.

PTLD in SCT patients is commonly donor derived. Proliferation of EBV-infected B cells occurs in the absence of normal T cell immune surveillance. If T cells are depleted from a marrow graft, as they are commonly in order to reduce the risk of graft vs. host disease (GVHD) while B cells remain, then the transformed B cells may escape from T cell surveillance and proliferate rapidly. PTLD is the most common malignancy complicating SOT. In contrast, PTLD accounts for a minority of second cancers following allogeneic SCT. The incidence of PTLD in this population is approximately 1% over 10 years, which is 30–50 times higher than in the general population. More than 80% of cases occur in the first year after transplant. Risk factors include the degree of T cell immunosuppression, EBV serostatus of the recipient, time after transplant, and recipient age and ethnicity.

The clinical manifestations are highly variable and depend on the type of PTLD and also the anatomic sites of involvement. Fever, weight loss, and fatigue (i.e., B symptoms) are common. Other manifestations include acute infectious mononucleosis like symptoms, lymphadenopathy, and dysfunction of involved organs. PTLD patients demonstrate marked elevation of the serum EBV viral load. PTLD may thus be detected early by monitoring the EBV serum PCR of patients at high risk. Because the majority of EBV-positive PTLD occurs in the first years after transplantation, it is reasonable to monitor high-risk patients more frequently during this period.

The diagnosis of PTLD requires a high index of suspicion. Radiology findings, unexplained anemia, thrombocytopenia, leukopenia or high serum level of lactate dehydrogenase (LDH), calcium, uric acid, or a monoclonal protein can be the first clues to the diagnosis of PTLD. The diagnosis, however, requires tissue biopsy with histological evaluation and is often supplemented by a PET scan. For PTLD, reduction of immunosuppression is the cornerstone of therapy. It is also important to give antiviral prophylaxis and to monitor the serum EBV PCR. Preemptive treatment of PTLD at the time of viral reactivation with the CD20 monoclonal antibody rituximab or reduced immunosuppression is also recommended. Chemotherapy, radiation therapy, or both may also be necessary. Adoptive immunotherapy with EBV-specific cytotoxic T cells is used in cases of disease that persists despite initial therapy.

Key Points/Pearls

- Consider PTLD with diffuse lymphadenopathy in an immunocompromised host after solid organ transplantation or allogeneic hematopoietic cell transplantation.
- PTLD is the most common malignancy complicating solid organ transplantation.
- Aggressive withdrawal and tapering of immunosuppressive agents are required for PTLD therapy.

- Preemptive treatment with the CD20 monoclonal antibody, rituximab, is recommended therapy for PTLD.
- The incidence of PTLD after solid organ transplants depends on the type of organ transplanted; incidence of PTLD is the highest in lung, heart-lung, and small bowel transplant, which require more profound immunosuppression to prevent organ rejection, while liver and especially kidney transplant recipients have a lower incidence of PTLD; kidneypancreas transplant recipient has an intermediate risk of PTLD.
- When lymphoproliferative disease develops within the transplanted organ, it is more likely to be in the lung or small bowel allograft.

Bibliography

1. Hanto DW. Classification of Epstein-Barr virus-associated posttransplant lymphoproliferative diseases: implications for understanding their pathogenesis and developing rational treatment strategies. Annu Rev Med. 1995;46:381–94.
2. Landgren O, Gilbert ES, Rizzo JD, et al. Risk factors for lymphoproliferative disorders after allogeneic hematopoietic cell transplantation. Blood. 2009;113:4992–5001.
3. Holmes RD, Sokol RJ. Epstein-Barr virus and posttransplant lymphoproliferative disease. Pediatr Transplant. 2002;6:456–64.
4. Straathof KC, Savoldo B, Heslop HE, Rooney CM. Immunotherapy for post-transplant lymphoproliferative disease. Br J Haematol. 2002;118:728–40.
5. European best practice guidelines for renal transplantation. Nephrol Dial Transplant. 2002;17(Suppl 4):1–85.
6. Allen U, Hébert D, Moore D, et al. Epstein-Barr virus-related post-transplant lymphoproliferative disease in solid organ transplant recipients, 1988-97: a Canadian multi-centre experience. Pediatr Transplant. 2001;5:198–203.

Papilledema in an HIV-Positive Patient

39

Eric Bhaimia and Nirav Shah

A 45-year-old male with human immunodeficiency virus (HIV) infection presented to the Emergency Department from the Ophthalmology Clinic with bilateral papilledema. He reported frontal headaches for the previous month and intermittent bilateral eye redness. He had recently been seen at an outside clinic, where he was given an unspecified antibiotic ophthalmic solution, which he reported using without relief. He also noted a decrease in his visual acuity during this time despite the use of new prescription glasses. This led him to make an appointment with an ophthalmologist, who noted papilledema of both eyes and referred him to the Emergency Department. The patient denied nausea, vomiting, or neck stiffness. He also denied fevers, chills, sinus congestion, molar pain, numbness, weakness, change in personality, weight loss, or night sweats.

Five months before, the patient's CD4+ T cell count was 436 cells/mm³ and his HIV viral load was undetectable. His CD4+ count had remained >200 cells/mm³ for the previous 6 years. His history was significant for treatment of latent tuberculosis infection with 9 months of isoniazid completed approximately 1 year prior to the current presentation, anxiety, depression, and LASIK eye surgery 9 years before. The patient reported that he was not then involved in a relationship, and he identified as a man who has sex with men (MSM). He was a former tobacco smoker and cocaine user (last use 2 years prior), and he reported consuming one glass of alcohol per week. He denied a history of recent travel, any recent exposure to sick contacts, or exposure to animals. He was adherent to his antiretroviral therapy (ART), comprised of atazanavir, ritonavir, and emtricitabine/tenofovir.

On physical examination, the temperature was 99.5 °F, blood pressure 113/66 mmHg, pulse 75 beats per minute, respirations 18 breaths per minute, and oxygen saturation 96% on room air. The patient appeared generally comfortable. His eye exam revealed non-icteric sclerae but significant bilateral conjunctival injection. The neck was supple and oropharynx without notable edema or tonsillar hypertrophy and sinuses were not tender to palpation. There was no appreciable lymphadenopathy in the cervical or occipital chains. Auscultation of the heart and lungs was normal. The abdomen was benign and the extremities were normal. Neurological exam revealed facial symmetry, intact cranial nerves, and normal sensation in all extremities. Assessment of the deep tendon reflexes and gait were normal. Ophthalmologic exam (performed prior to referral to the Emergency Department) revealed normal intraocular pressures with 2+ optic disc edema of

E. Bhaimia, D.O. • N. Shah, M.D., M.P.H. (✉)
Department of Medicine, NorthShore University HealthSystem, Evanston, IL, USA

University of Chicago Medicine, Chicago, IL, USA
e-mail: nshah2@northshore.org

© Springer International Publishing AG 2018
M. David, J.-L. Benoit (eds.), *The Infectious Disease Diagnosis*,
https://doi.org/10.1007/978-3-319-64906-1_39

the left eye and 3+ of the right eye. Initial laboratory studies, including basic metabolic panel and complete blood count, were without significant abnormality. CD4+ T cell count was 516 cells/mm^3. Prior laboratory studies revealed negative rapid plasma reagin (RPR), gonorrhea, and *Chlamydia* studies as recent as 5 months prior. Hepatitis B surface antigen, hepatitis B surface antibody, and hepatitis C antibody were negative 4 years before presentation. The *Toxoplasma* IgG was negative when checked 10 years prior to presentation.

Computed tomography (CT) of the head with and without contrast revealed soft tissue thickening of the nasopharynx, but was otherwise without acute intracranial abnormality. A magnetic resonance imaging (MRI) scan of the brain revealed bilateral enhancement of the nasopharyngeal soft tissue and faint bilateral enhancement of the internal auditory canals (Fig. 39.1). There was no evidence of venous sinus thrombosis on magnetic resonance venography (MRV). Lumbar puncture (LP) revealed cerebrospinal fluid (CSF) glucose of 53 mg/dL, protein of 42 mg/dL, and total cell count of 55 (21 WBC/µL with 7% PMNs and 34 RBC/µL). The opening pressure was not obtained due to the patient's position. CSF bacterial culture, fungal, and acid-fast bacilli (AFB) smears and cryptococcal antigen were all negative.

The patient's optic disc edema with associated changes in visual acuity supported the diagnosis of bilateral optic neuritis. The differential diagnosis for optic neuritis is presented in Table 39.1 [1]. The typical presentation consists of acute, often painful impairment of vision with monocular involvement. Symptoms develop over several days and generally peak within 2 weeks. Papillitis, or inflammation of the optic disc, with hyperemia and swelling of the disc is seen in one-third of patients with optic neuritis [2]. Papilledema, the term used to describe optic disc swelling that occurs secondary to elevated intracranial pressure, remained on the differential. It almost always presents as a bilateral phenomenon and may develop over hours to weeks, depending on the underlying etiology. Optic disc swelling occurs as a result of axoplasmic flow stasis with resultant intra-axonal edema [3]. This may occur as a complication of any space-occupying lesion within the central nervous system (CNS) or decreased CSF absorption (as occurs in the setting of venous sinus thrombosis, meningitis, and other inflammatory processes).

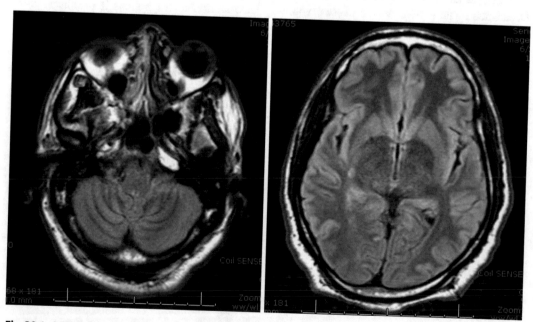

Fig. 39.1 MRI brain with and without contrast revealing bilateral enhancement of the nasopharyngeal soft tissue and faint bilateral enhancement of the internal auditory canals

Table 39.1 Differential diagnosis of optic neuritis [1]

Sarcoidosis
Multiple sclerosis
Systemic autoimmune disease (e.g., systemic lupus erythematosus, Sjögren's syndrome)
Meningitis (any cause)
West Nile virus
Syphilis (*Treponema pallidum*)
Lyme disease (*Borrelia burgdorferi*)
Cat scratch disease (*Bartonella henselae*)
Toxoplasmosis

Table 39.2 Laboratory results (from cerebrospinal fluid unless otherwise indicated)

Name of test (normal values in parentheses)	Test result
Opening pressure (10–25 cm H$_2$O)	22 cm H$_2$O
Glucose (45–80 mg/dL)	53 mg/dL
Protein (20–40 mg/dL)	42 mg/dL
White blood cells (0–5 cells/μL)	21 cells/μL
Neutrophils (<2 cells/μL)	7%
Lymphocytes (60–70%)	77%
Plasma cells (0%)	1%
Red blood cells (0 cells/μL)	34 cells/μL
Bacterial culture	Negative
Fungal culture	Negative
Acid-fast bacilli	Negative
Cryptococcus antigen	Negative
Epstein Barr virus (EBV) PCR	Negative
Cytomegalovirus (CMV) PCR	Negative
Herpes simplex virus (HSV) PCR	Negative
Varicella zoster virus (VZV) PCR	Negative
Angiotensin-converting enzyme (ACE)	Negative
Cytology	Negative for malignant cells
VDRL	Negative
FTA-ABS	Positive
RPR (serum)	Positive
RPR titer (serum)	1:512
FTA (serum)	Positive

FTA fluorescent treponemal antibody, *FTA-ABS* fluorescent treponemal antibody absorption, *PCR* polymerase chain reaction, *RPR* rapid plasma reagin, *VDRL* venereal disease research laboratory

The Neurology Service was consulted, and concern for bilateral papilledema was again raised based on fundoscopic examination. Also noted was mild ptosis and miosis of the left eye. Chest radiograph revealed diffuse, bibasilar airspace opacities suspicious for pneumonia, suggesting acute aspiration. The patient's headache persisted, but the conjunctival injection resolved. A repeat LP was performed with an opening pressure of 22 cm H$_2$O (normal range, 10–25 cm H$_2$O). Other CSF findings are detailed in Table 39.2. The serum RPR was positive with a quantitative titer of 1:512. Confirmatory serum and CSF fluorescent treponemal antibody (FTA-ABS) testing was positive, consistent with the diagnosis of probable neurosyphilis. Furthermore, the finding of optic disc edema in the setting of normal intracranial pressures is inconsistent with papilledema and supports the diagnosis of optic perineuritis secondary to acute syphilis infection.

The patient later endorsed unprotected sexual intercourse with multiple male partners over the previous 3 months. He also reported developing a painless rash on the penis that had spontaneously resolved. He was treated with intravenous penicillin G for 2 weeks and reported resolution of the headaches. Disc edema had improved on follow-up with the Ophthalmology Service and repeat LP revealed normal CSF cell counts.

39.1 Syphilis

Syphilis is an infection caused by the bacterial spirochete, *Treponema pallidum* (Fig. 39.2). Most new cases are sexually acquired. The protean clinical manifestations have garnered syphilis the designation of the Great Masquerader. Transmission occurs via direct contact with an infectious lesion, such as a primary chancre, mucous patch, or condyloma lata. From 2005 to 2014, the number of reported primary and secondary syphilis cases in the United States increased from 8724 to 19,999. During the same period, the annual incidence increased from 2.9 to 6.3 cases per 100,000 population [4]. Approximately 90% of syphilis cases occur in men and 61% of those cases occur in MSM.

Syphilis is divided into early and late infection. The signs and symptoms encountered correlate with the stage of infection. In the early stage, primary syphilis is characterized by the formation of a chancre approximately 21 days following infection. Syphilitic chancres are typically painless and indurated ulcers that spontaneously resolve within

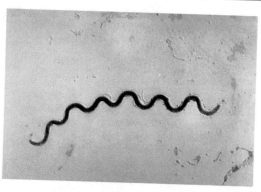

Fig. 39.2 *Treponema pallidum* bacterium shown under dark-field light microscopy. Source: Susan Lindsley, CDC https://phil.cdc.gov/phil/details.asp (image ID#; 14969, Accessed on May 4, 2017)

3–6 weeks, even in the absence of treatment. Despite resolution of the chancre, secondary syphilis develops within a few weeks to months in approximately 25% of individuals with untreated infection [5]. Patients develop a systemic illness which may consist of fever, headache, malaise, anorexia, sore throat, myalgias, and weight loss. Lymphadenopathy is also a common finding, and the enlargement of epitrochlear nodes is particularly suggestive of the diagnosis. Rash is the most characteristic finding. Although it may take any form, this rash is classically described as a diffuse, macular, or papular eruption involving the trunk and extremities as well as the palms and soles. Other dermatological diagnostic clues include alopecia, mucous patches, and condyloma lata, which are seen in a minority of patients. In HIV-infected patients, a more severe rash may rarely occur which is termed *lues maligna*, characterized by non-resolving, ulcerative skin lesions. Other potential findings in secondary syphilis include hepatitis, nephritis, synovitis, and neurologic and ocular signs and symptoms.

The transition to late syphilis occurs in approximately 25–40% of untreated individuals and is most commonly manifested by aortitis, gummas, and CNS involvement. Tertiary syphilis is the term used to describe patients with late syphilis who have symptomatic involvement of the cardiovascular system or gummatous lesions, which may occur on the skin, bones, or internal organs. The designation of latent syphilis is given to a patient with positive serology, yet without symptoms. This is further divided into early latent (if infection occurred within 12 months), late latent (if infection occurred earlier than 12 months prior), or latent syphilis of unknown duration (if the duration of infection is unknown).

39.2 Neurosyphilis

Neurosyphilis is the term used to describe *Treponema pallidum* infection of the CNS. Prior to antibiotics, neurosyphilis occurred in 25–35% of patients infected with syphilis [6]. Today, neurosyphilis is most frequently diagnosed in patients with HIV infection. The diagnosis is made by both serum nontreponemal and treponemal tests (see Table 39.3), with concomitant positivity of CSF studies. The CSF-VDRL test is considered highly specific but lacks sensitivity. If the CSF-VDRL is negative and suspicion for neurosyphilis remains, CSF FTA-ABS may be ordered because it is a more sensitive test [7]. However, CSF-FTA is poorly specific for neurosyphilis due to frequent contamination of CSF by blood during the lumbar puncture.

Early neurosyphilis may range from an asymptomatic state to symptomatic meningitis and meningovascular syphilis associated with meningitis and vasculitis causing strokes, with increased frequency in patients with HIV infection. Early neurosyphilis may also present as otosyphilis (a potentially partially reversible cause of sensorineural hearing loss) and ocular syphilis, the latter of which is described in the present case. Late features of neurosyphilis include general paresis, characterized as progressive dementia with associated personality change, and tabes dorsalis, most frequently associated with sensory ataxia and lancinating pains affecting the back, limbs, or face.

Ocular syphilis may involve any part of the eye, but most commonly presents as panuveitis or posterior uveitis, resulting in diminished visual acuity [8]. In 2016, the CDC reported a remarkable increase in cases of severe ocular neurosyphilis in the United States, with permanently

Table 39.3 Syphilis serologic testing

Serum nontreponemal tests
- Rapid plasma reagin (RPR)
- Venereal disease research laboratory (VDRL)

Serum treponemal tests
- Fluorescent treponemal antibody absorption (FTA-ABS)
- *Treponema pallidum* particle agglutination assay (TPPA)
- Syphilis enzyme immunoassays (EIAs)

decreased visual acuity often in HIV-infected persons [9]. Both ocular syphilis and neurosyphilis can occur at any stage of syphilis, including early syphilis.

Syphilitic optic perineuritis is yet another ocular manifestation characterized by swollen optic discs in the absence of increased intracranial pressure or visual disturbance. Optic perineuritis occurs due to inflammation of the optic nerve sheath and is often mistaken for papilledema or papillitis [10]. Reports of perioptic neuritis are usually associated with other manifestations of CNS involvement as evidenced by a CSF pleocytosis, elevated protein level, or positive CSF-VDRL. The clinical manifestation of optic perineuritis may aid in the diagnosis of syphilis and allow for early treatment before other features of neurosyphilis emerge.

Key Points/Pearls
- Clinical suspicion and CSF analysis are keys to the diagnosis of neurosyphilis.
- A positive CSF-VDRL associated with CSF leukocytosis confirms neurosyphilis but is not a sensitive test; CSF leukocytosis with a negative VDRL may indicate probable or possible neurosyphilis, depending on the clinical presentation.
- The presence of optic perineuritis may represent early neurosyphilis, permitting treatment and avoidance of further complications.
- Optic perineuritis is characterized by optic disc edema in the absence of increased intracranial pressure.
- Neurosyphilis should be treated with penicillin G (intravenous aqueous crystalline penicillin G or intramuscular procaine penicillin G

combined with oral probenecid) for a duration of 10–14 days.
- Desensitization to penicillin G may be required in patients with neurosyphilis who have a history of anaphylaxis to penicillin.
- Ocular syphilis is an ophthalmologic emergency as it can result in permanently decreased vision, especially in persons with HIV infection.
- Ocular syphilis can affect any part of the eye and may be associated with neurosyphilis.
- Secondary syphilis has protean manifestations, and it is in the differential diagnosis of nonspecific skin rashes, acute mononucleosis syndromes, and ocular or neurological clinical presentations.

References

1. Ray S, Gragoudas E. Neuroretinitis. Int Ophthalmol Clin. 2001;41(1):83–102
2. The clinical profile of optic neuritis. Experience of the Optic Neuritis Treatment Trial. Optic Neuritis Study Group. Arch Ophthalmol. 1991;109(12):1673–8.
3. Sinclair AJ, Burdon MA, Nightingale PG, Matthews TD, Jacks A, Lawden M, et al. Rating papilloedema: an evaluation of the Frisén classification in idiopathic intracranial hypertension. J Neurol. 2012;259(7):1406–12
4. Centers for Disease Control and Prevention. Sexually transmitted disease surveillance 2014. Atlanta: U.S. Department of Health and Human Services; 2015. http://www.cdc.gov/std/stats14/surv-2014-print.pdf. Accessed 3 May 2017.
5. Clark EG, Danbolt N. The Oslo study of the natural course of untreated syphilis: an epidemiologic investigation based on a re-study of the Boeck-Bruusgaard material. Med Clin North Am. 1964;48:613–23
6. Merritt HH, Adams RD, Solomon HC. Neurosyphilis. New York: Oxford; 1946.
7. Workowski KA, Bolan GA, Centers for Disease Control and Prevention. Sexually transmitted diseases treatment guidelines, 2015. MMWR Recomm Rep. 2015;64(RR-03):1.
8. Moradi A, Salek S, Daniel E, et al. Clinical features and incidence rates of ocular complications in patients with ocular syphilis. Am J Ophthalmol. 2015;159:334–43.e1.
9. CDC—Clinical Advisory: Ocular Syphilis in the United States [Internet]. [cited 12 Feb 2017]. https://www.cdc.gov/std/syphilis/clinicaladvisoryos2015.htm. Accessed 22 June 2017.
10. Meehan K, Rodman J. Ocular perineuritis secondary to neurosyphilis. Optom Vis Sci. 2010;87:E790–6

A Case of Fever and Rash After a Tick Bite

Jessica Ridgway

A 55-year-old man with a history of diabetes mellitus type 2 presented to the Emergency Department (ED) in May with 5 days of headache, fever to 104 °F, diffuse myalgias, and generalized weakness. He denied neck stiffness or photophobia. He also denied confusion, nausea, or vomiting.

The patient lived in rural Indiana. He frequently performed yardwork, and he had noticed a tick on his arm 10 days before. He removed the tick with tweezers and reported that it was not engorged. Three weeks prior to presentation, he went camping in the forest and slept in a cabin. He had a pet dog. He also had frequent contact with his 3-year-old granddaughter who had a recent febrile upper respiratory illness. For his diabetes he took metformin.

On physical examination, temperature was 38.7 °C, blood pressure 92/60 mmHg, heart rate 123 beats per minute, and respiratory rate 18 breaths per minute. In general, he appeared diaphoretic and uncomfortable. His cardiac exam revealed an irregularly irregular rhythm, pulmonary exam was clear, and abdominal exam was benign. He was alert and oriented, and his neurologic exam was grossly within normal limits. He had negative Kernig's and Brudzinski's signs.

In the ED, he received a dose of intravenous (IV) ceftriaxone, after which he developed an acute, diffuse, erythematous petechial rash on his trunk and extremities, including the palms of his hands (Fig. 40.1). Complete blood count showed a white blood cell (WBC) count of 8900/µL with 78% neutrophils and 14% bands, hemoglobin of 14.6 g/dL, and platelets of 25,000/µL (normal range,150,000–450,000/µL). His complete metabolic panel (electrolytes, liver tests, creatinine, and blood urea nitrogen) was unremarkable. A lumbar puncture was deferred due to thrombocytopenia and concerns for bleeding. Computed tomography (CT) of the head and magnetic resonance imaging (MRI) scan of the brain were unremarkable. An electrocardiogram (EKG) revealed that he was in atrial fibrillation. The patient became increasingly hypotensive, and he was intubated and mechanically ventilated, started on vasoactive agents, and transferred to the medical intensive care unit.

Microbiology studies drawn on admission are shown in Table 40.1. While he had positive serum IgG for cytomegalovirus (CMV) and Epstein Barr virus (EBV), indicating prior infection with these viruses, the rest of his microbiology results did not reveal a diagnosis. He was empirically treated with vancomycin, aztreonam, levofloxacin, acyclovir, and doxycycline to cover broadly for possible meningitis, encephalitis, and rickettsial disease. β-Lactam antibiotics were avoided as it was thought that ceftriaxone might have caused his rash. Five days into his admission, his platelet

J. Ridgway, M.D., M.S.
Section of Infectious Diseases and Global Health,
Department of Medicine, University of Chicago,
Chicago, IL, USA
e-mail: Jessica.Ridgway@uchospitals.edu

© Springer International Publishing AG 2018
M. David, J.-L. Benoit (eds.), *The Infectious Disease Diagnosis*,
https://doi.org/10.1007/978-3-319-64906-1_40

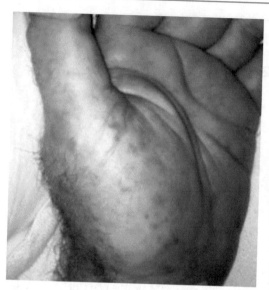

Fig. 40.1 Photograph of rash on patient's palm

Table 40.1 Patient's admission microbiology test results

Microbiology test (blood/serum unless noted)	Result
Blood culture	Negative
Urine culture	Negative
Human immunodeficiency virus (HIV) antibody	Negative
Respiratory viral panel[a]	Negative
Rickettsia rickettsii IgM, IgG	Negative
Rickettsia typhi IgM, IgG	Negative
Anasplasma phagocytophilum IgM, IgG	Negative
Ehrlichia chaffeensis IgM, IgG	Negative
Lyme disease (*Borrelia burgdorferi*) EIA	3.21 Lyme index units (normal range < 0.75)
Lyme Western blot IgM, IgG	Negative
Cytomegalovirus (CMV) IgM	Negative
CMV IgG	Positive
Epstein Barr virus (EBV) IgM	Negative
EBV IgG	Positive

[a]Polymerase chain reaction test for the following pathogens: adenovirus, coronavirus 229E, coronavirus HKU1, coronavirus OC43, coronavirus NL63, human metapneumovirus, human rhinovirus/enterovirus, influenza A, influenza A/H1, influenza A/H1–2009, influenza A/H3, influenza B, parainfluenza 1, parainfluenza 2, parainfluenza 3, parainfluenza 4, respiratory syncytial virus (RSV), *Bordetella pertussis*, *Chlamydophila pneumoniae*, and *Mycoplasma pneumoniae*

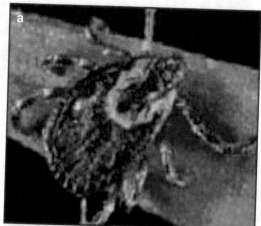

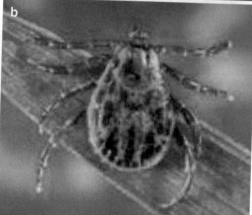

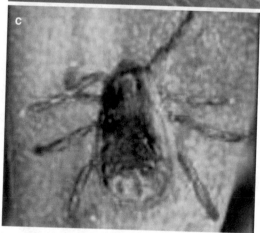

Fig. 40.2 Ticks that transmit *Rickettsia rickettsii* in the United States: (**a**) American dog tick (*Dermacentor variabilis*); (**b**) Rocky Mountain wood tick (*Dermacentor andersoni*); (**c**) brown dog tick (*Rhipicephalus sanguineus*). Source: Centers for Disease Control and Prevention. http://www.cdc.gov/ticks/geographic_distribution.html (Accessed on May 2, 2017)

count had improved to 120,000/μL, and a lumbar puncture was deemed safe and performed. It showed a total cell count of 18 cells/μL, with 10 WBC/μL, 8 red blood cells/μL, 14% neutrophils, 68% lymphocytes, and 16% monocytes. Protein was 54 mg/dL (normal range, <45 mg/dL), and glucose 106 mg/dL. In the cerebrospinal fluid (CSF), enterovirus polymerase chain reaction (PCR), herpes simplex virus (HSV) 1 and 2 PCR, varicella zoster virus (VZV) PCR, and West Nile virus (WNV) antibodies were negative.

The differential diagnosis for fever in a patient with a petechial rash includes meningococcemia, Rocky Mountain spotted fever (RMSF) and other rickettsial diseases, drug reaction, parvovirus B19 infection (fifth disease), and infectious mononucleosis (Table 40.2). The patient's his-

Table 40.2 Differential diagnosis of fever and maculo-papular and petechial rash

Disease	Pathogen
Infectious	
Rocky Mountain spotted fever	*Rickettsia rickettsii*
Murine typhus	*Rickettsia typhi*
Ehrlichiosis	*Ehrlichia chaffeensis*, *Ehrlichia ewingii*
Anaplasmosis	*Anaplasma phagocytophilum*
Scarlet fever	Group A *Streptococcus*
Meningococcemia	*Neisseria meningitidis*
Disseminated gonococcal disease	*Neisseria gonorrhoeae*
Fifth disease	Parvovirus B19
Roseola	Human herpesvirus-6 (HHV-6)
Enteroviral disease	Coxsackie virus, echovirus, etc.
Infectious mononucleosis	Epstein-Barr virus (EBV) infection
Mycoplasma pneumonia	*Mycoplasma pneumoniae*
Leptospirosis	*Leptospira* spp.
Noninfectious	
Kawasaki disease	
Drug reaction	
Thrombotic thrombocytopenic purpura (TTP)	
Stevens-Johnson syndrome	
Toxic shock syndrome	

tory of tick bite raises the concern for RMSF, human granulocytic anaplasmosis, or monocytic ehrlichiosis. This patient's severe illness and rash involving the palms is more characteristic of RMSF than ehrlichiosis.

One week after his initial presentation, the rickettsial serology was repeated and this time revealed a positive RMSF IgM titer (>1:256) with a negative IgG. Based on this result, he was diagnosed with RMSF. His antibiotics were narrowed to only doxycycline. He gradually recovered and was discharged to an acute rehabilitation facility.

40.1   Rocky Mountain Spotted Fever (RMSF)

RMSF is a tick-borne zoonosis caused by transmission of *Rickettsia rickettsii* to a human via the bite of an infected tick. The primary vector in the United States (US) is the American dog tick (*Dermacentor variabilis*), but the pathogen is also transmitted by the Rocky Mountain wood tick (*Dermacentor andersoni*) and the brown dog tick (*Rhipicephalus sanguineus*). RMSF occurs throughout the United States, but, despite its name, cases predominantly occur in the Midwest and Southeast [1].

The mean incubation period between exposure and onset of symptoms is 7 days, with a range of 2–14 days [2]. RMSF cases follow a seasonal pattern, with 90% of infections occurring between April and September. Clinical signs and symptoms include fever, myalgias, severe headache, as well as nausea, vomiting, and abdominal pain. A characteristic petechial or maculopapular rash that starts around the wrists and ankles and may involve the palms and soles appears 2–5 days after the onset of fever. Less common clinical presentations include myocarditis, pneumonia, acute kidney injury, and neurologic manifestations. RMSF often causes severe illness, with a case fatality rate of 5–10%.

The diagnosis of RMSF is based on clinical signs and symptoms in a patient with possible tick exposure. Treatment should not be delayed while awaiting laboratory confirmation of the diagnosis. Laboratory abnormalities include mild hepatic transaminitis, thrombocytopenia, hyponatremia, and mild lymphocytic pleocytosis in the CSF [3]. Immunohistochemistry performed on skin biopsy at rash onset may be useful to confirm a diagnosis. RMSF serology typically becomes positive 7–10 days after symptom onset. A fourfold increase in serum antibody titers or a convalescent titer >1:64 is diagnostic. There is possible cross-reaction between RMSF titers and other spotted fever group rickettsioses, especially *Rickettsia parkeri*, which is transmitted by the Gulf Coast tick *Amblyomma maculatum*, may have an eschar at the site of tick bite and usually causes a mild illness. The treatment of choice for RMSF is oral doxycycline 100 mg twice per day for 5–7 days, continuing at least 2–3 days after the patient defervesces. Chloramphenicol is an alternative treatment only used in cases of severe doxycycline allergy or during pregnancy if the illness is mild, but chloramphenicol is associated with increased mortality, is also associated with adverse effects, and is ineffective against other severe tick-borne infections in the differential diagnosis, i.e., human granulocytic anaplasmosis and human monocytic ehrlichiosis.

Key Points/Pearls

- Rocky Mountain spotted fever (RMSF) is a severe tick-borne zoonosis caused by *Rickettsia rickettsii* and transmitted by various ticks including the American dog tick, the Rocky Mountain wood tick, and the brown dog tick.
- Typical symptoms include fever and severe headache followed 2–5 days later by a maculopapular or petechial rash that starts around the wrists or ankles and may involve the palms and soles; skin biopsy may confirm the diagnosis when immunohistochemistry identifies *Rickettsia rickettsii* within the endothelium.
- The diagnosis of RMSF should be made clinically; serologic studies become positive 7–10 days after onset of symptoms.
- The treatment of choice for RMSF is doxycycline, even in children and during pregnancy.
- Severe rickettsioses to consider in the United States are RMSF, human granulocytic anaplasmosis, and human monocytic ehrlichiosis; in other regions of the world, Mediterranean spotted fever, epidemic typhus, and scrub typhus also can cause severe illness.
- In severely ill patients with fever and rash, one should consider the possibility of rickettsioses and the possible indication of adding doxycycline.

References

1. Parola P, Paddock CD, Socolovschi C, et al. Update on tick-borne rickettsioses around the world: a geographic approach. Clin Microbiol Rev. 2013;26(4):657–702
2. Dantas-Torres F. Rocky Mountain spotted fever. Lancet Infect Dis. 2007;7(11):724–32
3. Chapman AS, Bakken JS, Folk SM, et al. Diagnosis and management of tickborne rickettsial diseases: Rocky Mountain spotted fever, ehrlichioses, and anaplasmosis—United States: a practical guide for physicians and other health-care and public health professionals. MMWR Recomm Rep. 2006;55(RR-4):1–27

Fredy Chaparro-Rojas

A 62-year-old white man was readmitted to the hospital 2 days after he was discharged following single left lung transplantation for severe idiopathic pulmonary fibrosis. His posttransplant hospital course was unremarkable, and he left the hospital on prophylactic and immunosuppressive medications as per protocol. He presented to an outside hospital in respiratory distress and was transferred to our tertiary care hospital where he was found to have progressed to respiratory failure requiring emergent endotracheal intubation. A significant amount of bright red blood in the pulmonary secretions was seen during the intubation procedure.

His pretransplantation workup was negative for human immunodeficiency virus (HIV) 1 and 2 (ELISA) and *Toxoplasma* (IgG), and his serologies for herpes simplex virus (HSV) 1 and 2 IgG and cytomegalovirus (CMV) IgG were negative. The donor also tested negative for HIV, *Toxoplasma*, HSV-1 and 2 by plasma polymerase chain reaction (PCR), HSV-1 IgG, and CMV IgG. The donor's sputum was positive for methicillin-susceptible *Staphylococcus aureus*, and the patient therefore received a course of antibiotic therapy with linezolid. A wide differential diagnosis was initially considered, as shown in Table 41.1.

F. Chaparro-Rojas, M.D.
Delaware Valley Infectious Diseases Associates,
Wynnewood, PA, USA
e-mail: freddych6@yahoo.com

The patient was sedated and intubated. His vital signs were remarkable for a temperature of 35.4 °C, pulse of 58 beats per minute, respiratory rate of 28 breaths per minute, and blood pressure of 103/46 mmHg on a continuous infusion of intravenous (IV) dopamine. His examination showed an endotracheal tube in place and a scant amount of bloody material present in both the oral cavity and the endotracheal tube, but no ulcers or lesions were appreciated in his mouth. He had coarse breath sounds bilaterally. A left thoracotomy surgical wound was noted; it showed no evidence of inflammation or drainage and was healing properly. His skin examination was unremarkable.

The patient's white blood cell count on admission was 13,800/μL (normal range, 3500–11,000/μL) with a differential of 97% granulocytes (39–75%). His serum chemistries showed potassium of 5.7 mEq/L (3.5–5.0 mEq/L) and a creatinine of 1.2 mg/dL (0.5–1.4 mg/dL, baseline 0.8 mg/dL). A chest radiograph revealed fibrosis of his right (native) lung and "edema-like infiltrates in transplanted lung." A computed tomography (CT) scan of the chest with pulmonary embolism protocol was performed, showing no evidence of filling defects, making the diagnosis of pulmonary embolism unlikely. There were extensive interstitial and airspace opacities in the native right lung unchanged from his pretransplant scans, a moderate left pleural effusion, a small pneumothorax, and an edema-like abnormality demonstrated in the

Table 41.1 Differential diagnosis for acute respiratory distress and respiratory failure early after lung transplantation

Healthcare-acquired pneumonia
• *Pseudomonas aeruginosa* and other Gram-negative bacilli
• Methicillin-resistant *Staphylococcus aureus* (MRSA)
• *Legionella* spp.
• Influenza
Donor-derived infection
• Bacterial
– *Mycobacterium tuberculosis*
– Nontuberculous mycobacteria
– Bacteremia at the time of donation (many organisms)
• Viral
– Influenza
– Herpes viruses (cytomegalovirus [CMV], herpes simplex virus [HSV], varicella-zoster virus [VZV])
• Fungal
– *Aspergillus* spp.
– Endemic mycoses (*Histoplasma capsulatum*, *Coccidioides* spp., *Cryptococcus gattii*, *Cryptococcus neoformans*)
Acute rejection of transplanted organ
Opportunistic infection (bacterial, viral, or fungal)
Pulmonary embolism
Mechanical postoperative complications (e.g., pneumothorax, hemothorax)

transplanted lung (Fig. 41.1). A bronchoscopy with bronchoalveolar lavage (BAL) was performed; no gross abnormalities were evident other than mucosal erythema. The tissue biopsies showed no evidence of rejection. The BAL viral cultures were positive for HSV-1.

High-dose acyclovir therapy was begun after the positive viral cultures were reported. One week later, multiple vesicles were noted on the patient's lips, perioral skin, and oral mucosa. Cultures of these lesions were positive for HSV-1. The lesions continued to spread, involving larger segments of his face and mouth. The HSV-1 isolate was sent for genotyping and tested resistant to acyclovir (Fig. 41.2). CMX-001 (a liposomal formulation of cidofovir) was initiated

under an expanded access protocol. Initially, a down-trending plasma HSV-1 PCR assay was noted (Fig. 41.3.). However, physical examination demonstrated a persistent progression of the patient's skin lesions, with involvement of other anatomical areas, including his back and esophagus. These lesions were culture positive for HSV-1 and PCR-confirmed HSV-1 susceptible to cidofovir and foscarnet. Because of the progression of the HSV-1 lesions, CMX-001 was discontinued, and therapy with foscarnet was initiated. There was initially improvement in the lesions, but acute renal failure soon developed. His condition continued to deteriorate, and his course was complicated by *Pseudomonas* ventilator-associated pneumonia (VAP), bacteremia, and septic shock. The patient expired despite aggressive medical care.

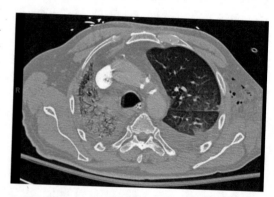

Fig. 41.1 CT scan of the lungs showing no filling defects suggestive of pulmonary embolus; extensive interstitial and airspace opacities in native right lung; moderate left pleural effusion, small pneumothorax, and an edema-like abnormality in the transplanted lung

	EC 50 µM	Result
ACV	70.6	Resistant
CDV	1.5	Sensitive
PFA	151	Sensitive

Fig. 41.2 HSV susceptibility studies by plaque assay, performed by the University of Alabama-Birmingham Virology Laboratory. *ACV* acyclovir, *CDV* cidofovir, *PFA* foscarnet phosphonoformate

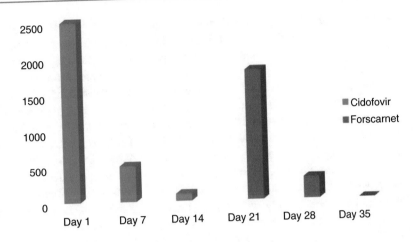

Fig. 41.3 Plasma HSV-1 viral load by PCR during antiviral therapy

41.1   Disseminated HSV Infection in a Lung Transplant Recipient

The incidence of herpesvirus (HSV-1, HSV-2, VZV, and CMV) infections after solid organ transplantation has declined over the last 20 years, mainly due to the generalized use of antiviral prophylaxis [1, 2]. Immunocompromised hosts are at risk for serious HSV infections, including disseminated disease, given their impaired cellular immunity [3]. In patients with HIV infection and in recipients of solid organ or bone marrow transplants, herpetic lesions can be extensive, tend to persist for longer periods, and have the potential to disseminate [4]. Studies in the pre-prophylaxis era revealed rates of pretransplant HSV seropositivity of more than 70% in liver and kidney recipients and 40% in heart-lung recipients, probably reflecting the younger age of the heart-lung recipients in the studied populations [5, 6]. The majority of HSV disease is due to reactivation of latent infection, usually during the first 6 months after transplantation in patients who were not receiving prophylaxis or during periods of augmented immunosuppression [5, 6]. Suspected pulmonary or hepatic involvement is a life-threatening emergency [7].

Nosocomial HSV infections have been described in healthcare personnel exposed to infectious patient secretions, most commonly manifested as a primary infection of the skin known as herpetic whitlow [8], as well as localized or disseminated disease in newborns contracted from maternal infections, nursery personnel, or monitoring equipment, representing cases of primary HSV infection [9]. Another common presentation of HSV infections is mucocutaneous disease and VAP in critically ill normal hosts. This usually represents a reactivation, probably induced by the stress of illness and/or intubation and ventilation [10].

Transmission of HSV to patients by healthcare workers is, in theory, possible given that reactivation of herpesviruses can result either in clinically evident disease or asymptomatic shedding of virus, mainly in saliva in the case of HSV-1. Oral HSV-1 shedding occurs frequently in virtually all seropositive subjects, including those with no history of symptomatic recurrences [11]. The role of asymptomatic viral shedding by healthcare workers and HSV infections in immunocompromised hosts is unknown, but, in our patient, given the absence of evidence of previous infection by HSV-1 in either the patient or the donor, this scenario might be considered. Another possible scenario is the transmission of HSV infections by a family member or visitor during hospitalization.

The prevalence of HSV infections with reduced susceptibility to acyclovir, as in our case, is higher in immunocompromised than in immunocompetent patients and varies from 2.5 to 10% in solid organ transplant recipients [11]. Acyclovir, penciclovir, and their respective prodrugs valacyclovir and famciclovir are selectively monophosphorylated only within virus-infected cells by viral thymidine kinase (TK). Thereafter, cellular kinases process the compounds to acyclovir, valacyclovir, or penciclovir triphosphate, which are the active form of the drugs. By competing with the natural nucleotide, deoxyguanosine triphosphate (dGTP), these triphosphorylated drugs inhibit HSV replication by selective inhibition of viral DNA polymerase and by termination of the growing viral DNA chain. The mechanisms for resistance to these medications involve mutations of the viral TK enzyme, expressed as TK negative (most common), TK partial/low producer, or TK altered, and are associated with mutations in the UL23 gene (Fig. 41.4). In our

case, the HSV isolate expressed resistance to acyclovir, demonstrating an IC50 (i.e., concentration of drug required for 50% inhibition of viral replication) of 3.8 µg/mL (ViroMed Labs, Minnetonka, MN).

Foscarnet (trisodium phosphonoformate) is an inorganic pyrophosphate analogue that inhibits HSV, as well as other viruses (e.g., CMV or VZV). Unlike acyclovir and penciclovir, foscarnet does not depend on viral TK for its activity. Instead, it directly inhibits herpesvirus DNA polymerase by reversibly blocking the pyrophosphate binding site of the viral polymerase in a noncompetitive manner. Cidofovir is a monophosphate, acyclic nucleoside analogue, TK-independent inhibitor of HSV, which acts as a competitive inhibitor and as an alternative substrate for DNA viral polymerase [12].

When acyclovir resistance is suspected, it is recommended that the dose of acyclovir be increased and that the clinical response be assessed. If there is no evidence of a favorable clinical response, it is recommended that therapy with foscarnet be considered and that the viral isolate be tested for susceptibility to acyclovir [4] (Fig. 41.5).

Fig. 41.4 HSV mechanisms of resistance. Adapted from [12]. *ACV* acyclovir

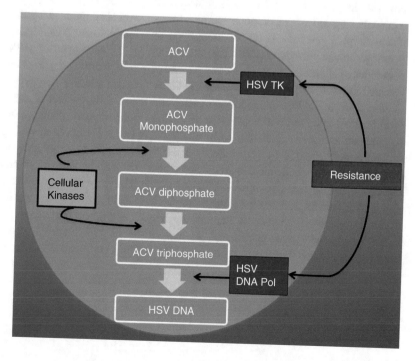

Fig. 41.5 Algorithm for the management of ACV-resistant HSV. Adapted from [4]. *ACV* acyclovir, *FCV* famciclovir, *FOS* foscarnet, *VACV* valacyclovir

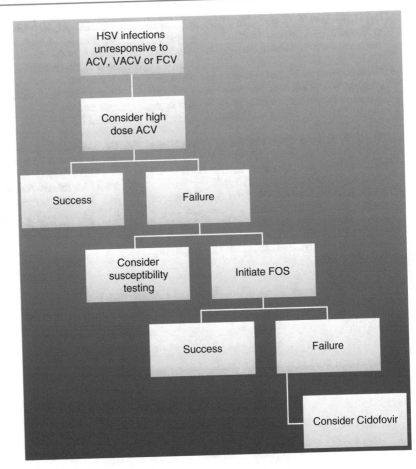

Key Points/Pearls

- Severe HSV infections should be suspected and promptly treated in immunocompromised patients with suggestive clinical findings.
- Infections by HSV resistant to acyclovir, penciclovir, and their prodrugs valacyclovir and famciclovir are uncommon, but the percentage of viral isolates resistant to these medications is higher in immunocompromised than in immunocompetent patients.
- In immunocompromised patients, HSV-associated lesions can be extensive, tend to persist for longer periods, and have the potential to disseminate.
- The majority of HSV disease reflects reactivation of latent infection, usually during the first 6 months after transplantation in patients who were not receiving prophylaxis or at times of augmented immunosuppression.

- Suspected pulmonary or hepatic involvement should be considered a life-threatening emergency.
- The role of asymptomatic viral shedding by healthcare workers and secondary HSV infections in immunocompromised hosts is unknown.

References

1. Subramanian AK. Antimicrobial prophylaxis regimens following transplantation. Curr Opin Infect Dis. 2011;24:344–9
2. Kotton CN, Kumar D, Caliendo AM, et al. International consensus guidelines on the management of cytomegalovirus in solid organ transplantation. Transplantation. 2010;89:779–95
3. Miller GG, Dummer JS. Herpes simplex and varicella zoster viruses: forgotten but not gone. Am J Transplant. 2007;7:741–7

4. Piret J, Boivin G. Resistance of herpes simplex viruses to nucleoside analogues: mechanisms, prevalence, and management. Antimicrob Agents Chemother. 2011;55:459–72

5. Singh N, Dummer JS, Kusne S, et al. Infections with cytomegalovirus and other herpesviruses in 121 liver transplant recipients: transmission by donated organ and the effect of OKT3 antibodies. J Infect Dis. 1988;158:124–31

6. Naraqi S, Jackson GG, Jonasson O, Yamashiroya HM. Prospective study of prevalence, incidence, and source of herpesvirus infections in patients with renal allografts. J Infect Dis. 1977;136:531–40

7. Smyth RL, Higenbottam TW, Scott JP, et al. Herpes simplex virus infection in heart-lung transplant recipients. Transplantation. 1990;49:735–9

8. Graman PS, Hall CB. Epidemiology and control of nosocomial viral infection. Infect Dis Clin North Am. 1989;3:815–41

9. Nahmias AJ, Keyserling HK, Kerrick GM. Herpes simplex. In: Remington J, Kelin J, editors. Infectious diseases of the fetus and newborn infant. Philadelphia: WB Saunders; 1983. p. 636–78.

10. Hanley PJ, Conaway MM, Halstead DC. Nosocomial herpes simplex virus infection associated with oral endotracheal intubation. Am J Infect Control. 1993;21:310–6

11. da Silva LM, Guimaraes AL, Victoria JM, Gomes CC, Gomez RS. Herpes simplex virus type 1 shedding in the oral cavity of seropositive patients. Oral Dis. 2005;11:13–6

12. Bush LM, Talledo-Thais K, Casal-Fernandez A, Perez MT. Resistant herpes simplex virus infection and HIV: a potential diagnostic and therapeutic dilemma. Lab Med. 2011;42:452–7

A Pain in the Back: A 50-Year-Old Man with Pancreatitis and a Fever

Vinny DiMaggio and Emily Landon

A 50-year-old man with a history of chronic pancreatitis was admitted after evaluation for jejunostomy tube (J-tube) placement for nutritional support. Due to complications from his chronic pancreatitis, the patient had required continuous supplemental nutrition by parenteral route. He stopped total parenteral nutrition (TPN) 10 days before this evaluation, on his own for unclear reasons. Upon further discussion, the patient endorsed a subjective fever and night sweats for the past month. He had no associated abdominal pain, nausea, vomiting, or diarrhea. He did, however, have a 10-lb weight loss over the 2 weeks prior to presentation. He also reported low back pain for 3 weeks. He was thus admitted for evaluation and subsequent J-tube placement.

The patient stated that he had had severe back pain in the lumbar region for the last 3 weeks. The pain was not positional, it radiated down both legs, and it caused him to limit his daily activities. He denied any trauma. The onset of pain was insidious and was not relieved by NSAIDs or muscle relaxants. He had no history of weakness or sensory loss. He had no bladder or bowel incontinence.

The patient had chronic pancreatitis due to alcoholism and was nutritionally dependent on

TPN due to recurrent pancreatitis. He also had a history of hepatitis C virus infection, which had never been treated. He had a positive partial protein derivative (PPD) test treated with isoniazid several decades earlier. Screening chest radiographs demonstrated a chronic lung mass that was unchanged over the course of a year, but the patient failed to follow up after this as recommended. His surgical history was only significant for bilateral knee arthroscopies.

As noted, the patient had a history of chronic alcohol abuse, but his last drink had been 6 months before his presentation. Also, he had a history of intravenous (IV) drug use, but at the time of his initial evaluation, he had not used IV drugs in 3 years. He was on methadone. He had a 50-pack-year history of tobacco use. He had previously been incarcerated. At the time of the evaluation, he was living with his wife and children. He had no pertinent family history.

On initial evaluation, he was afebrile with temperature of 37.7 °C, heart rate of 81 beats per minute, blood pressure of 103/62 mmHg, respiratory rate of 20 breaths per minute, and oxygen saturation of 94% while breathing room air. The patient had poor dentition and muddy sclerae. His pulmonary exam was normal. His cardiovascular exam demonstrated a normal heart rate with regular rhythm and no murmurs, rubs, or gallops. He had normal distal pulses. His abdomen was soft, not distended, and not tender, and he had normally active bowel sounds. He had no organomegaly.

V. DiMaggio, M.D. • E. Landon, M.D. (✉)
Department of Medicine, University of Chicago, Chicago, IL, USA
e-mail: Emily.Landon@uchospitals.edu

© Springer International Publishing AG 2018
M. David, J.-L. Benoit (eds.), *The Infectious Disease Diagnosis*,
https://doi.org/10.1007/978-3-319-64906-1_42

On rectal examination, he had normal tone without bleeding and negative fecal occult blood testing. While he had normal strength in all extremities and muscles with normal bulk and tone, he had diffuse tenderness in the lumbar musculature and vertebral body tenderness with percussion over the lumbar spine. There was no erythema or edema in the area of tenderness. He had no rashes on his skin and no lymphadenopathy.

The initial laboratory evaluation did not reveal any clear etiologies of the patient's presenting symptoms. The white blood cell count was 7300/μL with a normal differential, hemoglobin 9.1 mg/dL, and platelet count 314,000/μL. The basic metabolic panel demonstrated a low serum sodium of 129 mmol/L (normal range, 134–149 mmol/L). Coagulation studies were normal. The albumin was 2.7 g/dL (3.5–5.0 g/dL). Blood cultures were obtained.

Table 42.1 shows the differential diagnosis for a patient with lumbar pain and spinal tenderness accompanied by a fever. The differential includes a number of important infectious causes, including spinal osteomyelitis with or without epidural abscess due to pyogenic bacteria (most often *Staphylococcus aureus*), tuberculosis (Pott's disease), non-tuberculous mycobacteria, brucellosis, endemic fungi (especially blastomycosis and coccidioidomycosis), and rarely opportunistic fungi (including *Candida* spp. or *Aspergillus* spp.). The differential also includes noninfectious etiologies, such as malignancy (multiple myeloma, lymphoma, or metastasis) and osteoporosis with a compression fracture (though less likely given complaint of fever). Sometimes in cases of lumbar pain, the lesion is in the sacroiliac joint and not the spinal cord.

Given the patient's symptoms, signs, and objective findings, a magnetic resonance imaging (MRI) study of the lumbar spine was performed. Figure 42.1 shows a key image from the MRI, demonstrating the destruction of the L4 and L5 vertebral bodies and the intervertebral disk. The MRI findings were suspicious for an infectious etiology because bloodstream infections usually involve the disk first, then spread to the vertebral bodies above and below the infected disk (spinal discitis/vertebral osteomyelitis).

Table 42.1 Differential diagnosis of lumbar back pain, spinal tenderness, and fever

Hematogenous pyogenic bacterial spinal osteomyelitis/discitis:
- *Staphylococcus aureus*
- β-hemolytic streptococci
- Enterococci
- Gram-negative bacilli (enterics, *Pseudomonas*, *Salmonella*)
- May be complicated by epidural abscess with cord or cauda equina compression, paraspinal abscess, and psoas muscle abscess
- Endocarditis may be a complication or an etiology
- Post-procedural vertebral osteomyelitis (coagulase-negative staphylococci, *Propionibacterium acnes*)
- Contiguous spread vertebral osteomyelitis from soft tissue infection (such as in paraplegia or from extension of retropharyngeal abscess)

Brucellosis involving the spine or the sacroiliac joint
- Especially if older than 40 years of age
- More common in immigrants from highly endemic areas such as Mexico, Latin America, or the Middle East

Spinal tuberculosis (Pott's disease)
- Common in highly endemic countries

Spinal osteomyelitis due to non-tuberculous mycobacteria
- More common in the acquired immunodeficiency syndrome (AIDS)
- May rarely be seen in immunocompetent hosts
- *Mycobacterium avium* Complex
- Rapidly growing mycobacteria

Fungal spinal osteomyelitis
- Endemic fungi (especially blastomycosis and coccidioidomycosis)
- Opportunistic fungi (aspergillosis, *Scedosporium apiospermum*, zygomycosis, and phaeohyphomycosis)

Epidural/subdural abscess or paraspinal abscess complicating above infections

Meningitis

Pyelonephritis

Pyomyositis

Pancreatitis

Skin abscess/cellulitis

Prostatitis

Diverticulitis

Appendicitis

Varicella zoster virus

Sacroileitis in the setting of bacterial infection, brucellosis, or reactive arthritis associated with intestinal infection

Spinal stenosis

Mesenteric ischemia

(continued)

Table 42.1 (continued)

Rhabdomyolysis
Multiple myeloma
Lymphoma
Metastatic malignancy
Ankylosing spondylitis
Dermatomyositis
Other rheumatologic disease

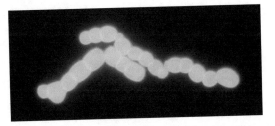

Fig. 42.2 Calcofluor stain of patient's blood culture demonstrating encapsulated zygomycetes

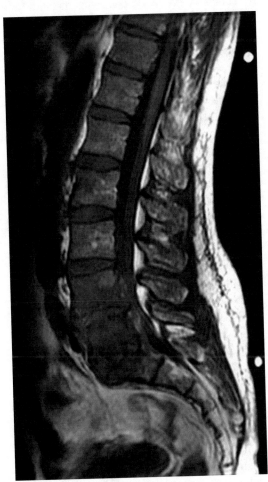

Fig. 42.1 MRI of the spine demonstrating destruction of L4 and L5 vertebral bodies

At this point in the work-up, blood cultures returned with a preliminary result of 1 of 2 positive for growth of "yeast." Figure 42.2 is the Calcofluor stain of a blood culture bottle specimen, which actually shows encapsulated buds of a zygomycete mold, later identified in culture as *Mucor*, a very rare cause of fungemia.

42.1   *Mucor* Fungemia

Mucor spp. are pathogenic zygomycetes. The four most important genera are *Rhizopus*, *Mucor*, *Rhizomucor*, and *Absidia*, but there are other genera rarely involved in human infections. The infections that zygomycetes cause is commonly called "mucormycosis" although the term "zygomycosis" may be more accurate. These molds have aseptate, hyaline, wide, irregular, ribbon-like hyphae that branch at straight angles in contrast to *Aspergillus*-like molds and are transparent (hyaline) in contrast to melanin-pigmented dematiaceous molds. Because the hyphae are nonseptate, zygomycetes may be difficult to recover in culture if the preparation is not handled carefully to avoid breaking the hyphae.

Mucor spp. cause infections in both immunocompromised and immunocompetent hosts. They are particularly known for causing necrotizing infections in hosts with diabetes mellitus, with neutropenia, or taking corticosteroids. Individuals with these conditions are at particular risk because of impaired ability to protect against fungal germination, which is mediated by granulocytes, specifically neutrophils and macrophages. To cause disease, *Mucor* spp. must scavenge sufficient iron for growth from the host, must evade host phagocytic defense mechanisms, and must access vasculature in order to disseminate.

In susceptible hosts, normal defense mechanisms break down. For example, in diabetic ketoacidosis (DKA), the acidic pH of the serum causes dissociation of free iron from sequestering proteins. This release of free iron allows rapid fungal growth. Defects in phagocytic defense mechanisms, for example, deficiency in cell number (neutropenia) or functional defects caused by corticosteroids or the hyperglycemia and acidosis of DKA, allow proliferation of the fungus. Finally, adherence to and damage of endothelial cells by the fungus allows fungal angioinvasion and vessel thrombosis leading to tissue necrosis and dissemination of the fungal infection.

Patients with diabetes mellitus tend to present with rhinocerebral mucormycosis whereas patients with neutropenia (specifically following stem cell transplantation) more commonly develop invasive pulmonary infection.

Mucormycosis fungemia is very uncommon. We identified only two reported cases of *Mucor* spp. fungemia at the time this case occurred. The first was a central venous catheter-associated infection in a patient who had received TPN; the infection was successfully treated with liposomal amphotericin. The second was a case of fungemia associated with severe, acute gastrointestinal infection, also successfully treated with amphotericin. Contemporary literature review to 2017 demonstrated no additional cases of blood-borne mucormycosis.

Mucormycosis causing osteomyelitis as a complication of fungemia is also an uncommon diagnosis, particularly infection of vertebral bodies. At the time of the present case, there were only two other documented cases of *Mucor* osteomyelitis in the literature; however, in both cases there was an external portal of entry.

Our patient was presumed to have hematogenous spread to vertebral bodies secondary to catheter-related *Mucor* spp. fungemia in the setting of chronic pancreatitis and TPN dependence. His peripherally inserted central venous catheter was removed, and he was started on therapy with liposomal amphotericin as well as vancomycin and ceftazidime given concern for bacterial coinfection. An appeal was made at the time for compassionate use of posaconazole, which had not yet been licensed by the United States Food and Drug Administration, given the substantial nephrotoxicity risk with the necessary long course of therapy with liposomal amphotericin. The patient entered a compassionate use trial, the neurosurgery service carried out the planned definitive debridement of his lumbar spine, and eventually the patient went on to have J-tube placed for nutritional support.

Key Points/Pearls

- *Mucor* spp. are zygomycetes responsible for invasive infections in immunocompromised and occasionally immunocompetent hosts in the United States.
- Patients with poorly controlled diabetes mellitus and acidosis are most likely to develop rhinocerebral mucormycosis and present with fever, unilateral facial swelling and pain, nasal or sinus congestion, headache, and nasal discharge; invasion of the orbit is common, with ptosis, proptosis, ophthalmoplegia, vision loss, and extension to the cavernous sinus; often, a necrotic eschar may be identified on the palate or inside the nose.
- Rhinocerebral mucormycosis is a life-threatening infection that must be treated with prompt, broad surgical debridement and amphotericin B.
- Patients with neutropenia, hematologic malignancy, or prolonged corticosteroid use may develop invasive pulmonary mucormycosis, with fever, cough, chest pain, dyspnea, and hemoptysis due to angioinvasion; angioinvasion may be demonstrated by the halo sign on CT imaging, and cavitary lesions are common.
- Patients with neutropenia, hematologic malignancy, or prolonged corticosteroid use can also present with rhinocerebral mucormycosis.
- Disseminated mucormycosis is often seen as a progression of pulmonary mucormycosis in immunocompromised neutropenic patients; however, *Mucor* can also cause catheter-related bloodstream infection, such as with TPN use; a catheter exit site infection with necrosis may be a clue in such cases.
- Cutaneous mucormycosis results from direct inoculation, and debridement may often be curative if undertaken quickly.
- Gastrointestinal mucormycosis more often affects neonates who ingest the fungus.
- Given an external point of entry, mucormycosis osteomyelitis has been reported, but as our case demonstrates, it can also be spread hematogenously.

- Zygomycetes use iron as growth factor; disseminated infection has been a complication of deferoxamine use as an iron chelator because the fungus can remove the iron from this drug.

Bibliography

1. Spellberg B, Edwards J, Ibrahim A. Novel perspectives on mucormycosis: pathophysiology, presentation, and management. Clin Micro Rev. 2005;18:556–69
2. Chayakulkeeree M, Ghannoum MA, Perfect JR. Zygomycosis: the re-emerging fungal infection. Eur J Clin Micro Infect Dis. 2006;25:215–29
3. Greenberg RN, Scott LJ, Vaughn HH, Ribes JA. Zygomycosis (mucormycosis): emerging clinical importance and new treatments. Curr Opin Infect Dis. 2004;17:517–25
4. Chen F, Lu G, Kang Y, et al. Mucormycosis spondylodiscitis after lumbar disc punture. Eur Spine J. 2006;15:370–6
5. Buruma OJS, Craane H, Kunst MW. Vertebral osteomyelitis and epidural abscess due to mucormycosis. Clin Neurol Neurosurg. 1979;81:39–44
6. Aboltins C, Pratt WAB, Solano TR. Fungemia secondary to gastrointestinal *Mucor indicus* infection [letter]. CID. 2006;42:154–5
7. Chan-Tack KM, Nemoy LL, Perencevich EN. Central venous catheter-associated fungemia secondary to mucormycosis. Scand J Infect Dis. 2005;37:925–7
8. Kontoyiannis DP, Lewis RE. Agents of mucormycosis and entomophthoramycosis. In: Mandell GL, Bennett JE, Dolin R, editors. Mandell's principles and practice of infectious diseases. 7th ed. New York: Elsevier/Churchill Livingstone; 2010. p. 3257–71.

A 9-Year-Old Boy with a Red Eye

43

M. Ellen Acree

A 9-year-old boy with no significant past medical history presented to the emergency department with 4 days of swelling just in front of his left ear and 1 week of "pink eye" on the left side. The patient had a fever 4 days prior to presentation and was taken to a local emergency department where he was given trimethoprim-sulfamethoxazole and cephalexin for "pink eye" and a "skin infection," according to the patient's mother. Given that the eye redness and left-sided facial swelling were not improving, the patient was taken to a different emergency department where he was given one dose of intravenous (IV) vancomycin and transferred to our pediatric tertiary care hospital.

On arrival, the patient was febrile to 39.7 °C. His physical examination was notable for a left-sided preauricular mass that extended to the outer canthus of the left eye. The mass was mildly tender, warm, erythematous, and indurated. No fluctuance was detected. Mild left-sided conjunctival injection was noted. The patient was also found to have left-sided submandibular adenopathy. The remainder of the examination was unremarkable.

A maxillofacial computed tomography (CT) scan was performed, which demonstrated mild, diffuse enlargement of the left parotid gland (see Fig. 43.1). No radio-opaque calculi were noted. Diffuse stranding of the overlying subcutaneous fat was seen. A lesion in the left temporal subcutaneous tissue was identified, which measured 9.5 mm and was believed to be a prominent lymph node. Laboratory studies included a comprehensive metabolic panel and a complete blood count, which were normal. Blood cultures were sent. The patient was started on IV clindamycin. After 24 h of therapy, he remained febrile and without any improvement in the left-sided facial swelling and tenderness.

The Pediatric Infectious Diseases service was consulted. The service recommended sending viral serologies for mumps, Epstein-Barr virus (EBV), cytomegalovirus (CMV), and Coxsackie A/B viruses. It was ascertained that the patient had a dog and a kitten at home although the patient's mother denied any known bites or scratches. There were no known risk factors for tuberculosis, and the patient had a negative purified protein derivative (PPD) screening test prior to entering school the previous year. He was fully vaccinated and had received two doses of the measles, mumps, and rubella vaccine. Blood cultures from admission showed no growth, and human immunodeficiency virus (HIV) testing was negative. EBV serologies were consistent with past infection. CMV and Coxsackie serologies were negative, as was the mumps IgM. *Bartonella henselae* serologies were obtained given his history of kitten exposure. A respiratory viral panel was negative. The differential diagnosis for parotitis is presented in Table 43.1.

M.E. Acree, M.D.
Section of Infectious Diseases and Global Health, Department of Medicine, University of Chicago, Chicago, IL, USA
e-mail: Mary.Acree@uchospitals.edu

© Springer International Publishing AG 2018
M. David, J.-L. Benoit (eds.), *The Infectious Disease Diagnosis*,
https://doi.org/10.1007/978-3-319-64906-1_43

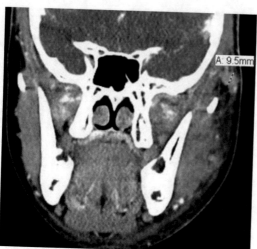

A: 9.5mm

Fig. 43.1 CT scan of the maxillofacial region. Mild diffuse enlargement of the left parotid gland is seen, along with stranding of the overlying fat. This is consistent with parotitis. The measured lesion is believed to be a prominent lymph node

Table 43.1 Differential diagnosis for parotitis

Infectious etiologies
Mumps virus
Human immunodeficiency virus (HIV)
Coxsackievirus A or B
Adenovirus
Lymphocytic choriomeningitis virus (LCV)
Gram-positive bacterial infection (including *Staphylococcus aureus*)
Bartonella species infection
Parinaud syndrome
Parainfluenza virus type 3
Influenza A virus
Epstein-Barr virus (EBV)
Parvovirus B19
Human herpesvirus-6 (HHV-6)
Atypical mycobacterial infection
Noninfectious etiologies
Sjögren's syndrome
Diabetes mellitus
Malnutrition
Parotid ductal obstruction by cyst or tumor
Sarcoidosis
Mikulicz's syndrome
Uremia
Laundry starch ingestion
Cirrhosis

The Pediatric Infectious Diseases service was concerned for *Bartonella henselae* infection given the conjunctivitis and ipsilateral preauricular adenopathy, a condition known as Parinaud oculoglandular syndrome, which is an uncommon manifestation of cat-scratch disease. The patient was started on azithromycin and his fevers resolved. After discharge, the results of the *Bartonella henselae* serologies returned, and both IgG and IgM were positive, indicating acute infection.

43.1 Bartonella henselae

Bartonella species are fastidious, facultatively intracellular Gram-negative bacteria. Of the 16 different species identified as human pathogens, *Bartonella henselae* is one of the most common. It is found all over the world. Cats are the reservoir and cat fleas transmit the bacterium between cats. Typically, *Bartonella henselae* is transmitted to humans via a cat scratch. Endocarditis, bacteremia, bacillary angiomatosis, and cat-scratch disease are potential manifestations of infection with *Bartonella* species. Bacillary angiomatosis, due to either *Bartonella quintana* or *Bartonella henselae*, is a disorder seen in immunocompromised patients, often with advanced HIV infection, who develop neovascular proliferation of the skin, in the form of nodules or papules, and regionally enlarged lymph nodes. It can also involve major organs, including the liver and spleen, a condition known as bacillary peliosis. Importantly, *Bartonella* species can cause prolonged bacteremia, culture-negative endocarditis, and fever of unknown origin in both immunocompromised and immunocompetent individuals.

43.2 Parinaud Oculoglandular Syndrome

Cat-scratch disease is caused by *Bartonella henselae*. Cats are a natural reservoir for this organism. Kittens, strays, and shelter cats are more likely than other cats to be bacteremic with *Bartonella henselae* and to transmit the organism with a scratch.

Typically, cat-scratch disease, marked by regional lymphadenopathy, develops in immunocompetent patients who are scratched by a cat and inoculated with *Bartonella henselae*. Fever and systemic signs of illness develop in approximately 30% of patients with cat-scratch disease. Since humans are often scratched on their hands or upper extremities, the most common site of lymphadenopathy is the axilla. Lymphadenopathy typically resolves spontaneously in 4–6 weeks. One quarter of patients with lymphadenopathy secondary to cat-scratch disease develop suppurative adenopathy.

Two to eight percent of patients with cat-scratch disease develop Parinaud oculoglandular syndrome, defined as unilateral conjunctivitis and ipsilateral preauricular lymphadenopathy, as occurred in the presented patient. It is caused by inoculation of *Bartonella henselae* into the eyelid conjunctiva, which can result from a cat (typically a kitten) scratch, rubbing the eyes after contact with a cat, a lick from the cat to the eye, or contact with feces from infected fleas that are feeding on the cat. The inoculation of the eyelid conjunctiva often causes eye redness, mild lid swelling, and a foreign body sensation approximately 2 weeks later. Granulomatous nodules may be seen on the bulbar and palpebral conjunctivae. As is typical of other manifestations of cat-scratch disease, regional adenopathy develops, which is most often in a preauricular location. Submandibular and cervical adenopathy can develop as well. Just as with the lymphadenopathy in typical cat-scratch disease, the conjunctivitis and preauricular swelling often spontaneously resolve without treatment.

Other infectious causes of Parinaud oculoglandular syndrome have been reported, including coccidioidomycosis, EBV, *Yersinia enterocolitica*, *Francisella tularensis*, herpes simplex virus, tuberculosis, syphilis, sporotrichosis, and *Chlamydia trachomatis*.

Serology is the cornerstone of diagnostic testing for cat-scratch disease and Parinaud oculoglandular syndrome. Seroconversion may be detected 3–5 days after inoculation. Most cases of Parinaud oculoglandular syndrome last 5–7 days. Azithromycin is the most commonly used therapy for cat-scratch disease and Parinaud oculoglandular syndrome caused by *Bartonella henselae*.

Key Points
- Parinaud oculoglandular syndrome secondary to infection with *Bartonella henselae* should be considered in patients with cat exposure, preauricular swelling, and conjunctivitis; everting the eyelids to evaluate for palpebral conjunctival nodules should be performed.
- Two to eight percent of patients with cat-scratch disease develop Parinaud oculoglandular syndrome, but other infectious etiologies have also been implicated in this syndrome.
- Cat-scratch disease is caused by *Bartonella henselae*.
- Kittens, strays, and shelter cats are more likely than other cats to be bacteremic with *Bartonella henselae* and to transmit the organism to humans.
- Bacillary angiomatosis and peliosis hepatis are seen in immunocompromised patients infected with *Bartonella quintana* or *Bartonella henselae*.
- A number of *Bartonella* species can cause culture-negative endocarditis or prolonged bacteremia.
- Cat-scratch disease may also manifest as a neuroretinitis (with a macular star in some cases) and an encephalopathy/encephalitis with delayed onset.

Bibliography

1. Arjmand P, Yan P, O'Connor MD. Parinaud oculoglandular syndrome 2015: review of the literature and update on diagnosis and management. J Clin Exp Ophthalmol. 2015;6:443
2. Ridder GJ, Boedeker CC, Technau-Ihling K, Sander A. Cat-scratch disease: otolaryngologic manifestations and management. Otolaryngol Head Neck Surg. 2005;132(3):353–8
3. Grando D, Sullivan LJ, Flexman JP, Watson MW, Andrew JH. *Bartonella henselae* associated with Parinaud's oculoglandular syndrome. Clin Infect Dis. 1999;28(5):1156–8
4. Rubin SA, Carbone KM. Mumps. In Kasper D, Fauci A, Hauser S, Longo D, Jameson JL, Loscalzo, J, eds. 2015. Harrison's principles of internal medicine. New York: McGraw-Hill, Medical Pub. Division.
5. Gandhi TN, Slater LN, Welch DF, Koehler JE. *Bartonella*, including cat-scratch disease. In Bennett JE, Dolin R, Blaser MJ, eds. 2015. Mandell, Douglas, and Bennett's principles and practice of infectious diseases, 8th ed. Philadelphia, PA: Elsevier/Saunders. pp. 2649–2663.

The Revolving (Bathroom) Door

44

Kathleen Mullane

An 87-year-old male with history of hypertension, diabetes mellitus, atrial fibrillation, recurrent kidney stones, and prostate cancer treated with radical prostatectomy 20 years ago was referred for recurrent *Clostridium difficile*-associated diarrhea. The patient's only gastrointestinal past medical history included an asymptomatic 5–8 mm tubular adenoma and diverticulosis noted on colonoscopy several years prior to presentation.

The patient initially presented with a urinary tract infection for which he received a 2-week course of ciprofloxacin. On day 10 of ciprofloxacin, he was brought to the emergency room in extremis with diarrhea, vomiting, fever, dehydration, and leukocytosis, and he was admitted to intensive care where he was found to have *C. difficile*-associated colitis. He was treated with intravenous metronidazole (500 mg every 8 h) and oral vancomycin (500 mg every 6 h) with resolution of diarrhea. He was then transitioned to and discharged on oral metronidazole (500 mg every 8 h) and vancomycin (125 mg every 6 h) to complete a 10-day course of therapy.

Eleven days after completing his oral metronidazole/vancomycin course, his diarrhea and fever recurred, and his stool again tested positive for *C. difficile* by polymerase chain reaction (PCR). He was restarted on oral vancomycin (125 mg every 6 h) to complete a 10-day course of therapy. His symptoms again resolved until 7 days after completion of oral vancomycin when he presented with 10–12 liquid stools per day for 72 h. He was prescribed a 30-day course of oral vancomycin (250 mg every 6 h for 10 days followed by a vancomycin "taper" [see Table 44.1]). He was seen in follow-up 1 week after completing his vancomycin taper and was symptom free. A stool specimen was tested for *C. difficile* by PCR and was negative. However, 3 days later symptoms recurred with eight liquid bowel movements over 6 h with associated cramping and bloating associated with his bowel movements. He presented immediately for evaluation. As the *C. difficile* PCR 3 days prior was negative, concern for a post-inflammatory colitis was considered in the differential. A repeat stool specimen was obtained for testing with plan to do a colonoscopy if the test returned negative. The patient had stable vital signs, and the results of testing would be available later that day;

Table 44.1 Vancomycin taper schedule in this case

Vancomycin 125 mg twice a day for 1 week
Vancomycin 125 mg once a day for 1 week
Vancomycin 125 mg every other day for 1 week
Vancomycin 125 mg every third day for 1 week

K. Mullane, D.O.
Section of Infectious Diseases and Global Health, Department of Medicine, University of Chicago, Chicago, IL, USA
e-mail: kmullane@medicine.bsd.uchicago.edu

© Springer International Publishing AG 2018
M. David, J.-L. Benoit (eds.), *The Infectious Disease Diagnosis*,
https://doi.org/10.1007/978-3-319-64906-1_44

therefore, *C. difficile*-directed antimicrobials were held pending these results. The repeat testing was positive, both by PCR and enzyme immunoassay (EIA) toxin methods.

The patient was offered three options: repeating vancomycin therapy followed by another vancomycin taper or fidaxomicin "chaser," fidaxomicin therapy followed by a fidaxomicin taper, or undergoing a fecal microbiota transplant (FMT). The patient opted for a FMT. He was started on vancomycin 125 mg four times daily for 10 days, and then the drug was withheld for 36 h. On the evening prior to the FMT, he was instructed to take one bottle (10 oz.) of magnesium citrate. He was then given an enema-delivered FMT and this was repeated 1 week later. On long-term follow-up, the patient remained free of *C. difficile*-associated diarrhea for 24 months.

44.1 *Clostridium difficile* Infection

C. difficile infection (CDI) is the leading cause of healthcare-associated infectious diarrhea [1]. The diagnosis of CDI should be based on clinical signs (passage of three or more unformed stools in 24 or fewer consecutive hours) and symptoms, combined with laboratory testing [2]. Cell cytotoxicity neutralization assay and toxigenic culture are regarded as the reference tests for diagnosing CDI [3, 4]. These tests take 2–3 days to perform, and therefore commercially available rapid tests whose performance is compared to reference tests have been developed. These tests include:

1. EIA tests that detect glutamate dehydrogenase (GDH), an enzyme produced by both toxigenic and nontoxigenic strains of *C. difficile*. Sensitivity of these tests ranges from 0.80 to 1.00 and specificity from 0.82 to 0.95.
2. EIA tests that detect the presence of toxins A and B in a stool specimen. Sensitivity of these tests ranges from 0.44 to 0.99 and the specificity from 0.87 to 1.00.
3. Nucleic acid amplification tests (NAAT) that detect the genes that produce toxins A and B. These include PCR tests that detect the gene

encoding toxin B (tcdB), Loop-mediated isothermal amplification (LAMP) testing that detects toxin gene tcdA, and a number of these tests that also look for the gene for tcdC, which is a putative negative regulator of toxins A and B, and the genes for binary toxin (*cdt*) [4]. Sensitivity of NAAT tests ranges from 0.83 to 1.0 with specificity of 0.91–0.98.

Because the toxin EIA tests have widely variable sensitivity, patients with active CDI may be missed by using these assays as a stand-alone test to diagnose CDI. However, neither the GDH nor the NAAT tests detect free toxin and may not distinguish patients with active CDI from patients colonized by or asymptomatically carrying a toxigenic strain. If these tests are used as stand-alone diagnostic testing, CDI may be diagnosed in patients who are carrying a toxin-producing *C. difficile* organism but who do not have active disease. Therefore it is strongly recommended that only patients with symptoms consistent with CDI be tested by these methods. It may be best to combine two tests in an algorithm (screen with GDH or NAAT and if positive follow with a toxin EIA) to optimize the diagnosis of CDI and reduce the number of false positive cases.

44.2 Guidelines for the Therapy of *Clostridium difficile*-Associated Diarrhea

There are currently five published guidelines for the treatment of CDI [2, 5–8]. For the first episode of CDI in mild to moderate cases, all of these guidelines recommend metronidazole 500 mg orally dosed every 8 h for 10–14 days. Four guidelines list vancomycin 125 mg dosed every 6 h as an alternative and two recommend fidaxomicin 200 mg dosed every 12 h for 10 days in those with known risk factors for recurrence (see Table 44.2). For patients with severe CDI (Table 44.3), vancomycin or fidaxomicin is recommended given superior outcomes in clinical trials [9–12]. Combination with metronidazole therapy may be considered, and in those with an ileus or fulminant colitis, vancomycin enemas

Table 44.2 Risk factors for recurrent CDI [9, 11, 15–17, 19–21, 34]

Disrupted colonic flora	Concomitant antimicrobials (during or after CDI therapy)
	Previous history of CDI
	10 unformed bowel movements per day
Altered immunity	Advanced age (age > 65 and especially >80)
	Inadequate antitoxin antibody response
	Peripartum women
	Leukopenia
Poor underlying health conditions	Chronic renal insufficiency (serum creatinine ≥1.2)
	Chemotherapy/underlying malignancy
	Concurrent bacterial infection
	Emergent hospitalization/ICU stay/prolonged or recurrent hospitalization(s)
	High comorbidity score (e.g., Horn's index 3–4)
	Low serum albumin
Other factors	Leukocytosis
	Proton pump inhibitors, H2 receptor blockers, antacids

Table 44.3 Criteria suggesting severe CDI [2, 3, 5–8]

Physical examination	Temperature > 38.5
	Rigors
	Abdominal tenderness
	Ileus
	Signs of peritonitis/perforation
	Hemodynamic instability
	Respiratory failure
	Mental status change
	Intensive care unit admission
Laboratory findings	Leukocyte count ≥15,000 cells/mm^3 or <2000 cells/mm^3
	Serum creatinine >1.5× baseline or acutely rising serum creatinine
	Albumin <2.5–3.0 mg/dL
	Lactate >2.2 meq/L
Imaging/colonoscopy	Megacolon/large intestinal distension
	Colonic wall thickening
	Pericolic fat stranding
	Pseudomembranous colitis

may be considered. If oral therapy is not possible, some guidelines recommend intravenous tigecycline 50 mg administered every 12 h [5, 8]. Bezlotoxumab (monoclonal antibodies directed against clostridial toxin B) has recently received FDA approval [13]. When combined with standard metronidazole or vancomycin therapy, a single dose of intravenous bezlotoxumab reduced the risk of recurrent CDI (rCDI) from ~27% to 16% ($p < 0.001$). Its place in therapy, however, has not yet been delineated [14].

44.3   Recurrent CDI (rCDI)

Recurrent *C. difficile* infection (rCDI) is the presence of symptoms along with a positive *C. difficile* stool assay within 2–8 weeks from the initial episode provided the symptoms from the previous episode resolved after completion of the initial treatment [2, 3, 5, 15–21]. Failure is considered when the patient has not had resolution of symptoms upon completion of a course of CDI therapy. Clinically, however, if a patient has persistent symptoms after 3–5 days of therapy, consideration of an alternative agent should be undertaken. Failure occurs in approximately 10–15% of cases. CDI recurs in nearly 15–35% of patients treated for the initial infection [22]. The relapse rate after therapy with metronidazole or vancomycin for the first occurrence of CDI has been shown in large clinical trials to be 25–35% [9–11, 13, 23]. The risk of relapse after therapy with fidaxomicin is 16% [9, 11]. After an initial recurrence, up to 65% of these patients will have a subsequent recurrence. For first recurrence, three of the five guidelines recommend repeating the same treatment as for the initial episode [2, 6, 7], while three guidelines recommend vancomycin or fidaxomicin for 10 days [3, 5, 6, 8]. In two large CDI clinical trials comparing vancomycin to fidaxomicin that enrolled patients with first relapse, fidaxomicin was superior to vancomycin in global clinical cure [9, 11].

For subsequent episodes after the first recurrence, there are no randomized controlled clinical trials (RCTs) evaluating therapies [24]. Vancomycin has been used in prolonged tapering regimens as was done in this case. Vancomycin treatment until resolution of diarrhea followed by fidaxomicin (a.k.a., "the fidaxomicin chaser"), fidaxomicin taper, and FMT have all been reported in the literature [22, 25–29].

If diarrhea persists and testing for *C. difficile* is negative after therapy, it is important to rule out primary inflammatory bowel disease, post-inflammatory colitis, collagenous colitis, microscopic colitis, or other possible etiologies for persistent diarrheal illnesses.

rCDI is postulated to arise from a disruption of the normal intestinal commensal microbiota [26, 29]. This may be due to antimicrobials, chemotherapeutic agents, age, and/or a suboptimal humoral immune response to *C. difficile* toxins. The colonic microbiome has been found to be less diverse, with increased Lactobacillaceae and Enterobacteriaceae and loss of Firmicutes and Bacteroidaceae, in those who develop rCDI compared to those who do not recur [30]. Disruption of the microbiota leads to loss of colonization resistance against *C difficile*. Also, disruption in the microbiota alters colonic bile acid composition resulting in the loss of secondary bile acids allowing a permissive inflammatory environment for *C. difficile* to survive and germinate [31].

44.4 Fecal Microbiota Transplant (FMT)

FMT is the introduction of feces from a healthy donor into the intestinal tract of an individual with a disrupted colonic microbiome in an effort to repopulate the colon with a "normal complement" of bacteria [26, 29]. In a double-blind RCT, cure rates were compared between colonoscopic administration of donor FMT and autologous FMT in patients who had at least three CDI recurrences [22]. After 10 days of standard vancomycin therapy, clinical cure was achieved in 90.9% of those receiving donor compared to 62.5% receiving autologous FMT at 8 weeks after the FMT. In the recipients of donor FMT, bacterial community diversity was restored with a composition resembling that of the donors. No difference has been shown in efficacy of FMT if the fecal microbiota suspension is made fresh just prior to transplantation or if it is stored frozen and thawed just prior to transplantation [32, 33].

There are multiple systematic reviews of uncontrolled case series and observational open-label studies that have reported success rates of 62–94% for FMT [26, 29]. Overall, administration by rectal enema or colonoscopy appears to be superior to nasogastric administration; related donor fecal microbiota (FM) may be more effective than unrelated donor FM; and >1 FMT appears to be superior to a single procedure.

In an unblinded study, duodenal infusion donor FMT following a 3-day course of vancomycin in individuals with rCDI in whom vancomycin had failed was compared with a 14-day course of vancomycin with or without bowel lavage [28]. At the study's first interim analysis, the cure rates in the study arm that received donor FMT were significantly higher (81%) than either of the vancomycin arms (31% vancomycin alone and 23% vancomycin plus bowel lavage). Because 2 weeks of oral vancomycin has been associated with a higher failure rate than vancomycin taper [18], an open-label RCT has been performed comparing the effectiveness of 14 days of oral vancomycin followed by a single FMT by enema 48 h after discontinuation of vancomycin with standard of care treatment (a 6-week taper of oral vancomycin) in patients experiencing an acute episode of rCDI [25]. The primary endpoint of the study was recurrence of CDI within 120 days after therapy. At the first a priori scheduled interim analysis, 56% of subjects who received FMT vs. 41.7% of those in the vancomycin taper group experienced rCDI. A futility analysis did not support continuation of the study.

More research is needed to standardize and optimize FMT including optimal timing for FMT (number of recurrences); donor choice vs. optimal "purified" bacteria/spore preparations; optimal pretreatment regimens; number of FMTs to risk of recurrence; and long-term consequences of alterations in the gut microbiome.

Key Points/Pearls

- *Clostridium difficile* is a common hospital-acquired pathogen that survives on environmental surfaces and on the hands of healthcare workers.
- To prevent the spread of *C. difficile*, hand hygiene is paramount before and after entering the patient's room; handwashing with soap and water is required to mechanically eliminate *C. difficile* spores on one's hands and is superior to hand hygiene with alcohol-based hand sanitizers.
- Careful cleaning of hospital rooms with bleach products between patients is also essential to prevent the spread of *C. difficile*.
- *C. difficile* is transmitted in community settings such as at home.
- *C. difficile* has become a more challenging pathogen in recent years due to the spread of isolates that produce high levels of toxins and are highly resistant to quinolone antibiotics; decreasing the unnecessary use of quinolones is useful in limiting the impact of *C. difficile* in hospitals and long-term care facilities.
- 10–15% of patients treated for CDI will not respond to initial therapy.
- 20–35% of patients who have a clinical cure at the end of CDI therapy will have recurrent CDI.
- Each recurrence of CDI increases the likelihood of relapse due to persistent alterations in the gut microbiome.
- Most published guidelines recommend 10–14 days of therapy with metronidazole or vancomycin for treatment of a first episode of mild to moderate CDI and vancomycin or fidaxomicin for treatment of severe CDI.
- For those with severe CDI and sepsis, IV metronidazole and oral/rectal vancomycin are recommended.
- A 10-day course of vancomycin or fidaxomicin is currently recommended for first relapse.
- When patients present with a second or greater relapse, vancomycin taper or fidaxomicin taper/chaser should be considered.
- For third or greater relapse, FMT should be considered.

References

1. Hall AJ, Curns AT, McDonald LC, Parashar UD, Lopman BA. The roles of *Clostridium difficile* and norovirus among gastroenteritis-associated deaths in the United States, 1999-2007. Clin Infect Dis. 2012;55(2):216–23.
2. Cohen SH, Gerding DN, Johnson S, et al. Society for Healthcare Epidemiology of America; Infectious Diseases Society of America. Clinical practice guidelines for *Clostridium difficile* infection in adults: 2010 update by the Society for Healthcare Epidemiology of America (SHEA) and the Infectious Diseases Society of America (IDSA). Infect Control Hosp Epidemiol. 2010;31(5):431–55.
3. Crobach MJ, Planche T, Eckert C, et al. European Society of Clinical Microbiology and Infectious Diseases: update of the diagnostic guidance document for *Clostridium difficile* infection. Clin Microbiol Infect. 2016;22(Suppl 4):S63–81.
4. Planche T, Wilcox M. Reference assays for *Clostridium difficile* infection: one or two gold standards? J Clin Pathol. 2011;64(1):1–5.
5. Debast SB, Bauer MP, Kuijper EJ, European Society of Clinical Microbiology and Infectious Diseases. European Society of Clinical Microbiology and Infectious Diseases: update of the treatment guidance document for *Clostridium difficile* infection. Clin Microbiol Infect. 2014;20(Suppl 2):1–26.
6. Sartelli M, Malangoni MA, Abu-Zidan FM, et al. WSES guidelines for management of *Clostridium difficile* infection in surgical patients. World J Emerg Surg. 2015;10:38.
7. Surawicz CM, Brandt LJ, Binion DG, et al. Guidelines for diagnosis, treatment, and prevention of *Clostridium difficile* infections. Am J Gastroenterol. 2013;108(4):478–98. quiz 499.
8. Trubiano JA, Cheng AC, Korman TM, et al. Australasian Society of Infectious Diseases updated guidelines for the management of *Clostridium difficile* infection in adults and children in Australia and New Zealand. Intern Med J. 2016;46(4):479–93.
9. Cornely OA, Crook DW, Esposito R, et al. Fidaxomicin versus vancomycin for infection with *Clostridium difficile* in Europe, Canada, and the USA: a double-blind, non-inferiority, randomised controlled trial. Lancet Infect Dis. 2012;12(4):281–9.
10. Johnson S, Louie TJ, Gerding DN, et al. Vancomycin, metronidazole, or tolevamer for *Clostridium difficile* infection: results from two multinational, randomized, controlled trials. Clin Infect Dis. 2014;59(3):345–54.
11. Louie TJ, Miller MA, Mullane KM, et al. Fidaxomicin versus vancomycin for *Clostridium difficile* infection. N Engl J Med. 2011;364(5):422–31.
12. Zar FA, Bakkanagari SR, Moorthi KM, Davis MB. A comparison of vancomycin and metronidazole for the treatment of *Clostridium difficile*-associated diar-

rhea, stratified by disease severity. Clin Infect Dis. 2007;45(3):302–7.

13. Wilcox MH, Gerding DN, Poxton IR, et al. Bezlotoxumab for prevention of recurrent *Clostridium difficile* infection. N Engl J Med. 2017;376(4):305–17.

14. Bartlett JG. Bezlotoxumab—a new agent for *Clostridium difficile* infection. N Engl J Med. 2017;376(4): 381–2.

15. Deshpande A, Pasupuleti V, Thota P, et al. Risk factors for recurrent *Clostridium difficile* infection: a systematic review and meta-analysis. Infect Control Hosp Epidemiol. 2015;36(4):452–60.

16. Fekety R, McFarland LV, Surawicz CM, Greenberg RN, Elmer GW, Mulligan ME. Recurrent *Clostridium difficile* diarrhea: characteristics of and risk factors for patients enrolled in a prospective, randomized, double-blinded trial. Clin Infect Dis. 1997;24(3):324–33.

17. Garey KW, Sethi S, Yadav Y, DuPont HL. Meta-analysis to assess risk factors for recurrent *Clostridium difficile* infection. J Hosp Infect. 2008;70(4):298–304.

18. McFarland LV, Elmer GW, Surawicz CM. Breaking the cycle: treatment strategies for 163 cases of recurrent *Clostridium difficile* disease. Am J Gastroenterol. 2002;97(7):1769–75.

19. McFarland LV, Surawicz CM, Rubin M, Fekety R, Elmer GW, Greenberg RN. Recurrent *Clostridium difficile* disease: epidemiology and clinical characteristics. Infect Control Hosp Epidemiol. 1999;20(1): 43–50.

20. Zilberberg MD, Reske K, Olsen M, Yan Y, Dubberke ER. Risk factors for recurrent *Clostridium difficile* infection (CDI) hospitalization among hospitalized patients with an initial CDI episode: a retrospective cohort study. BMC Infect Dis. 2014;14:306.

21. Zilberberg MD, Tabak YP, Sievert DM, et al. Using electronic health information to risk-stratify rates of *Clostridium difficile* infection in US hospitals. Infect Control Hosp Epidemiol. 2011;32(7):649–55.

22. Kelly CR, Khoruts A, Staley C, et al. Effect of fecal microbiota transplantation on recurrence in multiply recurrent *Clostridium difficile* infection: a randomized trial. Ann Intern Med. 2016;165(9):609–16.

23. Lee CH, Patino H, Stevens C, et al. Surotomycin versus vancomycin for *Clostridium difficile* infection: phase 2, randomized, controlled, double-blind, non-inferiority, multicentre trial. J Antimicrob Chemother. 2016;71(10):2964–71.

24. Crook DW, Walker AS, Kean Y, et al. Fidaxomicin versus vancomycin for *Clostridium difficile* infection: meta-analysis of pivotal randomized controlled trials. Clin Infect Dis. 2012;55(Suppl 2):S93–S103.

25. Hota SS, Sales V, Tomlinson G, et al. Oral vancomycin followed by fecal transplantation versus tapering oral vancomycin treatment for recurrent *Clostridium difficile* infection: an open-label, randomized controlled trial. Clin Infect Dis. 2017;64(3):265–71.

26. Kassam Z, Lee CH, Yuan Y, Hunt RH. Fecal microbiota transplantation for *Clostridium difficile* infection: systematic review and meta-analysis. Am J Gastroenterol. 2013;108(4):500–8.

27. Soriano M, Danziger L, Johnson S. The use of a fidaxomicin taper/pulsed chaser as effective salvage therapy for vancomycin-refractory, recurrent *Clostridium difficile* infections. Abstracts, *IDWeek* 2013, San Francisco, 2013.

28. van Nood E, Dijkgraaf MG, Keller JJ. Duodenal infusion of donor feces for recurrent *Clostridium difficile*. N Engl J Med. 2013;368(5):407–15.

29. Gough E, Shaikh H, Manges AR. Systematic review of intestinal microbiota transplantation (fecal bacteriotherapy) for recurrent *Clostridium difficile* infection. Clin Infect Dis. 2011;53(10):994–1002.

30. Seekatz AM, Rao K, Santhosh K, Young VB. Dynamics of the fecal microbiome in patients with recurrent and nonrecurrent *Clostridium difficile* infection. Genome Med. 2016;8(1):47.

31. Staley C, Weingarden AR, Khoruts A, Sadowsky MJ. Interaction of gut microbiota with bile acid metabolism and its influence on disease states. Appl Microbiol Biotechnol. 2017;101(1):47–64.

32. Lee CH, Steiner T, Petrof EO, et al. Frozen vs fresh fecal microbiota transplantation and clinical resolution of diarrhea in patients with recurrent *Clostridium difficile* infection: a randomized clinical trial. JAMA. 2016;315(2):142–9.

33. Youngster I, Sauk J, Pindar C, et al. Fecal microbiota transplant for relapsing *Clostridium difficile* infection using a frozen inoculum from unrelated donors: a randomized, open-label, controlled pilot study. Clin Infect Dis. 2014;58(11):1515–22.

34. Abou Chakra CN, Pepin J, Sirard S, Valiquette L. Risk factors for recurrence, complications and mortality in *Clostridium difficile* infection: a systematic review. PLoS One. 2014;9(6):e98400.

A Young Woman with Neurologic Symptoms

Jean-Luc Benoit

In early June, a 37-year-old African American female developed new paresthesias in her hands and feet, then progressive weakness in her hands and legs. She became so weak that she was unable to get up and stand, even for a few minutes. In late June, she needed help from her friends for most of her activities of daily living. Although she was not treated, her weakness began to improve spontaneously after 3–4 weeks.

In mid-July, a neurologist obtained magnetic resonance imaging (MRI) scans of the brain and cervical spine, which were normal. In late August, she was referred to neurology at the University of Chicago. She felt slightly weak in her legs, but by August, she had recovered quite well as she was able to walk without any assistive device. She denied any bowel or bladder problems or symptoms or any back pain. She still complained of tingling in her hands and feet, especially in her toes and fingers.

On physical examination, she was afebrile. Blood pressure was 139/77 mmHg, pulse rate 93 beats per minute, and respirations 16 breaths per minute. Her height was 172 cm and her weight 96 kg. Her examination was normal except for the neurological exam. She was awake and oriented, with normal attention, language, memory, and knowledge. Fundoscopy showed sharp optic disks without papilledema. Cranial nerves II to XII were intact. Motor function was 5/5 in both upper and lower extremities, with normal muscle bulk and tone. Deep tendon reflexes were decreased to 1+ in biceps, triceps, brachioradialis, patellae, and ankle jerks bilaterally. Plantar reflexes were down-going bilaterally. The sensory exam was normal to temperature, pinprick, and vibration. The Romberg sign was absent. However, her gait was hesitant and cautious. The neurologist reviewed the MRIs of the brain and C-spine and agreed that they were unremarkable.

An electromyogram (EMG) performed in late August, more than 2 months after her initial presentation, showed a mixed axonal and demyelinating polyneuropathy, suggesting that "given the subacute tempo, partial conduction block and segmental slowing of conduction velocities, an acquired cause such as chronic inflammatory demyelinating polyneuropathy (CIDP) or other inflammatory neuropathies should be considered" (see Table 45.1). However, the monophasic neurological presentation of the patient was also consistent with acute inflammatory demyelinating polyneuropathy (AIDP), otherwise known as Guillain-Barré syndrome (GBS; see Table 45.2). A number of important infections are associated with GBS (Table 45.3). A work-up was performed to confirm the diagnosis of GBS and identify the etiology (Table 45.4), revealing a positive test for human immunodeficiency virus (HIV) infection.

J.-L. Benoit, M.D.
Section of Infectious Diseases and Global Health, Department of Medicine, University of Chicago, Chicago, IL, USA
e-mail: jbenoit@medicine.bsd.uchicago.edu

Table 45.1 Presentation of chronic inflammatory demyelinating polyneuropathy (CIDP) [9]

Tempo	Either chronic or relapsing course
Symptoms and signs	Progressive weakness and impaired sensory function in both legs and arms
	Tingling or numbness (beginning in toes and fingers)
	Weakness of arms and legs
	Loss of deep tendon reflexes
	Fatigue
	Abnormal sensations

The patient had HIV-associated GBS, which may occur in three settings: (1) during acute HIV seroconversion syndrome (acute HIV), (2) within 3–6 months after starting antiretroviral therapy (ART) due to immune reconstitution inflammatory syndrome (IRIS) (i.e., IRIS-associated GBS), and (3) in chronic HIV infection, often with a relatively high CD4+ T cell count. Interestingly, HIV patients with GBS may or may not have cerebrospinal fluid (CSF) pleocytosis. They usually respond to standard GBS therapy with either intravenous immune globulin or plasma exchange therapy (PLEX).

Table 45.2 Presentation of Guillain-Barré syndrome (GBS) (i.e., acute inflammatory demyelinating polyneuropathy [AIDP]) [1, 2, 4, 9]

Tempo		
Epidemiology		Acute and monophasic
		Incidence 0.6–1.7 per 100,000/year
		Bimodal: peak at 15–35 years of age and again at 50–75 years of age
Symptoms and signs	General	No fever
		Pain in the lower back or hips, precedes weakness; severe in 15%
	Ascending, progressive weakness	Usually begins in the feet before involving all limbs
		Usually symmetric
		Arms: weakness is worse proximally
		Face: involved in 50%
		Ophthalmoplegia in <5%
		Oropharyngeal or respiratory: occurs in 40%; 1/3 of patients need mechanical ventilation
		Plateau of weakness after 2 weeks (50%) to 4 weeks (90%)
		Improvement in strength begins 1–4 weeks after plateau
	Sensory symptoms	Typically milder than motor symptoms
		Paresthesias usually in the distal limbs, often precede weakness by >1 day
		Proximal sensory changes if severe case
	Autonomic dysfunction (in 2/3 of cases)	Sinus tachycardia, postural hypotension
		Sweating dysfunction
		Urinary retention and constipation later
Diagnosis	Cerebrospinal fluid	Albumino-cytological dissociation
		Increase in protein beyond the first week
		Cell count <10 cells per mm³
	Electromyogram	Conduction slowing, block, and prolonged distal latency or F-wave latencies are strongly supportive (seen in 80%), but may be delayed for weeks
	Serology	Antiganglioside antibody may be present

Table 45.3 Infections associated with Guillain-Barré syndrome (GBS) [1, 2, 4, 9, 10]

Etiology	Comments
Respiratory or gastrointestinal infection	2/3 of patients with GBS give a history of either respiratory or gastrointestinal infection days to weeks before onset
Rarely post immunization	1976 swine flu vaccine was associated with an increased risk of GBS by 1/100,000; seasonal flu vaccine-associated GBS is 1/1,000,000
	GBS occurs rarely after rabies or MMR vaccines
Bacterial	*Campylobacter jejuni*: the most commonly recognized infection preceding GBS and GBS variants – molecular mimicry between ganglioside-like epitopes of *C. jejuni* lipopolysaccharide and peripheral nerve gangliosides
	Mycoplasma pneumoniae in children
Viral	Upper respiratory viral infection (e.g., influenza, Coxsackie virus)
	Acute Epstein-Bar virus (EBV) infection
	Acute cytomegalovirus (CMV) infection
	Acute Zika virus infection is high risk: GBS in 3/10,000
	Rare causes: rubella, measles, varicella zoster virus (VZV), hepatitis B virus, and hantavirus

These treatments were no longer indicated in our patient who had improved spontaneously [1, 2]. There is an important infectious differential diagnosis for GBS (see Table 45.5). The patient was informed of her HIV diagnosis over the telephone and was referred to the Infectious Diseases Clinic but did not keep her appointment. Social services attempted to reach her multiple times but she did not return their calls and was lost to follow up.

She presented again 20 months after her diagnosis of HIV infection, complaining of not feeling well, with chest pain, malaise, subjective fever, and chills. She denied cough, shortness of breath, weight loss, night sweats, diarrhea, and bleeding. She had not been on any medications. Her physical examination was significant for pale conjunctiva, tachycardia, lack of fever, and otherwise normal exam, except that she was noted to have a somewhat unusual affect with staring and delayed answers. Her laboratory tests were abnormal, demonstrating evidence of severe microangiopathic hemolytic anemia (MAHA) and also profound thrombocytopenia. There were many schistocytes (fragmented red blood cells) on blood smears, and the disseminated intravascular coagulation (DIC) work-up was negative. The patient was therefore diagnosed with HIV-associated thrombotic thrombocytopenic purpura (HIV-TTP), which was confirmed when the

Table 45.4 Initial diagnostic work-up in the present patient with Guillain-Barré syndrome (GBS)

Test	Result	Normal values
Complete blood count, peripheral	WBC, 2500/μL (ANC > 1000)	3500–11,000/μL
	Hemoglobin, 14.1 g/dL	13.5–17.5 g/dL
	Platelet count, 224,000/μL	150,000–450,000/μL
CSF (in late October, 4 months after presentation)	Glucose, 69 mg/dL	50–70 mg/dL
	Protein, 122 mg/dL	60–90 mg/dL
	Cell count, RBC 69, WBC 14 (93% lymphocytes, 7% monocytes)	0–30/μL total cell count
Rheumatology panel	ANA, 80 units	Negative
	ACE level, 10 u/L	8–53 u/L
	Otherwise negative	Negative
Antibodies	Antiganglioside antibody: negative	Negative
	Anti-MAG antibody: negative	Negative
Viral serologies	Hepatitis C serology: negative	Negative
	Hepatitis B surface antigen: negative	Negative
HIV testing	HIV screen: positive	Negative
	CD4+ T cell count, 189 cells/mm^3	365–1437 cells/mm^3
	CD4/CD3%, 14.9%	32–64%
	HIV viral load, 61,967 copies/mL	Undetectable

ACE angiotensin-converting enzyme, *ANA* antinuclear antibody, *ANC* absolute neutrophil count, *CSF* cerebrospinal fluid, *HIV* human immunodeficiency virus, *WBC* white blood cell count

Table 45.5 Differential diagnosis of patients suspected of having Guillain-Barré syndrome (GBS) [1, 2, 4, 9, 10]

West Nile virus (WNV) encephalitis	Often resembles poliomyelitis, but may resemble GBS
	Altered sensorium if encephalitis is present
Poliomyelitis	Asymmetric flaccid palsy (lower motor neuron syndrome) due to patchy spinal anterior horn viral infection
Botulism	Descending, symmetric paralysis that progresses rapidly
	4 Ds: dysphagia, diplopia, dysphonia, and dysarthria
	Clear sensorium
Myasthenia gravis	Muscular weakness with fatigability (worse after exercise or in the evening but improves with rest)
	Ptosis, oculomotor muscles, facial muscles, chewing, talking, and swallowing often involved
	Severe respiratory muscle involvement may occur
	Yellow fever vaccine may cause disseminated infection
	Avoid certain antibiotics (especially aminoglycosides, quinolones, telithromycin, azithromycin, and quinine)
Lambert-Eaton myasthenic syndrome (LEMS)	Muscular weakness that improves with exercise
	Association with malignancy, especially small cell lung cancer
	Autonomic symptoms are common (dry mouth)
Tick paralysis	Ascending paralysis
	Tick attached
	Usually children in the USA

(continued)

Table 45.5 (continued)

Tetanus (*Clostridium tetani*)	Painful muscle spasms triggered by small stimuli: trismus, risus sardonicus; dysphagia; muscle spasms in neck, abdominal wall, and spine with hyperextension of the spine (opisthotonos)
	Fever
	Sweats
	Hypertension
	Tachycardia
Ciguatera fish poisoning (CFP)	Gastrointestinal and cardiovascular symptoms within hours after ingestion of reef fish (barracuda, grouper, or snapper), followed by prolonged itching and neurological symptoms (paresthesia, pain, toothache, dysuria, weakness, fatigue, and characteristic inversion of heat and cold sensation)
Miller-Fisher syndrome	Triad of ophthalmoplegia, ataxia, and areflexia: *Campylobacter*
Autoimmune brainstem encephalitis	Bickerstaff brainstem encephalitis
	Responds to steroid therapy
Infectious brainstem encephalitis (rhombencephalitis): several etiologies	Herpes simplex virus type 1 (HSV-1)
	Listeria monocytogenes
	Rabies
	Enterovirus 71
	Monkey B virus (Herpes B)

level of ADAMTS 13 in the serum was found to be below 3% of normal, in the absence of an inhibitor (Table 45.6).

45.1 Thrombotic Thrombocytopenic Purpura (TTP)

Thrombotic thrombocytopenic purpura (TTP) is an acute prothrombotic disorder resulting from a

Table 45.6 Patient laboratory test results at time of her return to care

Test	Result	Normal value
White blood cell count	4600/μL	3500–11,000/μL
Hemoglobin	6.6 g/dL	13.5–17.5 g/dL
Mean corpuscular volume (MCV)	85.2 fL	81.6–98.3 fL
RBC distribution width	21.3%	11.9–15.5%
Platelet count	12,000/μL	150,000–450,000/μL
Creatinine	0.8 mg/dL	0.5–1.4 mg/dL
Total bilirubin	1.8 mg/dL	0.3–1.2 mg/dL
Nonconjugated bilirubin	1.3	0.3–1.0
Lactate dehydrogenase (LDH)	90 u/L	122–222 u/L
Haptoglobin	<20 mg/dL	30–200 mg/dL
COOMBS	Negative	Negative
Fibrinogen	405 mg/dL	200–393 mg/dL
Blood cultures, bacterial	No growth	No growth
CD4+ T cell count	47 cells/mm^3	365–1437 cells/mm^3
CD4/CD3%	4%	32–64%
HIV viral load	177,622 copies/mL	Undetectable
Genotype (RT, PR, IN)	Susceptible to all antiretroviral agents	Susceptible to all antiretroviral agents
Blood smear	Very few platelets; many schistocytes	N/A
ADAMTS 13	<3%	>70%
ADAMTS 13 inhibitor	None	None

IN integrase inhibitor, *PR* protease, *RT* reverse transcriptase

deficiency of the von Willebrand factor (VWF) cleavage protease ADAMTS 13, an enzyme that cleaves a peptide bond of the mature subunit of VWF and prevents interactions of the largest VWF multimers with platelets. In the plasma of patients with TTP, ultra-large VWF multimers (UL-VWF) cause widespread microvascular thrombosis.

The incidence of TTP is increased 15–40 times in HIV-infected persons as compared to the general population. HIV-TTP is an acquired form of ADAMTS 13 deficiency seen in patients with advanced HIV who have a low CD4+ T cell count and high HIV viral load. There is a strong female predominance. The pathogenesis of TTP is likely somewhat different when associated with HIV, but elucidating the precise pathophysiology will require more research. HIV-TTP may be the first manifestation of AIDS and appears much less frequently when patients have been on effective ART. Without treatment, HIV-TTP has a 90% mortality, and associated morbidities are severe, including neurological complications, renal failure, myocardial ischemia, bowel ischemia, retinal detachment, and bleeding from thrombocytopenia [3] (Table 45.7).

Table 45.7 Thrombotic thrombocytopenic purpura (TTP) pentad[a] [3, 5, 7, 9]

Microvascular platelet aggregation and thrombus formation	Profound thrombocytopenia
	Microangiopathic hemolytic anemia (MAHA) with fragmented red blood cells (schistocytes)
	Renal dysfunction
	Neurologic symptoms (intermittent)
	Fever

[a]The full pentad is present in a minority of patients

45.2 Patient Management

Management of TTP is shown in Table 45.8. The patient was hospitalized and started on PLEX for 2–3 h daily, trimethoprim-sulfamethoxazole (*Pneumocystis* prophylaxis) daily, and ART from the first day of admission, with administration of oral medications timed immediately after PLEX. The ART regimen was selected before any HIV genotype resistance data were available, for optimal efficacy and limited nephrotoxicity. A pharmacokinetic consult was obtained, but recommended standard daily dosages of the selected antiretroviral agents (darunavir 800 mg boosted with ritonavir 100 mg, lamivudine 300 mg and dolutegravir 50 mg) were administered daily.

With daily PLEX for 5 days, the serum level of ADAMTS 13 increased from <3% to 55% and the platelet count increased to 213,000/μL. The patient was afebrile and appeared well during the entire admission. She was closely monitored for complications of PLEX, which include bacterial superinfection and hypocalcemia. Her intravenous access was removed, and she was discharged on hospital day 6 with a very early follow-up in an infectious disease clinic approved by her health insurance for long-term HIV management.

Key Points/Pearls

- Current guidelines recommend HIV screening of all patients who are seen in a healthcare setting.
- Any patient with unexplained neurological symptoms should be screened for HIV.
- HIV is a neurotropic virus that can cause multiple central or peripheral nervous system manifestations including GBS, neuropathy, aseptic meningitis, acute encephalopathy, chronic HIV-associated encephalopathy and dementia, seizures, and cerebrovascular accidents.
- Complications of AIDS may affect the brain, causing either non-focal syndromes (e.g., meningitis due to *Cryptococcus neoformans*, *Coccidioides immitis*, or *Mycobacterium tuberculosis* or encephalitis due to cytomegalovirus) or focal syndromes (e.g., brain abscesses due to *Toxoplasma gondii* reactivation, primary central nervous system lymphoma due to Epstein-Barr virus, progressive multifocal leukoencephalopathy due to the JC polyomavirus [JCV], or meningovascular syphilis).
- Two-third of cases of GBS are preceded by an episode of respiratory or intestinal infection.
- *Campylobacter jejuni* is the pathogen most strongly associated with GBS, found in 25–50% of adults with GBS; an antibody response triggered by microbial antigens results in binding to the GM1 and GD1a gangliosides (molecular mimicry between microbial and human nerve antigens).
- Other infections clearly associated with GBS include HIV, cytomegalovirus (CMV), Epstein-Barr virus (EBV), influenza A, *Mycoplasma pneumoniae*, *Haemophilus influenzae*, the Chikungunya alphavirus, and the Zika flavivirus
- Vaccines have also rarely been associated with GBS, including the rabies vaccine and H1N1 influenza A vaccines [4].

Table 45.8 Management of thrombotic thrombocytopenic purpura (TTP) [3, 5, 7, 9]

Thrombotic thrombocytopenic purpura (TTP)	The initial diagnosis is clinical and treatment is urgent
	Plasma exchange (PLEX) should be started as soon as an access is established
	Measure both ADAMTS 13 and look for an inhibitor
	Serological tests for HIV, HBV, and HCV
	Pregnancy test
HIV-associated TTP (HIV-TTP)	Consider HIV-TTP with MAHA and thrombocytopenia
	PLEX and ART are started together on day one
	ART given daily immediately after PLEX completed
	Long-term ART continued to prevent TTP relapse
	With treatment, mortality decreases from 90% to 10–20%

ART antiretroviral therapy, *HBV* hepatitis B virus, *HCV* hepatitis C virus, *HIV* human immunodeficiency virus, *MAHA* microangiopathic hemolytic anemia

- Patients with HIV infection may develop severe thrombocytopenia due to HIV-associated immune thrombocytopenic purpura (ITP), thrombotic thrombocytopenic purpura (TTP), hemolytic-uremic syndrome (HUS), drugs, splenic sequestration associated with cirrhosis and portal hypertension, lymphoma and complications associated with opportunistic infections including disseminated intravascular coagulation (DIC), and hemophagocytic lymphohistiocytosis (HLH), for example, in disseminated histoplasmosis.

- The primary thrombotic microangiopathy (TMA) syndromes have common features: hemolytic anemia with the presence of schistocytes on blood smears (microangiopathic hemolytic anemia, MAHA), thrombocytopenia, organ injury, and microvascular thrombosis with consumption of platelets and fragmentation of red blood cells; the TMA syndromes include TTP (ADAMTS 13 deficiency-mediated TMA), diarrhea-associated HUS (Shiga toxin-mediated HUS), complement-mediated TMA (which responds to eculizumab), and a number of other syndromes [5].

- TTP is classically described as a clinical pentad of fever, MAHA, thrombocytopenia, acute kidney injury, and neurological manifestations, but the full pentad is only seen in a minority of patients.

- TTP is due to a deficiency in the ADAMTS 13 von Willebrand factor-cleaving protease and is associated with microthrombi that include platelets and ultra-large von Willebrand factor multimers anchored to the endothelium [6].

- HUS is classically described as a triad of MAHA, thrombocytopenia, and prominent acute renal failure; in HUS, the renal manifestations are prominent, and most patients do not have systemic symptoms.

- HUS may be associated with infectious etiologies; Shiga toxin HUS (ST-HUS) is due to endothelial injury by absorbed Shiga toxin produced by enteric pathogens, often enterohemorrhagic *Escherichia coli* in North America although *Shigella dysenteriae* type 1 causes the same complication mostly abroad.

- Like TTP, HUS is associated with HIV [7].

- The secondary TMA syndromes include infection, cancer, malignant hypertension, systemic sclerosis, systemic lupus erythematosus, antiphospholipid syndrome, stem cell or solid organ transplant, and complications seen in the third trimester of pregnancy (pre-eclampsia/eclampsia and HELLP syndrome, i.e., hemolysis, elevated liver enzyme levels, and low platelet) [5].

- Although advanced HIV disease causes severe CD4+ T cell lymphopenia-associated immunodeficiency, people living with HIV may often develop autoimmune conditions [8].

References

1. Afzal A, Benjamin M, Gummelt K, et al. Ascending paralysis associated with HIV infection. Proc (Bayl Univ Med Cent). 2015;28:25–8
2. Brannagan TH III. HIV-associated Guillain–Barré syndrome. J Neurol Sci. 2003;208:39–42
3. Meiring M, Webb M, Goedhals D, Louw V. HIV-associated thrombotic thrombocytopenic purpura—what we know so far. Eur Oncol Haematol. 2012;8:89–91
4. Willison HJ, Jacobs BC, van Doorn PA. Guillain-Barré syndrome. Lancet. 2016;388:717–27
5. George JN, Nester CM. Syndromes of thrombotic microangiopathy. N Engl J Med. 2014;371:654–66
6. Lopes da Silva R. Viral-associated thrombotic microangiopathies. Hematol Oncol Stem Cell Ther. 2011;4:51–9
7. Jin A, Boroujerdi-Rad L, Shah G, et al. Thrombotic microangiopathy and human immunodeficiency virus in the era of eculizumab. Clin Kidney J. 2016;9(4):576–9
8. Virot E, Duclos A, Adelaide L, et al. Autoimmune diseases and HIV infection: a cross-sectional study. Medicine. 2017;96:e5769
9. Medical knowledge self-assessment program (MKSAP), 17th ed. American College of Physicians;2017.
10. Bennett JE, Dolin R, Blaser MJ. Mandell, Douglas, and Bennett's principles and practice of infectious diseases. 8th ed. New York: Elsevier/Saunders; 2015.

A Woman with a History of a 2-Year Stay in Gabon and Onset of a Cyclical Fever More Than 1 Year Later

Jean-Luc Benoit

A 23-year-old female medical student presented with fever every other day for 1 week, which she believed was a cyclical fever highly suggestive of malaria. After graduating from college, she spent 1 year as a volunteer in Gabon, West Africa, before starting medical school. She had not traveled to a malaria-endemic area since leaving Gabon 13 months before.

She was healthy until 1 week prior to presentation, when she developed fever up to 102.5 °F, with chills and sweats. The symptoms only occurred every other day. Associated symptoms included myalgia, headache, profuse sweats with defervescence of the fever, and intense fatigue. She denied nasal or sinus congestion, sore throat, odynophagia, cough, chest pain, shortness of breath, abdominal pain, nausea, vomiting, diarrhea, dysuria, urinary frequency, or vaginal discharge. The patient's past medical history was otherwise unremarkable.

During the year spent in Gabon, other than a few episodes of watery diarrhea, she did not develop any illness. She had not swum in freshwater (no risk of exposure to schistosomiasis), and she had taken weekly mefloquine malaria prophylaxis during her stay and until 4 weeks after returning to the United States (US). Since

J.-L. Benoit, M.D.
Section of Infectious Diseases and Global Health, Department of Medicine, University of Chicago, Chicago, IL, USA
e-mail: jbenoit@medicine.bsd.uchicago.edu

returning to the USA, she had remained in good health with no febrile illnesses. She was very active physically including running a few times a week. She had one sexual partner. She considered that they were in a monogamous relationship and were both at very low risk of HIV or other sexually transmitted infection (STI). She never had an STI herself and was followed regularly by a primary care physician who last did her cervical PAP smear about 3 months prior. She last had a negative HIV screening test 1 year prior to presentation.

She had never had a blood transfusion. She took no prescription drugs and was not taking a contraceptive pill. She had no drug allergies. The patient resided in Illinois and had traveled extensively within the USA including to the Upper Midwest and to New England. She reported never noting any tick bites. She had traveled abroad to the Caribbean, Israel, and Jordan, but she had not been in a malaria-endemic area since her stay in Gabon.

On physical examination, the patient was not in any acute distress. She was afebrile but stated that she had a fever to 102.5 °F the night before. Her blood pressure and pulse and respiratory rate were normal. Her conjunctivae appeared a bit pale but her sclerae were anicteric. She had no rash. The oral exam was normal, and she had no cervical or axillary lymphadenopathy. The heart rhythm was regular, without any murmur or abnormal sound. The lungs were clear to

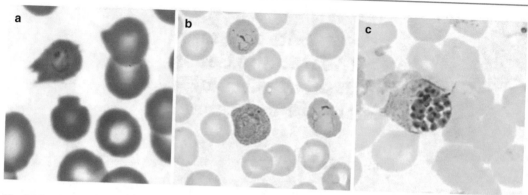

Fig. 46.1 *Plasmodium ovale* on thin blood smear: large ring form with fimbriated red blood cell cytoplasm (**a**), amoeboid trophozoites (**b**), and schizont with brown pigment (**c**). Source: U.S. Centers for Disease Control and Prevention (CDC), DPDX Laboratory Identification of Parasites of Public Health Concern. https://www.cdc.gov/dpdx/resources/pdf/benchAids/malaria/Povale_benchaidV2.pdf (Accessed June 27, 2017)

Fig. 46.2 *Plasmodium vivax* on thin blood smear: intracytoplasmic Schüffner's dots; young ring forms are about one third of the diameter of an RBC; amoeboid trophozoites. Source: U.S. Centers for Disease Control and Prevention (CDC), http://phil.cdc.gov/phil_images/20021230/12/PHIL_2720_lores.jpg (Accessed June 27, 2017)

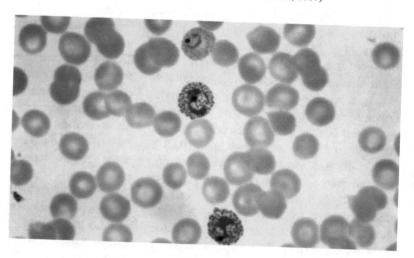

auscultation. The abdomen was soft and without hepatomegaly or splenomegaly. There was no suprapubic or costovertebral tenderness. A pelvic exam was unremarkable.

Laboratory tests were notable for hemoglobin 11.0 g/dL, white blood cell count 4000/μL (60% neutrophils, 30% lymphocytes, 8% monocytes, and 2% eosinophils), and platelet count 80,000/μL (normal range, 150,000–450,000/μL). Iron studies, liver enzymes, kidney function tests, and urinalysis were normal. Blood cultures were negative. A chest radiograph was normal.

The differential diagnosis was broad as it included infections acquired in the USA and abroad as well as a few noninfectious etiologies (see Table 1). However, because of the cyclical nature of her febrile illness, malaria was considered much more likely than other etiologies, although a cyclical fever is not pathognomonic of malaria. Thin and thick blood smears were obtained and reviewed carefully.

Thin blood smears showed intraerythrocytic plasmodia-like protozoa including ring forms, older trophozoites, and schizonts, with a parasitemia of about 2%. Older parasites had brown pigment. Infected red blood cells had intracytoplasmic dots and were enlarged, often with an oval shape. No gametocytes were identified but they may be difficult to recognize.

Babesiosis was ruled out due to the lack of tetrads, polymorphism, or vacuoles and the presence of brown pigment in older protozoa. *Plasmodium falciparum* malaria was also ruled

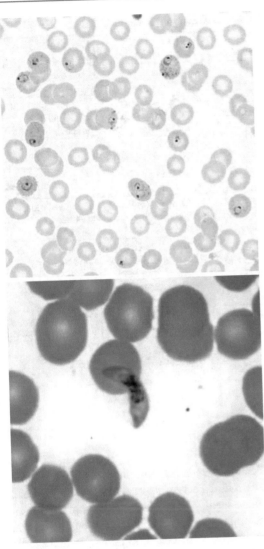

Table 46.1 Differential diagnosis of cyclical fever and abnormal blood smear in a woman with a history of living in Gabon, West Africa

Malaria due to *Plasmodium falciparum*
Hypnozoite relapse of malaria with either *Plasmodium ovale* or *Plasmodium vivax*
Chronic malaria due to *Plasmodium malariae*
West African trypanosomiasis due to *Trypanosoma brucei gambiense*
Babesiosis due to *Babesia microti* acquired in the USA through the bite of *Ixodes scapularis* or *Ixodes pacificus* blacklegged deer ticks
Tick-borne relapsing fever acquired in the Western USA through the bite of *Ornithodoros* species soft ticks
Mononucleosis syndrome due to acute infection by Epstein-Barr virus (EBV), cytomegalovirus (CMV), human immunodeficiency virus (HIV), *Toxoplasma gondii*, or *Treponema pallidum* (secondary syphilis)
Brucellosis (*Brucella* spp.)
Infective endocarditis
Endemic fungal infection
Tuberculosis (*Mycobacterium tuberculosis*)
Amoebic liver abscess
Noninfectious etiologies: In a young woman, consider systemic lupus erythematosus, sarcoidosis, and lymphoma

Fig. 46.3 *Plasmodium falciparum* on thin blood smear: (*top*) only delicate, young ring forms with small cytoplasm and 2 chromatin dots; very high parasitemia; multiply infected RBCs; accolé forms; no pigment; (*bottom*) banana-shaped gametocytes appear only about a week after the onset of illness, but may persist in asymptomatic persons (i.e., the human reservoir). Source: U.S. Centers for Disease Control and Prevention (CDC), DPDX Laboratory Identification of Parasites of Public Health Concern. https://www.cdc.gov/dpdx/resources/pdf/benchAids/malaria/Pfalciparum_benchaidV2.pdf (Accessed June 27, 2017)

out because in this infection only tiny, young ring forms with two dots of chromatin and a scant cytoplasm are identified on blood smear, with at times a few banana-shaped gametocytes [1]. Maturing *P. falciparum* induces the formation of knobs rich in *P. falciparum* erythrocyte membrane protein 1 (PfEMP-1) on the surface of red blood cells (RBC), with binding of PfEMP-1 to endothelial receptors on post-capillary venules, so that older parasites are trapped in the microcirculation [2–4].

Non-falciparum malaria was therefore diagnosed as all *Plasmodium* stages were identified, including young ring forms, older trophozoites, and schizonts. There are three non-falciparum plasmodia to consider. *P. malariae* can cause minimally symptomatic chronic malaria but is not common. In *P. malariae* infection, the parasitemia is very low, infected RBCs are of normal size, and typical trophozoites called band forms are recognized. *P. vivax* and *P. ovale* are quite similar on blood smears. In both of these, infected RBCs are enlarged, with the presence of intracytoplasmic Schüffner's dots; young ring forms are large, about one third of the diameter of an RBC; and ameboid trophozoites are recognized. It is difficult to differentiate between the

Table 46.2 Morphological comparison of *P. falciparum*, *P. ovale*, *P. vivax*, and *P. malariae* [2–5]

	Plasmodium falciparum	Plasmodium vivax	Plasmodium ovale	Plasmodium malariae
Number of plasmodia per RBC	Multiple	Only one	Only one	Only one
Parasitemia	Often high as all RBCs can be infected	Low to moderate; only young RBCs infected	Low to moderate; only young RBCs infected	Very low; only old RBCs can be infected
Size and shape of infected RBCs	Normal	Enlarged Spherical	Enlarged Oval	Normal
Cytoplasmic Schüffner's dots	None	Present	Present	None
Stages seen on blood smear	Only young trophozoites	Young and older trophozoites, schizonts	Young and older trophozoites, schizonts	Young and older trophozoites, schizonts
Trophozoites: shape, size, and location within RBC	Small rings with two dots of chromatin; scant cytoplasm; at the periphery of RBC	Larger trophozoites, some with filaments in their cytoplasm, called **amoeboid trophozoites**	Larger trophozoites, some with filaments in their cytoplasm, called **amoeboid trophozoites**	Trophozoites with **band forms**
Schizonts	Not seen	Multiple nuclei and brown pigment	Multiple nuclei and brown pigment	Multiple nuclei and brown pigment
Brown pigment	None	Yes	Yes	Yes
Gametocytes	Banana shaped; seen in longer infections	Spherical	Spherical	Spherical

RBC red blood cell

two species, but *P. ovale* tends to cause infected, enlarged RBCs to have an oval shape (see Table 46.2) [1–4].

Both *P. vivax* and *P. ovale* cause late relapses of malaria due to activation of dormant liver forms, called hypnozoites in the US literature. *P. ovale* is not as prevalent as *P. vivax*, except in Western Africa because local populations lack the Duffy blood type that is the major receptor for *P. vivax* entry into RBCs [2–4]. Our patient had therefore acquired *P. ovale* malaria in West Africa despite being on malaria prophylaxis there. She remained asymptomatic for more than a year when a hypnozoite activated and caused a relapse of malaria. The patient was treated for *P. vivax* malaria with chloroquine phosphate 1000 mg once, followed by 500 mg 6 h, 24 h, and 48 h later. Her glucose-6-phosphate dehydrogenase (G6PD) level was normal, allowing her physicians to prescribe safely primaquine 30 mg a day for 14 days to eradicate hypnozoites and to prevent further relapses of malaria [5].

46.1 Malaria

Female *Anopheles* mosquitoes transmit malaria at night, injecting sporozoa when they take a blood meal. Plasmodia are Apicomplexa, protozoa that use an apical complex of organelles and microtubules to penetrate into cells. Plasmodia infect hepatocytes (exoerythrocytic schizogony) first, then reach the blood, and infect RBCs (erythrocytic schizogony). There are four species of human plasmodia.

P. falciparum is highly lethal, causing about 95% of malaria-related mortality. Because the parasite infects all RBCs regardless of their age, it can cause very high parasitemia. Because it induces RBCs to grow PfEMP-1 knobs on their surface with resulting entrapment of the mature protozoa in the microcirculation, tissue injury is much more severe in falciparum malaria, with manifestations including cerebral malaria, placenta infection with adverse effects on pregnancy, and pulmonary edema or the acute respiratory distress syndrome (ARDS) [2–4]. Uncomplicated falciparum malaria manifestations include fever (every day initially, especially in travelers without prior semi-immunity; with prior semi-immunity, a fever every other day is often seen) and many associated symptoms (e.g., headache, nausea, vomiting, abdominal pain, and profuse sweats). The complete blood count usually shows anemia, thrombocytopenia, and a normal white blood cell count. Even uncomplicated falciparum malaria can progress rapidly to severe illness. *P. falciparum* can result in a large number of complications (see Table 46.3), and treatment is considered an emergency. Because *P. falciparum* has acquired drug resistance to multiple antimalarial agents, including chloroquine, sulfadoxine/pyrimethamine, mefloquine, quinine, and recently artemisinin derivatives, treatment always includes two different agents, and choice of therapy depends on the severity of illness. Acutely ill patients are best treated in the intensive care unit with rapidly acting intravenous agents, such as quinidine, quinine, or artesunate, plus a second

active drug (doxycycline or clindamycin). Patients who are stable and can take oral therapy usually receive one of three combinations: atovaquone/proguanil, artemether/lumefantrine, or a combination of quinine plus either doxycycline or clindamycin [2–5].

P. vivax is highly prevalent, including previously in North America and Europe. It only infects young RBCs, resulting in lower parasitemia (1–2%). It requires the Duffy receptor on the surface of RBCs and therefore is rare in most of sub-Saharan Africa, although common in the horn of Africa and in Madagascar. Liver hypnozoites allow the parasite to survive cold winters. Chloroquine resistance has been described in Papua New Guinea and Indonesia. Patients present initially with daily fever and then get febrile paroxysms every 48 h (benign tertian fever). Splenic rupture is a rare complication.

P. ovale causes malaria that is clinically indistinguishable from *P. vivax* malaria and is also associated with late relapses due to the activation of hypnozoites. It is most prevalent in western Africa.

P. malariae is a minor species causing chronic malaria of low severity, as it only infects old cells with very low parasitemia. It may cause nephrotic syndrome due to chronic immune complexes [2–4].

P. knowlesi causes malaria in long-tailed and pig-tailed, crab-eating macaques found over a wide range of Southeast Asia from Myanmar to Timor. It causes zoonotic human malaria in Malaysia (especially Borneo), with cases reported elsewhere (Thailand, Myanmar, Singapore, and Philippines). Blood smears show tiny ring forms (like *P. falciparum*) and band forms (like *P. malariae*, with which it is confused). It results in a higher mortality than non-falciparum malaria, and chloroquine is an effective therapy [1–5].

Table 46.3 Complications of *Plasmodium falciparum* malaria [2–4]

Cerebral malaria: seizures, altered mental status, sequelae
Hypoglycemia: due to malaria itself or quinidine release of insulin from islet cells
Severe anemia: hemolysis and splenic clearance; ineffective erythropoiesis
Severe thrombocytopenia
Pulmonary edema and acute respiratory distress syndrome (ARDS)
Hypotension and shock: increase fluids, rule out bleeding, rule out Gram-negative sepsis, avoid epinephrine, and use dopamine
Acute renal failure: prerenal, microvascular injury, intravascular hemolysis (hemoglobinuria), acute tubular necrosis (ATN)
Blackwater fever: macroscopic hemoglobinuria and renal failure due to intravascular hemolysis, may be associated with quinine therapy with or without G6PD deficiency
Bilious remittent fever: abdominal pain, vomiting, diarrhea, and painful hepatomegaly with icterus
Lactic acidosis: major role in death from severe malaria
Bacterial superinfection with sepsis
Symmetrical peripheral gangrene

G6PD glucose-6-phosphate dehydrogenase

Key Points/Pearls

- *P. falciparum* smears only show young ring forms, but no mature trophozoites or schizonts because these are entrapped in the microcirculation.
- Banana-shaped gametocytes are pathognomonic of *P. falciparum*, but are not seen in recently infected travelers; gametocytes

appear late and are seen alone in non-ill persons in endemic areas.

- Relapsing malaria only occurs with *P. vivax* and *P. ovale*; the term "relapse" in malaria has a specific meaning: the appearance of blood-stage parasites originating from a dormant liver stage of the parasite, called a hypnozoite.
- Malaria relapses occur in 50% of persons infected with *P. vivax* or *P. ovale*, for up to 1–3 years after infection.
- Only primaquine (30 mg base a day for 14 days) kills hypnozoites, but there is a risk of severe intravascular hemolysis in patients with G6PD deficiency.
- Proper malaria prophylaxis in most areas is mefloquine taken weekly or either atovaquone/proguanil or doxycycline taken daily; malaria prophylaxis is continued after returning to a non-endemic area for 1 week with atovaquone/proguanil and for 4 weeks with either doxycycline or mefloquine.

References

1. U.S. Centers for Disease Control and Prevention (CDC), DPDX Laboratory Identification of Parasites of Public Health Concern. http://www.dpd.cdc.gov/dpdx/HTML/Babesiosis.htm. Accessed 27 June 2017.
2. Bennett JE, Dolin R, Blaser MJ. Mandell, Douglas, and Bennett's principles and practice of infectious diseases. 8th ed. New York: Elsevier/Saunders; 2015.
3. Farrar J, Hotez PJ, Junghanss T, et al. Manson's tropical infectious diseases. 23rd ed. New York: Elsevier/Saunders; 2013.
4. Guerrant RL, Walker DH, Weller PF. Tropical infectious diseases principles, pathogens & practice. 3rd ed. New York: Elsevier/Saunders; 2011.
5. CDC Guidelines for Treatment of Malaria in the United States. https://www.cdc.gov/malaria/resources/pdf/treatmenttable.pdf. Accessed 27 June 2017.

An Infectious Malignancy

47

Kathleen Mullane

An 82-year-old Cantonese-speaking woman presented with her daughter complaining of a rapidly enlarging, painless mass on her right breast. The patient noted the mass approximately 6 months before she told her daughter of its presence and prior to the initial evaluation by her primary care provider. A chest x-ray was obtained which was negative for intrapulmonary findings, but due to concern for malignancy, a magnetic resonance imaging (MRI) scan was obtained. The MRI showed a large, subpectoral right chest wall mass measuring 9 × 4.5 × 6.8 cm that extended into the anterior mediastinum through the proximal sternum. Post-contrast images demonstrated thick peripheral enhancement of the mass with a central region of non-enhancement consistent with necrosis and concerning for malignancy. Incidentally noted were bilaterally enlarged thyroid gland lobes and two sub-centimeter, non-enhancing lesions within the right lobe of the liver. This was followed by a computerized tomography (CT) scan of the chest, abdomen, and pelvis that showed a large mass in the ascending colon, likely representing a primary colonic malignancy as well as the large chest wall mass described on the recent MRI. The chest wall mass was read as being consistent with a site of osseous metastatic disease to the sternum that had broken through the bony cortex and extended into the soft tissues of the chest. A metastatic lesion was also reported in the left iliac body with cortical breakthrough, but no clear soft tissue extension was observed. There were many other areas of ill-defined increased density in the marrow spaces suspicious for sites of metastatic disease.

The patient was referred for a colonoscopy, and referral to an oncologist was also recommended. The ascending colon mass was biopsied. Pathologic examination demonstrated a tubulovillous adenoma as well as multiple adenomatous polyps. The colonic mucosa also showed multiple non-caseating granulomas with negative silver and acid fast stains. The pathologist commented that it was unclear if the tubulovillous adenoma was harboring a malignancy given the large size of the polyp/mass and recommended surgical resection for optimal pathologic evaluation.

The patient's family brought her to our medical center for further evaluation. She denied fevers, rash, headaches, dizziness, throat pain, dysphagia, odynophagia, night sweats, weight loss, cough, shortness of breath, or hemoptysis. She denied abdominal pain, change in her stool color or caliber, blood in stool, diarrhea, or constipation. She denied dysuria, hematuria, or vaginal discharge but did complain of menopausal

K. Mullane, D.O.
Section of Infectious Diseases and Global Health, Department of Medicine, University of Chicago, Chicago, IL, USA
e-mail: kmullane@medicine.bsd.uchicago.edu

© Springer International Publishing AG 2018
M. David, J.-L. Benoit (eds.), *The Infectious Disease Diagnosis*,
https://doi.org/10.1007/978-3-319-64906-1_47

"hot flashes." A chest x-ray showed increased opacity over the right upper lobe, at the site of the patient's known chest wall mass with no signs of pulmonary metastasis. A positron emission tomography (PET) scan was obtained and was read as showing a large, hypermetabolic mass in the right upper chest wall consistent with a malignancy. Also reported were extensive nodal metastasis in the neck, mediastinum, lung hila, bilateral axillary regions, abdominal cavity and pelvis; osseous metastases in the T12 vertebral body and left iliac bone; and soft tissue metastases in the left upper arm and left lower chest wall.

She underwent a biopsy of the chest mass 2 months after initial presentation to her primary care provider (6 months after she initially reported noticing the mass). The pathology of the mass showed necrotizing and non-necrotizing granulomas. Acid fast stain showed rare acid fast bacilli within the granulomas; silver stain was negative; and PCR was negative for *Mycobacterium tuberculosis* complex. As it was believed that she was undergoing biopsy for malignancy, no tissue cultures were obtained. An interferon-gamma release assay (IGRA) was obtained and was negative. A second biopsy was obtained, and the patient was then started on rifampin, isoniazid, pyrazinamide, and ethambutol (RIPE) therapy. The tissue culture was positive for *M. tuberculosis* complex. Two months later susceptibilities returned. The organism had low-level resistance to isoniazid and was susceptible to ethambutol, pyrazinamide, and rifampin.

47.1 Isoniazid-Resistant Extrapulmonary Tuberculosis

M. tuberculosis infection may have many different presentations including latent infection and pulmonary and extrapulmonary disease. The World Health Organization (WHO) estimated that in 2014 approximately 8.6 million new cases of tuberculosis occurred and 1.5 million died from this disease [1]. WHO estimated that there were 2–3 billion persons latently infected with tuberculosis. In the United States (US), there were 9412 cases of active infection reported in 2014 with 66% of these occurring in foreign-born persons. An estimated 11 million persons in the USA were infected with tuberculosis, representing a large reservoir of latently infected individuals. Individuals with latent tuberculosis have a 4–15% lifetime risk of developing active tuberculosis, with half of these cases occurring following recent exposure.

The majority of infections affect the lungs. However, worldwide it is estimated that between 10 and 25% of infections occur outside of the lungs [2]. Extrapulmonary tuberculosis results from hematogenous and lymphatic spread of the *M. tuberculosis* bacillus [3]. The most common forms of extrapulmonary tuberculosis are lymphadenitis, pleurisy, bone and joint infections, and infections of the brain. Rarely, tuberculosis can present at other sites including the abdominal cavity, kidneys, genitourinary tract, pericardium, and skin. Depending upon the country of residence, extrapulmonary tuberculosis represents 20–50% of cases. Diagnosis of extrapulmonary tuberculosis should trigger evaluation for pulmonary tuberculosis as well, given concern for communicability, and testing for the human immunodeficiency virus (HIV). It is often difficult to establish a diagnosis in extrapulmonary disease because clinical symptoms and diagnostic testing may be inconclusive. Diagnosis of cutaneous lesions may be difficult, as they resemble many other dermatological conditions. Tuberculosis is often difficult to identify by culture, pathology, or molecular techniques [4].

Immune protection against tuberculosis is primarily achieved by cell-mediated immunity. Risk factors for reactivation of latent tuberculosis include HIV infection, organ transplantation, silicosis, immunosuppression by tumor necrosis factor-α (TNF-α) blockers, steroids and other drugs, chronic renal failure requiring dialysis, and close contacts of individuals with active tuberculosis. In the elderly population, approximately 90% of cases are due to reactivation of primary infection [5]. An estimated 57% of tuberculosis-related deaths occur among people older than 50 years with half of these deaths in those aged 65 and above [6]. Aging is associated with reduced T cell production by the thymus, reduced capacity for T cell proliferation (immune senescence), reduced capacity to produce cytokines and other effector molecules (immune exhaustion), as well as reduced macrophage production of tumor necrosis factor (TNF) and reduced phagocytosis. Ex vivo stimulation of mononuclear cells from elderly people with *M. tuberculosis* antigens generated lower interferon-γ (INF-γ) responses than in those from younger persons. These age-related changes in the immune system may compromise immunological tests for evidence of latent or active infection with tuberculosis [7, 8]. Two-step tuberculin skin testing (TST) has been advocated in the elderly to improve sensitivity for diagnosis of latent tuberculosis although this method is not more predictive in active tuberculosis [9].

Although the lungs are the most common site of tuberculosis infection in elderly persons, extrapulmonary disease is more common with advancing age, including tuberculous meningitis and renal, bone, and joint infection [8]. Elderly patients may not exhibit the classic features associated with tuberculosis including cough, hemoptysis, fever, night sweats, and weight loss [10–14]. Symptoms may mimic age-related illnesses such as reduced functional capacity, chronic fatigue, cognitive impairment, anorexia, back pain, compression fractures, and fever of unknown origin. Elderly patients commonly have other comorbid conditions that increase the risk of active tuberculosis including poor nutrition, diabetes mellitus, chronic obstructive pulmonary disease, malignancies, and rheumatic conditions necessitating immune-modulating therapies [15–18]. With treatment elderly patients are more likely to develop adverse drug reactions including increased risk of hepatotoxicity from isoniazid and acute kidney injury from rifampin [19].

Chemotherapy for extrapulmonary tuberculosis is initiated with rifampin, isoniazid, pyrazinamide, and ethambutol (RIPE) for an initial 2-month phase. At the time the *M. tuberculosis* isolate is found susceptible to both rifampin and isoniazid (susceptible tuberculosis), ethambutol is discontinued. After 2 months of therapy, for extrapulmonary tuberculosis caused by susceptible strains, pyrazinamide is also discontinued, and isoniazid and rifampin continued for 6–9 months (based upon clinical evidence of resolution of infection). However in tuberculous meningitis, the optimal duration of therapy has not been established through randomized controlled trials: most experts and society guidelines recommend 12 months of treatment [20].

Drug-resistant tuberculosis has been increasingly reported over the past 20 years. Multidrug-resistant tuberculosis (MDR-TB) (i.e., resistance to isoniazid and rifampin) has been reported in 500,000 cases from 127 countries. Extensively resistant tuberculosis (XDR-TB) (i.e., resistance to isoniazid and rifampin plus any fluoroquinolone and at least one of three injectable second-line agents, amikacin, kanamycin, or capreomycin) has been reported from 105 countries. Resistance to isoniazid is classified as low level (MIC 0.2–1 μg/mL) or high level (MIC > 2 μg/mL). Treatment of high-level resistant strains with only first-line drugs has resulted in suboptimal outcomes [21]. Treatment requires discontinuation of isoniazid and use of other agents to which the organism is susceptible for an extended period of time. Isoniazid may be included in treatment regimens for low-level resistance as resistance may be overcome when high serum concentrations can be achieved.

The patient in our case completed 1 year of therapy. The chest wall mass shrunk to near disappearance on physical exam. Follow-up PET scans showed total resolution of all noted enhancing lesions. The patient had a repeat colonoscopy with no evidence of malignancy. She continues to live independently.

Key Points/Pearls

- Infectious disease experts always consider tuberculosis in their differential diagnosis, recognizing its protean manifestations and the difficulties in reaching the diagnosis in many cases.
- Elderly patients are at high risk of reactivation tuberculosis and have a higher likelihood of presenting with extrapulmonary tuberculosis.
- TST and IGRA (e.g., Quantiferon gold) screening may miss latent tuberculosis and active disease in the elderly.
- Elderly patients may not present with classic signs and symptoms of tuberculosis.

- Inappropriate treatment of tuberculosis is common worldwide, due to a lack of consistent performance of culture and susceptibilities in both new cases and relapses, poor adherence to or early discontinuation of therapy, limited availability of second-line drugs, and sometimes inappropriate recommendations for the retreatment of drug-resistant tuberculosis. This unfortunately has led to an epidemic of drug-resistant tuberculosis.
- Directly observed therapy (DOT) is essential to decrease the risk of acquired resistance.
- MDR-TB (multidrug-resistant tuberculosis): resistance to isoniazid and rifampin.
- XDR-TB (extensively resistant tuberculosis): resistance to isoniazid and rifampin plus any fluoroquinolone and at least one of three injectable second-line drugs (amikacin, kanamycin, or capreomycin).
- Low-level isoniazid resistance may be treated with an isoniazid containing combination antimycobacterial regimen.
- The most effective management of isolated high-level isoniazid resistance is still unsettled and controversial, but the WHO-recommended regimen of 2 months of rifampin, isoniazid, pyrazinamide, and ethambutol followed by 4 months of rifampin, isoniazid, and ethambutol has been associated with a high risk of failure and further acquired resistance.
- Re-treatment of tuberculosis in the setting of high-level resistance to isoniazid should be discussed with experts.

References

1. World Health Organization. Global tuberculosis report 2015. Geneva: World Health Organization; 2015.
2. World Health Organization. Global tuberculosis control: epidemiology, strategy, financing. WHO report 2009. Geneva: World Health Organization. p. 2009
3. Fisher D, Elwood K. Nonrespiratory tuberculosis. In: Canadian Thoracic Society, Canadian Lung Association, and the Public Health Agency of Canada, eds. Canadian tuberculosis standards. 7th ed. Ottawa: Canadian Thoracic Society;2013.
4. Frankel A, Penrose C, Emer J. Cutaneous tuberculosis: a practical case report and review for the dermatologist. J Clin Aesthet Dermatol. 2009;2(10):19–27
5. Rajagopalan S. Tuberculosis in older adults. Clin Geriatr Med. 2016;32(3):479–91
6. Global, regional, and national incidence and mortality for HIV, tuberculosis, and malaria during 1990–2013: a systematic analysis for the Global Burden of Disease Study 2013. 2014. Institute for Health Metrics and Evaluation. http://www.healthdata.org/gbd. Accessed 26 June 2017.
7. Dorken E, Grzybowski S, Allen EA. Significance of the tuberculin test in the elderly. Chest. 1987;92(2):237–40
8. Perez-Guzman C, et al. Does aging modify pulmonary tuberculosis?: a meta-analytical review. Chest. 1999;116(4):961–7
9. Chan-Yeung M, et al. Tuberculin skin test reaction and body mass index in old age home residents in Hong Kong. J Am Geriatr Soc. 2007;55(10):1592–7
10. Byng-Maddick R, Noursadeghi M. Does tuberculosis threaten our ageing populations? BMC Infect Dis. 2016;16:119
11. Morris CD. Pulmonary tuberculosis in the elderly: a different disease? Thorax. 1990;45(12):912–3
12. Negin J, Abimbola S, Marais BJ. Tuberculosis among older adults—time to take notice. Int J Infect Dis. 2015;32:135–7
13. Rajagopalan S. Tuberculosis and aging: a global health problem. Clin Infect Dis. 2001;33(7):1034–9
14. Schluger NW. Tuberculosis and nontuberculous mycobacterial infections in older adults. Clin Chest Med. 2007;28(4):773–81
15. Brode SK, et al. Increased risk of mycobacterial infections associated with anti-rheumatic medications. Thorax. 2015;70(7):677–82
16. Dixon WG, et al. Drug-specific risk of tuberculosis in patients with rheumatoid arthritis treated with anti-TNF therapy: results from the British Society for Rheumatology Biologics Register (BSRBR). Ann Rheum Dis. 2010;69(3):522–8
17. Jeon CY, Murray MB. Diabetes mellitus increases the risk of active tuberculosis: a systematic review of 13 observational studies. PLoS Med. 2008;5(7):e152
18. Tubach F, et al. Risk of tuberculosis is higher with anti-tumor necrosis factor monoclonal antibody therapy than with soluble tumor necrosis factor receptor therapy: the three-year prospective French Research Axed on Tolerance of Biotherapies registry. Arthritis Rheum. 2009;60(7):1884–94
19. Perrin P. Human and tuberculosis co-evolution: an integrative view. Tuberculosis (Edinb). 2015;95(Suppl 1):S112–6
20. Nahid P, et al. Official American Thoracic Society/Centers for Disease Control and Prevention/Infectious Diseases Society of America clinical practice guidelines: treatment of drug-susceptible tuberculosis. Clin Infect Dis. 2016;63(7):e147–95
21. Gegia M, et al. Treatment of isoniazid-resistant tuberculosis with first-line drugs: a systematic review and meta-analysis. Lancet Infect Dis. 2017;17(2):223–34

Appendix: Differential Diagnosis Index to All Cases

Index

© Springer International Publishing AG 2018
M. David, J.-L. Benoit (eds.), *The Infectious Disease Diagnosis*,
https://doi.org/10.1007/978-3-319-64906-1